F

The Doctors' Vitamin and Mineral Encyclopedia

SHELDON SAUL HENDLER, M.D., Ph.D.

Board of Medical Advisors

JOE GRAEDON, M.S.

ALEX MERCANDETTI, M.D.

ROBERT NAGOURNEY, M.D.

DEBORAH U. WATERS, M.D.

A Fireside Book
Published by
Simon & Schuster

New York   London   Toronto   Sydney

Tokyo   Singapore

Fireside

Rockefeller Center
1230 Avenue of the Americas
New York, New York   10020

First Fireside Edition 1991

FIRESIDE and colophon are registered trademarks
of Simon & Schuster Inc.

Designed by Liney Li
Manufactured in the United States of America

20   19   18   17   16   15   14   13   12   11   Pbk.

Library of Congress Cataloging in Publication Data

Hendler, Sheldon Saul, date.
    The doctors' vitamin and mineral encyclopedia / by Sheldon Saul Hendler.
        p.   cm.
    Includes bibliographical references.
    Includes index.
        1. Vitamins—Dictionaries.   2. Minerals in human nutrition—
Dictionaries.   3. Dietary supplements—Dictionaries.   I. Title.
    QP771.H363   1990
    613.2—dc20   89-26367
                                                                                  CIP

ISBN 0-671-66784-X
ISBN 0-671-74092-X Pbk.

Acknowledgments

This book was conceived over twenty years ago but would not have been born without the invaluable assistance of my literary agent, David Michael Rorvik, of Proteus, Inc.

Special thanks:
   To my wife, Joyce, for her constant love, support and friendship.
   To Alan Kapuler, who always reminds me that the study of nutrition should be the most important work of the biologist and the physician.
   And to Robert Nagourney, who makes talking about science and medicine so much fun.

My gratitude to Jeffrey Blumberg, Donald R. Davis, Yasuo Hotta, Junda Liu, A.M. Michelson, Michael Neuschul, Forrest Nielson, Karl Ransberger, Gerhard Schrauzer, Austin Shug and Julian Spallholz for sharing with me their most interesting papers, and to Herbert Boynton and Mark McCarty for inspiring conversations.

For my sons, Ross and Seth,
who I hope will read this book

Contents

PART THREE A FORTUNE IN FORMULAS FOR BETTER HEALTH *391*

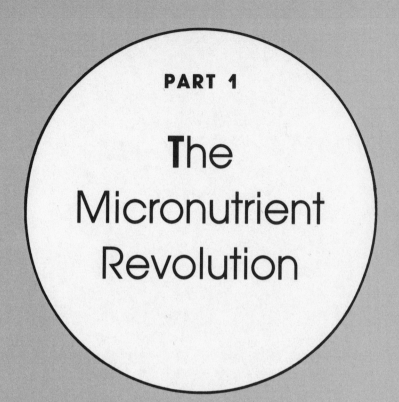

PART 1

The Micronutrient Revolution

ONE

What This Book Can Do for You That No Other Book Can

YOUR GUIDE TO THE BENEFITS OF THE NUTRITION REVOLUTION
(From Home-Remedy to High-Tech)

This book will help you reap the benefits of an extraordinary "revolution" that is rapidly gaining momentum in our midst. This is a revolution in information and thinking, one in which more and more people feel empowered to exert control over and take more responsibility for their own health. Nutrition is central to all of this, including "micronutrition," the vitamins, minerals and other health-giving components of our food. We are discovering that through the manipulation of nutrition, and especially micronutrition, we can not only treat but, in many cases, *prevent* the ills that we once accepted as inevitable. And we can often do so without always having to resort to costly and, not infrequently, ineffective medications that come freighted with adverse side effects.

This is a revolution in which we are at last heeding the counsel of Hippocrates, who, centuries ago, said, "Let thy food be thy medicine."

We are making exciting new discoveries every day related to the micronutrient components of our food—with the result that, in the United States alone about *half* of the entire population is now taking micronutrient supplements, convinced that diet itself, given the kind of polluted and stressful world we live in, is inadequate to supply all the nutrients that are needed, convinced that these supplements will help prevent and treat disease, as well as boost energy, promote a feeling of physical and mental well-being and prolong life.

Even some of the more conservative bastions of the medical "establishment" are finally joining this revolution. At first there was massive resistance to this, but now the data in support of prudent nutritional supplementation are becoming so overwhelming that the resistance is fading. The National Cancer Institute, the American Cancer Society, major medical journals and medical schools are all involved in research related to nutritional supplements and/or have already acknowledged the very significant benefits some of these supplements can confer.

The supplement marketplace is rapidly moving from its old "home remedy" roots to its "high tech" future. This book can guide you to that future *today,* so that you can *immediately* begin benefiting from the very best and very latest research findings and breakthroughs related to micronutrition.

Congratulations on joining the most significant health movement in history. Congratulations on reading this book. I believe you will find it your best possible guide. The reasons for this are explained below.

1) MORE AUTHORITATIVE/MORE OBJECTIVE/BETTER DOCUMENTED

Not all vitamin/mineral supplement guides are equal. They can—and do—differ enormously in real value to the consumer. Some, though published recently, are woefully out of date; some others are full of scientific and medical misinformation and mistakes. Most are still poorly documented. Many are obviously biased—designed either to knock the whole idea of taking supplements or to praise, indiscriminately, every supplement that comes along.

For many years, friends, patients and fellow doctors, familiar with my background as a biochemist, researcher and medical doctor with a strong interest in human metabolism, diet, nutrition, and experimental and preventive medicines, have asked me where they could get objective, well-documented information on vitamins, minerals, amino acids and other food supplements. Among their questions were these: Which supplements, if any, are worth taking? Is there *good* evidence suggesting that these supplements are really helpful? Which substances are safe and in what doses? Which are the best forms in which to take these supplements? What are the optimal combinations? What results can be expected? Who should take supplements—and when? Should all of us be taking the same things or should people in different age groups and life situations follow regimens specific to their needs? Can any of these substances really have *significant* impact on health and longevity; can they do anything to *reverse,* as well as *prevent,* disease?

Several years ago I set out methodically to answer these questions. My focus at that time was on aging and the degenerative processes that accompany aging. I wanted to know if nutritional supplements could have any measurable impact on the degenerative diseases that accompany aging. I studied very carefully the information that was typically being provided the general public *and* most physicians. I was distressed by what I discovered. It was as if the "experts" had formed up in two teams and were doing fierce battle with each other. On one side were what I call the old-line nutritional "academic conservatives" who doggedly insist that "the great American diet" provides everything anyone could possibly need in the way of nutrition. And on the other side were what I call the nutritional "true believers," those who proclaim every new supplement to be a "miracle cure" for one dire ill or another and sometimes for just about *every* ailment known.

The trouble with the nutritional conservatives is that they are sadly out-of-date, badly out-of-tune with new research findings. The "great American diet," far from providing optimal nutrition, has just about done us in, contributing not to health but to obesity, heart disease, cancer and premature aging and death. As a nation we are overfed and often seriously undernourished. Calories we've got—in excess. But they are calories too often devoid of real nutritional value. Dietary/nutritional imbalances and deficiencies contribute significantly to the premature deaths of *millions* of Americans annually. And our changing world has placed new demands on our bodies, exposing them to environmental and psychological stresses and insults that were not previously so prevalent, stresses that deplete our tissues of protective and regulatory nutrients as never before.

As for the "true believers," the trouble there is obvious. This side, as much as the other, has impeded nutritional research with its often uninformed and excessive claims. (As noted later, the true believers, even while making insupportable claims, often overlook real benefits that are sometimes more remarkable than the ones they have focused on.)

In between these two warring factions I found few and generally only feeble voices of reason. So I set out to research and write a book that would, without any axe to grind, without any products to sell or any vested interests to protect, systematically and objectively analyze *all* of the available scientific and medical data for each of the substances for which anti-aging claims had been made. That project resulted in *The Complete Guide to Anti-Aging Nutrients* (Simon and Schuster, 1984; Fireside, 1986). I wanted the book to serve as a bridge between the two opposing camps and hoped that it would bring the investigation of nutritional supplements onto a higher plane, where the consumer would be better served.

In large part I feel rewarded for my effort, as that book managed to garner strong support in both camps, drew both closer to the center and brought many serious researchers, previously alienated by the extremes on both sides, into the supplement arena. Even two Nobel Laureates, who told me they had previously dismissed out-of-hand most claims being made for nutritional supplements, took a new interest in the field after reading my book. The book garnered excellent reviews in both the medical and popular press and won a "Best Book" award from *Self-Care* magazine. It was subsequently cited as a major source in a number of best-selling diet, nutrition, and other health books.

Encouraged by that response, I have now updated and vastly expanded that book, to embrace the whole nutritional marketplace. The result is this book, and it is, I believe, the most objective and best documented book ever published on this important topic. My conclusions are based upon my own biochemical insights, my own laboratory and clinical research and an exhaustive study of the relevant worldwide research literature. I have, in the course of preparing this book, analyzed literally *thousands* of research papers.

I believe I have succeeded in being as objective and pragmatic as possible. I have sought always to be guided by the best possible evidence. If something works, I say so. If there are no data (nor any good rationale) to support a particular claim, I don't hesitate to say that, either. In some cases I am compelled to say we simply don't know, that more research is warranted or required before we can declare a particular substance safe and effective.

2) MORE *NEWS* AND MORE *GOOD* NEWS

I am convinced that this book delivers more genuine nutritional news than any other and, in fact, more *good* news than any other. You might expect a book that sticks to the *facts* and leaves the wishful thinking to others to be short on positive news—but that expectation is wrong. The more we really understand the vitamins, minerals and other food substances the more good we discover can be said about them.

Over and over I find supplements being touted for all the wrong reasons—entirely or largely without scientific support. Meanwhile, really wonderful uses to which these substances could be applied (as suggested by sound research data) get entirely overlooked. Thus the consumer gets cheated twice: first by being given an erroneous "indication" or reason for using a supplement, second by *not* being told about a *real* indication for using the substance. This has far-reaching ramifications. The reason *why* someone takes a supplement has, logically, a great deal to do with *who* should take it, *when* it should be taken, *how much* should be taken, *with what* it should be taken and so on. It is vitally important, therefore, to know, first and foremost, whether the claimed indications or reasons for using any given substance are valid.

This book focuses sharply on those "indications." It highlights the "good news"—but only the good news that is genuinely supported by the best, most reliable scientific findings. If there's bad news the book will tell you that, too. Even that, however, is good news for the discriminating consumer. Knowing what *won't* help you or might even harm you is, in many ways, just as useful as knowing what will help.

The wonderful thing about this rapidly expanding field is that, if you know how to find it and apply it, there is so much that is exciting and promising that even the most ardent supplement enthusiast need not resort to exaggeration in order to deliver plenty of very good news. The *facts* are exciting enough in their own right. Let's *insist* on those facts. That's the only way the excesses and oversights of the true believers can be vanquished and the skepticism of the academic conservatives, who still control much of this research, can be overcome. (For a preview of "good news" specifics, see the following chapter.)

3) MORE COMPREHENSIVE, UNDERSTANDABLE AND HELPFUL

This book is unique in its organization and the scope of its coverage. It analyzes *all* the vitamins and minerals that have any genuine relevance as nutritional supplements. It does the same for the amino acids and many other substances. Each analysis is structured so that you can quickly and easily determine what the nutrient is, what it does—and doesn't—do, who it's good for, what ailments it can help treat or prevent, what amounts it should be taken in, what it should be taken with, what precautions apply and so on. This book provides more consumer guidance than any other currently on the market.

It also covers many substances that are overlooked by or are unknown to other authors of supplement guides. These include the most important nucleic acids and their derivatives, lipids and their derivatives, *all* of the significant medicinal herbs, a variety of miscellaneous food supplements and a number of often exciting "biologicals," pharmaceuticals and other potentially therapeutic chemicals which are, increasingly, being used as adjuncts in nutritional and alternative therapies.

This book combines information in one place that was, previously, available, if at all, only in diverse texts and research papers. It is a compilation and analysis of the most exciting "medicine" of our time.

4) MORE UP-TO-DATE (AND AHEAD-OF-DATE)

This book provides not only the most comprehensive, authoritative supplement information available, it also provides you with the most up-to-date information available. In fact, some of this information is "ahead-of-date," since, in some instances, it tells you about exciting, newly emerging substances that can be expected to enter the marketplace in the near future—or that are already in experimental use. Since I am personally involved in a number of laboratory and clinical research efforts related to nutritional and other therapeutic substances, I have a lot of "inside" preview data I am, in some instances, at liberty to share with you.

5) MORE PRESCRIPTIVE

Many health-related books *describe;* few *prescribe.* In this book, I not only describe the most exciting nutritional and supplemental substances available, I also tell you how to use them, both *individually* and in a variety of *combinations* designed to meet specific needs and different lifestyles. In the analysis of each substance you will find information on the illnesses and disorders for which that substance might be used, the doses that have been reported effective and other helpful information, including any relevant precautions. In Part Three of this book you will find formulas specifically designed for such purposes as:

losing weight
lowering cholesterol quickly without dieting
building stamina and endurance
protecting your heart
fighting cancer
dealing with "female troubles"
resisting pollutants
boosting immunity
fighting colds, flu, allergies
protecting against cigarette smoke
fighting arthritis

I'd like to introduce you now to some of the specific benefits that are in store for you. In the following chapter, I will give you a summary review of some of the most significant and beneficial discoveries that have been made to date with respect to a number of micronutrients and other therapeutic substances.

TWO

Medical "Miracles"

From Micronutrients and

Other Substances

The word "miracle" is so often abused that I sometimes need to place it in quotation marks. But, in fact, there are properties in many of the micronutrients and other substances discussed in this book that are every bit as miraculous as those found in some of our most highly touted "wonder" drugs. In this chapter, I want to introduce you to some of those remarkable properties, to give you a sampling of what is to come. Bear in mind, this *is* only a *sampling*. And, remember, too, that you should read the complete analysis of each nutrient and sub- stance before using it. There may be some specific precautions you need to know about.

Now let's look at some of the most exciting medical discoveries of our time.

VITAMINS

VITAMIN A/BETA-CAROTENE—These substances, much in the news a few years ago for their anti-cancer properties, are now generating excitement anew—this time for their immune-stimulating effects and the ability of some of their derivatives to help renew aging skin and to treat diseased skin.

VITAMIN B$_1$ (THIAMIN)—There are more American adults deficient in this vitamin than in any other, largely because of the high rate of alcohol consumption. Alcohol markedly depletes thiamin reserves; supplementation with this vitamin is crucial for those who regularly consume alcohol. Thiamin has also been shown to be a protector against lead poisoning—highly significant in view of the widespread lead pollution in so many public water systems.

VITAMIN B$_3$ (NIACIN)—Niacin is proving to be one of the most potent cholesterol-lowering substances around. Used *properly,* it can be more effective—and safer—than the commonly prescribed cholesterol-lowering drugs.

VITAMIN B$_6$—This vitamin can boost immunity in some very important ways. It has been effective against some cancers, including melanoma.

VITAMIN B$_{12}$—It turns out that this oft-maligned vitamin may really boost energy, after all. It's also been showing some anti-cancer effects, among other things.

BIOTIN—For those with "cowlicks" or the "uncombable hair syndrome," biotin can be miraculous, indeed.

FOLIC ACID—Recent research reveals anti-cancer effects and some good news for smokers.

PANTOTHENIC ACID AND PANTETHINE—There is finally some evidence to support the persistent claim that pantothenic acid can boost athletic endurance. Pantethine, a metabolite of pantothenic acid, now also available as a supplement, may help lower cholesterol and triglycerides and may also be useful in alcohol detoxification.

VITAMIN C (ASCORBIC ACID)—A great deal of research now makes it clear that even though vitamin C cannot reduce the number of colds one gets, it *can* reduce their duration and severity. On the other hand, it does not appear to be an effective cancer *treatment,* but it *is* a powerful cancer *preventive.* And, a new wrinkle: it appears that the vitamin may be useful in the treatment of some mental disorders.

VITAMIN D—Exciting new discoveries are being made that indicate that vitamin D may be quite useful in both preventing and treating some cancers.

VITAMIN E—Though long touted as a great protector against heart disease, vitamin E, the latest and best research suggests, may actually be far more important as an immune stimulator and nervous-system protector.

MINERALS

CALCIUM—Apart from the significant impact calcium can have on preventing osteoporosis, it now also appears to have properties protective against colorectal cancer and high blood pressure.

FLUORINE—This mineral can prevent more than dental cavities; recent research suggests it may also help prevent (and treat) osteoporosis and some forms of heart disease.

GERMANIUM—Though not "the most important healing substance on the planet," as someone recently claimed, germanium may have some immune-stimulating, anti-cancer and anti-viral properties.

IODINE—Protective against some forms of radioactive fallout and possibly effective in the treatment of fibrocystic breast disease.

MAGNESIUM—There is good evidence that this mineral can significantly increase the survival rate of those who have heart attacks. It is emerging as an important therapeutic agent in medicine and is useful for the treatment of many cardiac arrhythmias and certain forms of angina (heart pain).

POTASSIUM—Of great importance in controlling blood pressure and can help protect against strokes.

SELENIUM—A potent protector against cardiovascular disease and cancer; can detoxify a number of major pollutants and seems to inhibit *all* of the degenerative processes related to aging.

ZINC—A powerhouse that has been showing major immune-boosting effects and may even be helpful in aborting the common cold. Recently zinc was demonstrated to be an effective treatment in stopping a disease that is a major cause of blindness.

AMINO ACIDS

L-ARGININE—Showing considerable promise as an immune booster and cancer fighter. *May* be able to build muscle and burn fat.

L-ASPARTIC ACID—May be useful in the treatment of chronic fatigue and opiate withdrawal.

BRANCHED-CHAIN AMINO ACIDS—Can help restore muscle mass in those who have been ill or have undergone surgery. An exciting preliminary study indicates these nutrients may have a beneficial effect in ALS (amyotrophic lateral sclerosis), a disease that has previously resisted all attempted treatments.

L-CYSTEINE—Significantly extended life spans in experimental animals; has potent detoxifying effects.

L-HISTIDINE—Showing promise in the treatment of rheumatoid arthritis.

L-LYSINE—The best study to date indicates a real anti-herpes effect.

L-TRYPTOPHAN—May be a useful mood controller and has suppressed food, alcohol and amphetamine cravings. However, has recently been found to be associated with severe side effects in some people.

L-TYROSINE—May, studies suggest, be a good anti-depressant and psychic energizer; useful in drug detoxification; may improve performance under stress.

NUCLEIC ACIDS AND DERIVATIVES

DNA AND RNA—Evidence, at last, that *oral* supplementation with these substances may be beneficial; specific immune-stimulating effects noted in recent animal experiments.

ADENOSINE—Excitement over adenosine's benefits in congestive heart failure, in reducing the death rate from recurrent heart attack and in the treatment of herpes zoster.

ISOPRINOSINE—Notable immune stimulator, useful in herpes and possibly in chronic fatigue syndrome and AIDS.

LIPIDS AND DERIVATIVES

AL 721—Lipid formulation making waves for its apparent immune-stimulating and possible anti-aging effects; being used by some AIDS and chronic fatigue patients.

FISH OILS—Expanding their sphere of influence to include arthritis, hypertension, psoriasis, some forms of cancer and kidney disease.

LECITHIN/PHOSPHATIDYLCHOLINE—Exhibiting very useful effects in a number of neurologic, psychiatric and infectious diseases and disorders.

HERBS

ASTRAGALUS—Shows real promise as an immune enhancer and adjuvant therapy in some cancers.

BUTCHER'S BROOM—May have circulatory benefits.

CAPSICUM/HOT PEPPERS—Looks good for inhibiting dangerous blood clots and may be useful as a pain killer.

COMFREY—Speeds skin ulcer healing.

ECHINACEA—Significant immune-stimulating properties.

FEVERFEW—Effective for the treatment of migraine headaches and may alleviate some arthritis symptoms.

GINKGO—Recent research indicates ginkgo may be quite helpful in some serious circulatory disorders and may improve mental functioning in some elderly people. One of the herb's constituents has prolonged survival of organ transplants in experimental animals.

LICORICE—Showing value for treating a variety of ulcers, chronic viral hepatitis and some other viral infections. A constituent of the herb has inhibited the AIDS virus in test-tube studies. The same constituent also has anti-depressant effects.

MILK THISTLE—Has remarkable detoxifying and liver-protective effects.

OATS—Decoctions of fresh oat plants have reduced the craving for nicotine.

SAINT JOHN'S WORT—Showing potent antibiotic and anti-viral effects in recent studies. Strongly inhibits the AIDS virus in test-tube work. (Very toxic if not used properly.)

WHEAT GRASS/BARLEY GRASS—May be protective against radiation, some cancers and various toxins.

YOHIMBINE—Appears to have *some* genuine aphrodisiac effects.

OTHER SUPPLEMENTS

BIOFLAVONOIDS—Making strong comeback by showing notable anti-allergy, anti-inflammatory and anti-viral effects in recent research.

BREWER'S YEAST—New interest in this old standby due to findings that one of its constituents, skin respiratory factor, may increase collagen production and could, therefore, be useful in smoothing out wrinkles.

COENZYME Q$_{10}$—May strengthen muscle and boost immunity.

L-CARNITINE—Helpful in the treatment of various forms of cardiovascular disease.

SEAWEEDS AND DERIVATIVES—Showing great promise as detoxifiers, wound healers and as anti-cancer and anti-viral substances.

OTHER SUBSTANCES

ASPIRIN—Looking better than ever as a clot-inhibitor and now also as a possible immune stimulant and anti-viral agent.

CHARCOAL—Not only a great "de-gasser" but also a good "de-cholesterolizer."

DHEA AND ANALOGUES—Preliminary cancer work underway; DHEA *may* protect against degenerative diseases linked to aging.

FRUIT ACIDS—These fascinating substances may soon be giving Retin A, the "anti-wrinkle" drug, a run for its money.

HYALURONIC ACID/CHONDROITIN SULFATE—These sulfated polysaccharides may have cell-rejuvenating qualities, anti-viral properties and various other impressive therapeutic credentials.

MEMORY ENHANCERS—A number of "smart pills" are showing promise in sharpening the mind and memory.

SOD AND LIPSOD—Superoxide dismutase (SOD) may be another of the real anti-aging substances; could affect favorably *all* of the degenerative processes.

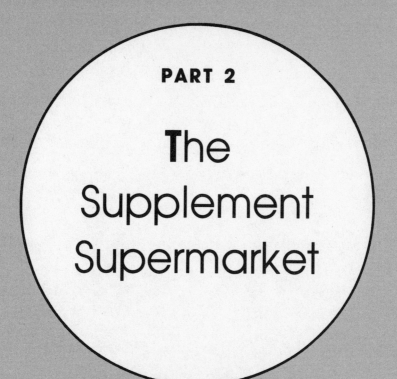

PART 2

The Supplement Supermarket

THREE

How to Use This Part

of the Book

In the following chapters, you will learn about the preventive and therapeutic benefits of vitamins, minerals, amino acids, nucleic acids, lipids and their derivatives, herbs and a variety of other supplements and substances ranging from acidophilus to wheat germ, aspirin to transfer factor. In many cases, you will find each supplement or substance analyzed in the following manner:

Overview—A summary statement of the supplement's/substance's origins, functions, preventive and therapeutic pros and cons.

Positive Claims—A list of the benefits that have been claimed for the supplement/substance.

Negative Claims—A list of the adverse effects that have been attributed to the supplement/substance.

Evidence Related to Positive Claims—A discussion and evaluation of the research that supports each positive claim.

Evidence Related to Negative Claims—A discussion and evaluation of the research that supports each negative claim.

Recommendations—These cover appropriate doses, the best source and form for each supplement/substance, when and with what each supplement should be taken and, when needed, appropriate precautions to observe (including drug/nutrient interactions and conditions that may make use of certain supplements inadvisable.)

Please read each analysis in its entirety so that you learn about any possible risks, as well as the benefits, of supplement use. Note that most nutrients should be used in combination with others. Refer to Part Three for the "formulas" that will tell you how to combine nutrients properly for different circumstances.

You will frequently encounter the abbreviation "RDA" as you read about the vitamins and minerals. RDA stands for "Recommended Daily Dietary Allowance." The RDAs for vitamins and minerals have been established by the Food and Nutrition Board of the National Academy of Sciences and the Food and Drug Administration (FDA). The RDAs set by the two groups have only minor differences. The RDAs that you will find listed on the labels of vitamin and minderal products are those of the FDA. They are often referred to as "U.S. RDA."

There is a lot of confusion among consumers and even doctors and nutritional researchers concerning the RDAs. The RDAs are the levels of essential nutrients that the two organizations named above believe are *adequate* to meet the nutritional needs of *healthy* individuals.

You should be aware, however, that there can be a big difference between "adequate" and *optimal*. The amounts of vitamins, minerals and other nutrients needed for optimal/maximal health and longevity have *not* been established, but the research you will learn about as you read this book indicates that in some cases these amounts *exceed* the RDAs.

FOUR

Vitamins

Vitamins are a group of chemically unrelated organic (carbon-containing) nutrients that are essential in small quantities for normal metabolism, growth and physical well-being. These nutrients must be obtained through diet since they are either not synthesized in our bodies or are synthesized in inadequate amounts. Our bodies use vitamins to make substances that are vital participants in many of the chemical reactions in our cells, reactions essential for the proper functioning of cells.

Vitamins are traditionally divided into two categories: the fat-soluble vitamins, which can be stored in the body, and the water-soluble vitamins, which are not stored in significant quantities. Some vitamins are fundamental participants in the energy-producing reactions of our bodies. Vitamins themselves, however, are insignificant sources of biological energy.

The fat-soluble vitamins are vitamins A, D, E and K. Vitamin D is derived both from dietary sources and from reactions occurring in sun-exposed skin. The active forms of most vitamins, that is, the substances formed within our cells from dietary vitamins, participate in cellular metabolism (chemical reactions of the cell) as cofactors for enzymes (biological catalysts). In contrast, the active form of vitamin D is a hormone important for the regulation of the body's calcium and the production of white blood cells, among other things. Vitamin K is derived from dietary sources and also is produced by some of the bacteria residing in our intestines.

The water-soluble vitamins comprise the B vitamins and vitamin C (ascorbic acid). The B vitamins essential for humans are: B_1, or thiamin; B_2, or riboflavin; niacin, which includes both nicotinic acid and nicotinamide; B_6, which encompasses pyridoxine, pyridoxal and pyridoxamine; B_{12}, or cobalamin; folic acid; pantothenic acid; and biotin.

The chemical structures of all of the vitamins essential to humans are now known, and whether one consumes a natural or synthetic version of a vitamin, the active principle is identical.

There are other substances that are occasionally considered to be essential vitamins for humans; their vitamin status, however, has not been established. These substances include: choline; lipoic acid; para-aminobenzoic acid (PABA); inositol; coenzyme Q_{10}, or ubiquinone; bioflavonoids; and L-carnitine. It has been established that some of these substances do in fact have vitamin activity in some animals other than humans.

Although many biochemical and physiological roles for the vitamins are already known, there is much that we do not understand about them. It is often difficult to reconcile deficiency states of some of the vitamins with their known biochemical functions. It is anticipated that the vitamins will continue to be a rich area for both basic and clinical investigation and that new roles for known vitamins will be discovered. And there may be vitamins that we are not yet aware of.

Although consumption of the so-called well-balanced diet is still thought by some to supply all the vitamins we need in quantities sufficient for the maintenance of good health, there are many situations that place people at an increased risk for vitamin-insufficiency states. Among those at risk are people on low-calorie diets, alcoholics, pregnant women, the elderly in general, surgical patients, users of certain medications and strict vegetarians. Vitamin supplementation is prudent in those and other cases that will be identified in subsequent chapters.

Recently there has been in increasing tendency to use "megadose" quantities (greater than ten times the RDA) of certain vitamins for several reasons: to help with the stress of daily life, to protect against colds, to increase sexual prowess, etc. Evidence for and against mega-dosing will be presented in the analyses of each of the vitamins. There are defined indications for the use of megadose vitamins as pharma-ceutical agents in the treatment of certain pathologic conditions, but megadosing in these situations requires a physician's supervision. These conditions include: the use of megadose nicotinic acid to lower blood cholesterol levels; the treatment of certain skin disorders with vitamin A and synthetic vitamin A derivatives; the use of vitamin B_6 to prevent seizures if one takes an overdose of INH, a drug used for the treatment of tuberculosis.

Evidence is gradually accumulating that even well-fed individuals can profit—in terms of optimizing health—by taking vitamin supple-ments in prudent amounts. In addition to their role in metabolism, certain vitamins are antioxidants and as such protect tissues against toxic oxygen damage. This protection helps establish a preventive role for vitamins with respect to a number of degenerative diseases.

VITAMIN A/BETA-CAROTENE

I. OVERVIEW: The "Miracle" Vitamin

Vitamin A, among nutrients, continues to be the real newsmaker, grab-bing headlines everywhere. Some decades ago it was already being called "the anti-infective vitamin." A few years ago it generated excite-ment anew as its anti-cancer properties began to emerge from studies being conducted around the world. More recently still it has attained even greater prominence as its immune-stimulating effects in the body and its curative and restorative effects in the skin have been confirmed.

In 1988 news that a vitamin A derivative could "improve photoaged skin" had a galvanizing effect on the public. Even some normally con-servative medical researchers and publications began using the word "miracle" with an ease that had previously eluded them. Overnight "Retin A"—the vitamin-A derivative drug—became a household word. Doctors everywhere were swamped with calls from patients wanting prescriptions, hoping that they, too, could erase some of their wrinkles and undo some of the damage of sun and time.

It's safe to say that the makers of Retin A were not particularly ruffled by all this attention, for Retin A had long enjoyed a reputation for the miraculous, at least among the millions of sufferers of acne vulgaris, the skin disorder that marred most of our teenage lives. Retin A has been remarkably successful in alleviating this particular adolescent agony.

Also much in the news these days are two other vitamin-A-derived drugs, Accutane and Tigason. Even the most serious (cystic) form of acne, which can be severely disfiguring, has yielded to Accutane, and Tigason has provided a powerful treatment for psoriasis, one of the most vexing skin disorders around.

That vitamin A is essential for human health is well established. We get varying amounts of it in our diet—either as preformed vitamin A or as provitamin A. The preformed variety (technically known as retinol or retinyl esters) is found in some of the meats and animal products we eat. Provitamin A includes such precursor substances as beta-carotene, which get converted to vitamin A once inside the body; these are typically found in carrots, sweet potatoes and many other fruits and vegetables. It's the beta-carotene that makes carrots and many other plant foods yellow/orange.

Vitamin A is essential for, among other things, vision (especially night vision), regulation of cell development, reproduction and immunity. Deficiencies often result in alterations in skin and mucous membranes that resemble precancerous conditions. This finding has led to increased research into vitamin A as a possible anti-cancer agent or cancer preventive.

All vitamin A substances seem to protect against cancer-causing agents. There is a difference, of course, between protection/prevention and direct anti-cancer effects once malignancy is established. But even here evidence is mounting that vitamin A and its derivatives may prove useful. Such effects have already been demonstrated in laboratory animals.

Some 22,000 physicians are currently playing guinea pig in a particularly ambitious, long-term study under the supervision of the Department of Medicine at Harvard. Results, due in 1991, will give us some indication of just how effective long-term use of beta-carotene is in terms of reducing the incidence of human cancer.

We do know from large population studies that low intakes of beta-carotene are associated with higher incidence of cancer. And it appears likely that beta-carotene exerts a protective effect through its unique antioxidant properties. It appears likely that it is especially good at trapping a very toxic form of di-oxygen, called singlet oxygen, that contributes to the malignant process in tissues. Researchers studying this antioxidant effect have called beta-carotene "the most efficient quencher of singlet oxygen thus far discovered."

Equally exciting is vitamin A's role in immunity, a role which almost certainly contributes to its anti-cancer properties. It appears that many of the hopes that were raised for vitamin A as the "anti-infective vita-min" more than fifty years ago are now being realized. Studies in third-world populations have demonstrated the enormous power of this vitamin in boosting resistance to infection and reducing the related mortality. Recently researchers in this country have suggested a possi-ble role for vitamin A in the treatment and prevention of AIDS.

Although high doses of preformed vitamin A can have toxic effects, beta-carotene is mercifully devoid of most toxicity. Even among pa-tients using extremely high doses of beta-carotene (300 milligrams or 500,000 IUs daily) for prolonged periods there was no significant tox-icity.

Vitamin A, even in the wake of all its "miracles," continues to be the most feared vitamin. It is surprising how many physicians still warn patients to stay away from vitamin A, neglecting to mention that beta-carotene, available for several years now without prescription, has the same benefits as preformed vitamin A and almost none of its adverse side effects.

II. CLAIMS

Positive:
1) Boosts immunity; 2) has anti-cancer effects; 3) fights skin disor-ders and prevents/reverses aging of the skin; 4) improves vision; 5) speeds wound healing.

Negative:
1) Highly toxic; 2) may cause birth defects if taken during pregnancy; 3) may cause bone disease among those with chronic kidney failure.

III. EVIDENCE

Related to Positive Claims:
1) Boosts immunity—Both human population and animal studies have shown that vitamin A deficiencies are associated with higher rates of

infection. Giving vitamin A supplements, in various forms, has boosted immunity in a variety of lab animals. These boosting effects have included increased antibody activity, faster rejection of skin grafts and accelerated production of various disease-fighting cells.

Vitamin A deficiencies appear to make the linings of the digestive tract, respiratory tract and hollow organs more vulnerable to attack by infectious agents. Giving vitamin A supplements in those cases fortifies the cells of those linings and makes them more resistant to agents that cause respiratory infections, diarrhea and other ills. The measles virus, for example, targets these cells when they are weakened. Giving vitamin A supplements to children in third-world countries where measles continues to be a major problem has cut the death rate among young children by at least 35 percent in some populations.

Increases in cellular immunity have been reported among lung cancer patients given very high doses of vitamin A for three weeks. And depression of immune function has been blocked in surgical patients given high doses of vitamin A. Supplementation was given just before surgery and for a few days afterward. In the case of the cancer patients, 1.5 million IUs were given daily, and in the case of the surgical patients, the daily dose was 300,000 to 450,000 IUs. Those doses require medical supervision and cannot be tolerated for long periods. Similar studies using the relatively non-toxic beta-carotene have not yet been reported.

It is also now well established that very high doses of the preformed vitamin A can significantly reduce the immune-depressive effects of radiation treatment and cancer chemotherapy. But once again the doses of preformed vitamin A required to achieve these results are much too high and too toxic for prolonged use. In this case, however, researchers *have* tried beta-carotene—to see if similar benefits could be realized. They were rewarded for their efforts, demonstrating that the addition of beta-carotene enabled them to increase dosages of radiation and chemotherapy in laboratory animals sufficiently to get complete regression of tumors in most cases. Some 92 percent of the animals remained cancer-free fourteen months after treatment. Results of human studies have not yet been reported.

Some particularly exciting research has shown that supplemental beta-carotene in high but still non-toxic doses of 180 milligrams per day can increase the number of very important immune cells (T-lymphocyte "helper" cells). The subjects of this study were healthy males with normal immune function. After only two weeks of supplementation, there was a 30 percent increase in T-helper cell numbers among this group.

It is quite possible that even more dramatic increases might be achieved among individuals who are immune compromised. It has been suggested by those involved in this work that beta-carotene supplementation, used in conjunction with other therapies, might be quite helpful in AIDS patients and in some cancer patients.

Another group of researchers has also proposed looking into the use of vitamin A/beta-carotene in the treatment of AIDS. They have noted that, in test-tube work, beta-carotene can stimulate immune cells so that they are better able to fight off such infections as *Candida albicans* (yeast infections commonly known as "thrush"), the sort that often multiply in AIDS patients. They found that they could more than double the kill rate of *Candida* when beta-carotene was added to suspensions of immune cells called neutrophils.

2) Has anti-cancer effects—Studies of large populations make it clear that vitamin A has anti-cancer effects. In one study of 8,000 men who were monitored over a five-year period, those with the lowest intake of beta-carotene were found to be at the greatest risk of getting lung cancer. In an even longer term study of 2,000 men, it was shown that smokers with the lowest intake of beta-carotene were several times more likely to develop lung cancer than smokers with the highest intake of beta-carotene. This study did not find a similarly protective effect from preformed vitamin A.

The results of many other studies suggest the cancer-protective effects of beta-carotene related to numerous human cancers, including those of the bladder, larynx, esophagus, stomach, colon/rectum and prostate.

In addition to the population studies, there are literally hundreds of papers demonstrating that vitamin A, primarily in the preformed variety, can suppress the malignant behavior of cultured cells adversely transformed by radiation, chemicals or viruses, can delay the development of transplanted tumors and can even completely prevent malignancy in animals exposed to various potent cancer-causing substances. Some of these results, it should be noted, have been obtained with doses of preformed vitamin A far too high and too toxic for general, preventive use. Experiments of the same sort with the far less toxic beta-carotene, meanwhile, appear promising, but are still few in number.

The drug derivatives of vitamin A are also showing promise in the fight against cancer. Accutane, for example, has been shown to be of benefit in the treatment of cutaneous T-cell lymphoma, a blood cancer that affects the skin. There is also emerging evidence of Accutane's usefulness in the treatment of myelodysplastic syndrome, a premalignant condition with leukemia-like characteristics. Accutane has, in addition, been able to shrink dramatically and, in some cases, completely eradicate oral leukoplakia, precancerous lesions found on the lips and inside the mouth.

Both preformed vitamin A and beta-carotene, either in combination or alone, are capable of shrinking and sometimes eradicating these leukoplakias, particularly common among smokers. They are particularly good at *preventing* the development of new leukoplakias, which resemble white spots or patches.

The same vitamin A derivative that is used in Retin A has been used in experiments that suggest this substance may help prevent cervical cancer. In one study, 50 percent of possibly precancerous cervical lesions disappeared completely after treatment with the vitamin A derivative Tretinoin.

The various modes of action by which vitamin A and its derivatives inhibit cancer may include the immune-enhancing factors and the singlet-oxygen-quenching capabilities discussed earlier, as well as retinol's role in regulating the growth and differentiation of cells.

3) Fights skin disorders and prevents/reverses aging of the skin— Though preformed vitamin A itself is capable of clearing up various forms of acne, it takes huge doses to do the job; that means toxicity, and once the vitamin A is withdrawn the acne usually comes back. The vitamin A derivatives discussed earlier do a far better job. Accutane is effective against cystic acne. Tretinoin (the active ingredient in Retin A) is now the treatment of choice for acne vulgaris, the commonest form of acne, and Tigason (etretinate) is showing remarkable promise in the treatment of psoriasis.

Etretinate has been found to clear up psoriasis in 80 percent of patients who take it daily for three to four months, making it remarkably better than any drug previously approved for the treatment of this frequently severe disorder. Once clearing has been achieved, the patient is typically put on a much smaller dose of the drug and is sometimes cycled on and off it. Some may require maintenance treatment for life.

Both Accutane and etretinate have caused concern because of their ability to produce birth defects if taken by women during pregnancy. Neither should be taken by any woman of childbearing age who is pregnant or not using birth control. Both require close medical supervision. Etretinate should not be used by women of childbearing age at all because even after its use is discontinued, traces of it potent enough to potentially cause birth defects remain in the body for two years or more. Etretinate derivatives that clear the body much more quickly are currently under development; one or more of these suitable for use by women of childbearing age may soon be available. Accutane clears the body in a week or less.

The Accutane/etretinate controversies have posed a special dilemma for the Food and Drug Administration, as well as for the many physicians who are called upon to prescribe these drugs. On the one hand, of course, there is the real concern about birth defects. But counterbalancing that concern is the empathy physicians—and the FDA—feel for the many thousands of sufferers of severe acne and psoriasis, disorders that are frequently so uncomfortable and so disfiguring that those who suffer from them have even resorted to suicide. These new drugs have transformed a once seemingly hopeless situation into one that many rightly label as "miraculous." The results these vitamin A derivatives get are frequently nothing short of astonishing.

For now the FDA has properly tightened controls on these drugs but has also quite properly refrained from banning them as some have demanded.

There has also been controversy over another vitamin A derivative—Retin A, the "miracle" skin restorer. Originally developed—and approved—for the treatment of acne, this substance has now found a potentially far larger market among those who want to prevent or retard the aging of their skin. Claims that it could do just that were made by researchers in 1988; "before-and-after" photos that accompanied their reports seemed to support the idea that this substance, applied topically to the skin, can roll back the years and undo damage caused by the accumulation of years and exposure to the sun.

Other researchers, however, were quick to find fault with these reports that produced headlines around the world. Some said the photos exaggerated the amount of improvement that actually took place by placing the subjects in different lights and exposures in the before-and-after pictures. The truth of the matter, when the bulk of the evidence is carefully examined, is that, yes, Retin A *does* "improve" sun-damaged (photoaged) skin—but not with the consistency or to the extent that some enthusiasts claimed. The improvement is, overall, fairly modest in most cases, limited to reducing fine surface wrinkles. Some claim, however, that more prolonged use (a year or longer) can produce more striking effects. This remains to be convincingly demonstrated, and no one is sure yet what the long-term effects (both good and bad) might be.

Retin A is, in any case, a genuine "breakthrough" drug, the first of what promise to be a long succession of "cosmeceuticals" that will be introduced in the near future. Other, perhaps far more effective, vitamin A derivatives are likely to be among them.

4) Improves vision—No one disputes the idea that vitamin A plays a crucial role in helping to *maintain* good vision. Real deficiencies in vitamin A will result in night blindness, still a prevalent problem in some third-world countries. There is no good evidence, however, that vitamin A, in any form, can restore eyesight once it begins to fade, unless it is fading because of a frank vitamin A deficiency. Most common vision problems are unrelated to how much vitamin A you consume.

5) Speeds wound healing—Supplemental beta-carotene has been shown to speed wound healing in laboratory animals. In cases where the animals were vitamin A deficient to begin with this acceleration was quite significant. Human diabetics and surgical patients are noted for having slow-healing wounds, and some researchers, extrapolating from their studies of diabetic and other test animals, believe these individuals can be helped with supplemental vitamin A. This seems likely but remains to be confirmed.

Related to Negative Claims:
1) Highly toxic—Preformed vitamin A is unquestionably toxic in high doses, although these usually have to be maintained for long periods before signs of toxicity begin to appear. There is a high degree of variability from one individual to another. Some take 50,000 IUs of vitamin A daily for years without apparent difficulty, while a few may react adversely to a single 20,000 IU capsule. Signs of toxicity include headaches, blurred vision, nausea, hair loss, itchy eyes, aching bones and sores on the skin. These symptoms usually subside rapidly once

vitamin A intake is reduced or discontinued. Beta-carotene, on the other hand, has extremely low toxicity. Vitamin A derivatives that are being marketed as prescription drugs have some of the same toxicity as preformed vitamin A but, when properly administered under the supervision of a physician, can usually be tolerated sufficiently well to achieve the desired therapeutic effects.

2) May cause birth defects if taken during pregnancy—Preformed vitamin A has been linked to birth defects in various animals. In humans, a few cases of defects linked to daily intake of 40,000 IUs (or more) have been reported. There is no evidence that beta-carotene, at any dose level, produces birth defects. Pregnant women, however, should not take any drug, vitamin, mineral or food supplement without first consulting their physicians. Accutane and etretinate, as previously discussed, can produce birth defects and must not be used under any circumstances by pregnant women or those women of childbearing age who are not using contraception. Women of childbearing age are advised not to use etretinate at all since it remains in the body long after its use is discontinued.

3) May cause bone disease among those with chronic kidney failure—Kidney patients who are undergoing dialysis may be at special risk of developing one particular form of vitamin A toxicity: a bone disease that results from increased resorption of bone leading to high levels of calcium in the blood. This hypercalcemia, associated with a high intake of preformed vitamin A, is relatively rare in normal individuals. The higher-than-expected frequency of bone fractures in *polar bears,* by the way, is related to their high dietary intake of preformed vitamin A. Patients with chronic kidney failure should consult their physicians before taking vitamin A.

IV. RECOMMENDATIONS

A) *Suggested Intake:* The U.S. Recommended Daily Allowance for vitamin A is 5,000 IUs. Some "megavitamin" advocates have recommended taking up to 50,000 IUs daily—a dose that definitely could be hazardous in many cases. The U.S. RDA 5,000, on the other hand, may be insufficient for many people, particularly those who smoke, those who live on junk foods or otherwise have poor nutrition, those who are hospitalized, those who are recovering from surgery, those who are diabetic, those who are fighting infections, those who are exposed to high levels of toxic chemicals and pollutants. The U.S. RDA is based on the assumption that vitamin A will be derived in whole or part from preformed vitamin A, the potential toxicity of which, in high doses, is established. Even where preformed vitamin A is concerned, however, there is virtually no evidence that daily supplementation with up to 15,000 IUs will pose any real risk, even in children.

With the recent advent of inexpensive and readily available beta-carotene supplements, and with the accumulation of evidence suggesting that this vitamin A precursor can confer many of the same and perhaps even additional benefits, there is *no reason to take preformed vitamin A supplements at all,* except under certain doctor-prescribed circumstances. Instead, you should eat at least some foods rich in vitamin A on a daily basis (for example, one average-sized carrot gives you a full 5,000 IUs of beta-carotene) and, as a potential preventive against some of the diseases discussed previously, take a daily supplement of 5,000 to 25,000 IUs of beta-carotene. This amount can safely be used by children as well as adults. Beta-carotene in those quantities is safe for pregnant women too, but, as noted, all pregnant women should consult with their physicians about any drugs, vitamins, minerals or other food supplements they are considering. Pregnant women should definitely avoid taking more than 5,000 IUs of *preformed* vitamin A daily during pregnancy.

B) *Source/Form:* Fish-liver oil, meats and animal products are the richest sources of preformed vitamin A. Half a pound of calf's liver contains almost 75,000 IUs of preformed vitamin A. Carrots, sweet potatoes, broccoli, spinach, collards, turnip greens, kale, cantaloupe, winter squash, mustard greens, beet greens, papayas, apricots, watermelons, tomatoes and lettuce are among the foods rich in beta-carotene. A single sweet potato contains nearly 10,000 IUs of beta-carotene. As for supplements, there are numerous beta-carotene preparations on the market today. Most of these appear to be of about equal value. Compare prices.

C) *Take With:* Try to incorporate beta-carotene into a well-balanced vitamin/mineral regimen. Be aware that high intake of vitamin E (apparently in amounts greater than 600 IUs daily) has been shown to interfere with beta-carotene absorption and utilization.

D) *Cautionary Note:* Discontinue taking vitamin A, in any form, if signs of toxicity arise, such as persistent headaches, blurred vision, nausea, hair loss, aching bones, skin lesions. Toxicity is *highly* unlikely with beta-carotene supplementation. If you are taking preformed vitamin A (retinol), limit the dosage to 15,000 IUs daily. Discontinue taking *preformed* vitamin A or cut back to no more than 5,000 IUs daily if you are a pregnant woman or a woman using the birth-control pill. The Pill has been shown to increase blood levels of retinol independent of supplementation. Beta-carotene, however, *has not* been shown to have an adverse interaction with the birth-control pill. Also, as noted before, do not take more than 600 IUs of vitamin E daily with the recommended beta-carotene. Vitamin E, in high doses, has been shown to interfere with beta-carotene absorption.

Note that those with hypothyroidism and some with diabetes may not be able to efficiently convert beta-carotene to vitamin A and may thus assume a yellowish pigmentation even at lower doses. This pigmentation is not harmful in itself and will fade once beta-carotene intake is stopped or reduced. Those who note yellowish pigmentation while taking beta-carotene in the dose ranges suggested here and who have not previously been diagnosed as diabetic or as having hypothyroidism should be tested for these conditions. I've seen a number of cases where low-dose beta-carotene supplementation has unmasked these diseases.

VITAMIN B_1
(Thiamin)

I. OVERVIEW: Protects Against Some Symptoms of Alcoholism

There are probably more adults deficient in this vitamin than any other. That is true in most developed countries for one reason—the high rate of alcoholism. Alcohol interferes with all nutrients but especially with thiamin, vitamin B_1.

Thiamin plays a major role in the conversion of blood sugar (glucose) into biological energy. It is involved in some key metabolic reactions, in nervous tissue, in the heart, in the formation of red blood cells and in the maintenance of smooth and skeletal muscle.

Thiamin deficiency is known as beriberi (from the Singhalese language meaning extreme weakness). "Dry" beriberi occurs when the deficiency affects the nervous system, producing symptoms of mental confusion, visual disturbances, paralysis of some of the eye muscles, staggering gait, foot drop and decreased sensation in the feet and legs. "Wet" beriberi involves the heart and circulatory systems. The most extreme manifestation of wet beriberi is shoshin beriberi. Shoshin is Japanese for damage to the heart which is characterized by severe heart failure due to the accumulation of lactic acid in the blood, a condition that, if not promptly treated, leads to death 100 percent of the time.

In addition to alcoholics, the very young and the elderly with grossly unbalanced diets are also at higher risk of having thiamin deficiencies sufficient to produce symptoms of beriberi.

II. CLAIMS

Positive:
1) Protects against metabolic imbalances caused by alcohol; 2) beneficial in the treatment of heart disease; 3) useful in neurological disorders; 4) helpful in the treatment of anemia; 5) capable of detoxifying lead; 6) improves mental ability and IQ; 7) helps control diabetes; 8) protects against sudden unexplained death syndrome (SUDS); 9) useful in the treatment of herpes and other infections; 10) repels fleas and other insects.

Negative:
1) Toxic.

III. EVIDENCE

Related to Positive Claims:
1) Protects against metabolic imbalances caused by alcohol—Thiamin is particularly vulnerable to alcoholic assault. Alcohol produces a thiamin deficiency by interfering with intestinal absorption of the vitamin, by impairing the ability of tissues to store the vitamin and by decreasing the conversion of thiamin to its active form. Making matters even worse is the fact that alcoholics typically eat very unbalanced diets, limiting intake of vitamin B_1 to begin with.

Most alcoholics suffer from symptoms of beriberi, especially mental confusion, visual disturbances and paralysis of some of the eye muscles. These and such other symptoms as staggering gait and decreased sensation can usually be prevented and often successfully treated with supplemental B_1. The doses needed in alcoholics are large—up to 100 milligrams daily.

2) Beneficial in the treatment of heart disease—When there is too little thiamin in the body the heart suffers. B_1 deficiencies can result in disturbed heart rhythm, shortness of breath, swelling of the feet and legs, low blood pressure, chest and abdominal pain, kidney failure, cardiac failure and, if not corrected, death. All of these symptoms can be prevented or treated by making up for the deficiency with additional thiamin.

The biologically active form of thiamin—thiamin pyrophosphate or cocarboxylase—has recently proved useful in the treatment of heart attacks in experiments with dogs. Intravenous injection of this form of thiamin increased strength of contractions of the injured hearts while decreasing oxygen demand. Russian researchers have reported similar benefits in human heart attack sufferers. These intriguing results certainly warrant further investigation. Thiamin itself should also be studied in this regard.

It is not unlikely that the events leading to heart attacks create localized deficiencies of thiamin and cocarboxylase in the heart. Such deficiencies have, in fact, been detected in patients with cardiac failure who otherwise exhibit normal levels of thiamin.

3) Useful in neurological disorders—The many adverse effects thiamin deficiency can have on the nervous system have already been discussed. Some of these symptoms come about because of the role thiamin plays in the function of both smooth and skeletal muscles. B_1 deficiencies frequently result in generalized skeletal muscle weakness with resulting paralysis, especially in the eye muscles. Where neurological problems are caused by frank B_1 deficiency, supplementation with the vitamin is an effective treatment. There is no basis, however, for claims that B_1 can help alleviate symptoms of neurological disorders unrelated to thiamin deficiency, such as multiple sclerosis, Bell's palsy, myasthenia gravis and Meniere's disease.

4) Helpful in the treatment of anemia—Even though anemia is not one of the consequences of thiamin deficiency, there is a type of anemia that responds well to large doses of the vitamin—the so-called thiamin-

responsive anemia syndrome. Even those who have this disorder have normal thiamin levels—yet their disease responds to high-dose supplementation. Most likely there is some impairment of the conversion of thiamin to its active form in these individuals. I believe it warranted to treat those with unexplained anemias with a therapeutic trial of high-dose thiamin (up to 100 milligrams daily).

5) Capable of detoxifying lead—Given the fact that lead continues to be the most important industrial pollutant, it is surprising and unfortunate that more attention has not been given to a study showing that thiamin can potentially exert a very powerful protective effect against this toxin. Cattle were injected with twenty times their usual intake of thiamin, a treatment that effectively blocked toxic symptoms from orally administered lead and greatly reduced lead deposition in their brains, livers, kidneys and all other tissue examined.

6) Improves mental ability and IQ—In frank deficiency states, supplemental thiamin can help clear up mental confusion. This is true in many alcoholics and some of the elderly, especially when they are put under the stress of surgery, which further depletes their thiamin stores.

As for the claim that supplemental vitamin B_1 can increase IQ, this grew out of a study in which a small number of mentally retarded children, treated with thiamin and other nutrients (as well as thyroid in many cases), were said to gain 11 to 24 IQ points. This study attracted worldwide attention but, unfortunately, failed to be confirmed in no less than seven follow-up studies.

7) Helps control diabetes—Abnormal glucose tolerance, similar to that found in diabetes, appears to be part of the clinical picture of thiamin deficiency. Correction of the deficiency corrects the problem in these cases. Diabetics who have normal B_1 levels, however, will not be helped with thiamin supplementation.

8) Protects against sudden unexplained death syndrome (SUDS)—It was recently postulated that the sudden deaths of Southeast Asian refugees (120 of these deaths since 1977) in this country might be due to thiamin deficiency. At this time, however, there is still no convincing evidence to support this idea.

9) Useful in the treatment of herpes and other infections—There was a report many years ago that intramuscular injections of thiamin could

clear up herpes zoster (shingles). There has never been any confirmation of this report; it's possible no one has ever tried to reproduce this finding.

Supplementary thiamin doesn't seem to boost immunity in humans, except in one instance. There is a rare disorder in which the neutrophils, white blood cells involved in immunity, are subpar. Giving thiamin stimulates the neutrophils, in this case, making them more energetic and efficient in killing bacteria.

10) Repels fleas and other insects—A lot of people say that thiamin supplements help them and their pets ward off attack by fleas, mosquitoes and other biting insects. This idea has never been tested scientifically, although it has been hypothesized by researchers that the odor associated with the excretion of the vitamin via perspiration may repel the insects. Even without the addition of thiamin it appears that there is a complex and unique chemistry to each of our bodies which may either attract or repel various insects—a phenomenon that possibly accounts for some people saying biting insects "love" them, while others say they never have problems with these pesky creatures. If you're the type that insects love, you may want to give thiamin—in doses up to 100 milligrams daily—a try, especially during those periods when mosquitoes are swarming or fleas are particularly troublesome.

Related to Negative Claims:

1) Toxic—Following reports several years ago that the water-soluble vitamin B_6 could, in high doses, lead to neurological toxicity, some worried that other water-soluble vitamins, such as thiamin, might likewise have toxic effects. To date no toxicity has been reported by those taking large doses of vitamin B_1 over prolonged periods of time.

IV. RECOMMENDATIONS

A) *Suggested Intake:* The RDA for thiamin is 1.2 to 1.5 milligrams of thiamin daily for males. The RDA for adult women is 1.0 to 5 milligrams daily with an addition of 0.4 milligrams daily for pregnant women and 0.5 milligrams daily for nursing mothers.

Chronic alcoholics are particularly vulnerable to thiamin deficiency and may require 10 to 100 milligrams daily to maintain the proper balance.

Others at risk of getting too little thiamin include those on weight-loss diets, those who are heavy coffee or tea drinkers, the elderly on less than adequate diets, the elderly following surgery, those who use furosemide (Lasix), digoxin, antacids and those who consume foods containing bisulfite preservatives, which destroy thiamin. For these, supplementation from 1.5 to 10 milligrams of B_1 daily is advisable.

Intake for those suffering from acute alcohol toxicity sufficiently severe to require hospitalization: this situation requires special care and can mean the difference between life and death; alcoholics in this situation should be *injected* with 100 to 250 milligrams *before* they are given any intravenous glucose. Alcoholics are already building up lactic acid due to thiamin deficiency. If glucose is given without first giving thiamin then acid accumulation accelerates—fast enough and severely enough in some cases to cause serious neurologic and cardiac symptoms and even death.

Those with marginal nutritional deficiencies who are *not* alcoholic but who are being fed intravenously may also experience life-threatening crises if given glucose without also getting sufficient B_1 intravenously.

B) *Source/Form:* All plant and animal foods contain thiamin. Good sources are whole-grain products, brown rice, seafood and beans. Highly milled foods (such as polished white rice) are low in thiamin. Beriberi was first recognized in those whose diets consisted mainly of polished rice. As a supplement, vitamin B_1 is mostly available in the forms of thiamin hydrochloride and thiamin mononitrate, either individually or in combination with other vitamins and minerals. Either form is acceptable.

C) *Take With:* Best taken in a well-balanced vitamin/mineral preparation.

Vitamin B_2
(Riboflavin)

I. OVERVIEW: The Exerciser's Friend

Riboflavin, like thiamin, is crucial in the production of body energy. It is involved with an enzyme called glutathione reductase, which helps maintain glutathione, a major protector against free-radical damage.

And B_2 itself also has antioxidant qualities. Thus riboflavin is pivotal both in the inner breathing of our cells where energy is produced and also in the quenching of the toxic exhausts of that inner, energy-producing cell respiration.

Riboflavin is water soluble and so is not stored in significant quantities in the body. It must be replaced continuously through diet or supplementation to avoid deficiency. The most common cause of riboflavin deficiency is unbalanced diet. (The richest sources of the vitamin are milk, cheese and yogurt.) It is not uncommon to find deficiencies in the elderly, who often subsist on such things as tea, coffee, toast and cookies.

Riboflavin deficiency is common in alcoholics, as well. It is also associated with some psychotropic drugs (such as tranquilizers), hypothyroidism and borate toxicity.

People who indulge in a lot of physical exercise often need extra riboflavin—particularly women. Vigorous exercise raises the daily requirement for the vitamin.

Riboflavin deficiency mainly affects skin and mucous membranes. Symptoms include cracks in the corners of the mouth, cracks on the lips, reddening of the tongue associated with a burning sensation and eczema of the face and genitals. When there is a deficiency of riboflavin there is usually a lack of the other B vitamins, too.

II. CLAIMS

Positive:
1) Protects exercisers from antioxidant damage and boosts athletic performance; 2) protects against cancer; 3) protects against anemia.

Negative:
1) Toxic in high doses.

III. EVIDENCE

Related to Positive Claims:
1) Protects exercisers from antioxidant damage and boosts athletic performance—While there is no evidence that B_2 boosts athletic performance, there is no doubt that those who indulge in heavy physical activity need more of this vitamin to protect their energy-making mechanisms from free-radical damage. A study has confirmed that women who exercise a lot, in particular, need more riboflavin.

2) Protects against cancer—Riboflavin deficiencies have been linked to esophageal cancer in some areas of the world. A recent study indicates that supplementation with B_2 reduces the number of possibly precancerous cells in the esophagus. More definitive studies will have to be done, however, before riboflavin can be said to have a role in preventing or treating cancer.

3) Protects against anemia—riboflavin and iron deficiency not uncommonly occur at the same time in humans. And since riboflavin is believed to enhance iron absorption, there may be some link, yet to be clearly demonstrated, between riboflavin deficiency and anemia. A study needs to be done to see whether riboflavin supplementation will enhance red blood cell response to iron treatment.

Related to Negative Claims:
1) Toxic in high doses—There is no evidence that high doses have adverse effects.

IV. RECOMMENDATIONS

A) *Suggested Intake:* The U.S. RDA for adults is 1.7 milligrams of vitamin B_2 daily. Those who exercise, pregnant women and nursing mothers probably require from 2 to 2.5 milligrams daily. Those at risk for riboflavin deficiency include alcoholics, the elderly who eat unbalanced diets, those on weight-loss diets, those with hypothyroidism, users of boric acid or borates which bind B_2 (found in some eye products, mouthwashes and supplements—see boron under Minerals), users of such medications as chlorpromazine, imipramine (Tofranil), amitriptyline (Elavil), the antimalarials chloroquine and quinacrine, the anti-cancer drug doxorubicin and chronic users of soluble fibers such as psyllium (which also binds B_2). For these, supplementation with from 1.7 to 10 milligrams daily is advisable.

B) *Source/Form:* Good sources of riboflavin are milk, cheese, yogurt, green leafy vegetables, fruits, bread, cereals and meats (especially organ meats). Milk is probably the best source. One quart of milk contains 1.7 milligrams of B_2. (Milk is seldom sold in clear bottles anymore because sunlight can destroy most of the riboflavin within a few hours.) Riboflavin is widely available in supplement form, either individually or in vitamin/mineral preparations.

C) *Take With:* Best taken in a well-balanced vitamin and mineral formula.

VITAMIN B$_3$
(Niacin)

I. OVERVIEW: The Best Cholesterol-Lowering Agent

Nicotinic acid, one of the forms of niacin (vitamin B$_3$), after decades of neglect by the medical establishment, is abruptly coming to be regarded as one of the substances of choice for lowering blood levels of cholesterol, edging out multimillion dollar drugs that were designed for that purpose but which do the job less well, have more side effects and cost the consumer up to forty times as much!

It is also clear now that nicotinic acid significantly reduces the risk of death among those who have previously had heart attacks.

On another front, nicotinic acid has achieved a sort of cult status in the supplement underground, first for its claimed benefits in preventing or even curing schizophrenia, more recently for its claimed efficacy as a detoxifying agent, a substance that can cleanse the body of all manner of toxins, pollutants and even many narcotic drugs.

The term niacin is commonly used to refer to the two forms of vitamin B$_3$, nicotinic acid and nicotinamide.

II. CLAIMS

Positive:

1) Lowers cholesterol and protects against cardiovascular disease; 2) protects against and detoxifies pollutants, alcohol, narcotics; 3) prevents or cures schizophrenia and some other mental disorders; 4) may be of benefit in diabetes; 5) relieves migraine headaches; 6) alleviates arthritis; 7) stimulates the sex drive; 8) reduces high blood pressure.

Negative:

1) Toxic in high doses.

III. EVIDENCE

Related to Positive Claims:

1) Lowers cholesterol and protects against cardiovascular disease—Beginning in the 1950s, researchers reported that nicotinic acid could lower blood levels of cholesterol and triglycerides, both of which contribute to the fatty deposits that narrow the arteries and lead to heart attacks and strokes. At first it appeared that huge doses were required to achieve these results, but now favorable outcomes have been reported with doses in the neighborhood of 2 grams per day and even with as little as 1,200 milligrams per day. The 1975 Coronary Drug Project Research Group, in a major study, found that nicotinic acid markedly reduces cholesterol levels and reduces the recurrence rate for heart attacks by almost 30 percent.

A follow-up on the landmark Coronary Drug Project study has more recently revealed that those who got nicotinic acid, rather than placebos, have a significantly lower mortality rate in *every* cause-of-death category analyzed: coronary, other cardiovascular diseases, cancer and all "other" causes. Even more surprising to the researchers was the finding that those who got the nicotinic acid supplements during this long-term study were also far less likely to die from any cause than were those who were treated with several of the major cholesterol-lowering drugs. These other drugs, in fact, were shown to be no better than the placebo in keeping people alive.

Other studies have confirmed the cholesterol- and triglyceride-lowering capabilities of nicotinic acid. One five-year follow-up study found reduced illness and death among nicotinic acid-treated patients suffering from heart disease, when compared with those who did not receive the vitamin. Another study, involving people who were genetically predisposed to high blood levels of cholesterol, has provided preliminary evidence that nicotinic acid may be capable of actually *reversing* some atherosclerosis. Cholesterol reductions as high as 22 percent and triglyceride lowering as great as 52 percent have been reported.

The daily dose of nicotinic acid used in the Coronary Drug Project ranged up to 7 to 8 grams, high enough to cause frequent adverse side effects. More recently other researchers have obtained significant decreases in total cholesterol by using only 2 grams per day. This dose was sufficient in most of the patients studied to increase the so-called good cholesterol (HDL) by 33 percent. HDL helps carry cholesterol out of the body. More recently still, another researcher reported comparable benefits using only 1,200 milligrams of nicotinic acid daily. An 800-milligram dose, however, was found to be ineffective. It appears that for many patients relatively modest doses of niacin can achieve significant results, but there is a wide variability in requirements from one individual to the next. Incidentally, nicotinamide, the other form of niacin, does not have the cholesterol-lowering capability of nicotinic acid.

2) Protects against and detoxifies pollutants, alcohol and narcotics— These claims have persisted for some time and, in fact, have been amplified in recent years. There have been anecdotal reports that nicotinic acid can vanquish "bad trips" induced by LSD and other recreational drugs. Others claim that it can detoxify everything from heroin to Agent Orange.

Several years ago there were reports in the press that Narconon, a Los Angeles drug-rehabilitation program, was using nicotinic acid to detoxify thousands of individuals addicted to a variety of drugs. Some Vietnam veterans, participating in that same program, claimed to have been cleansed of residues from the toxic defoliant Agent Orange. The Los Angeles-based Foundation for Advancement in Science and Education reportedly did a follow-up study on 103 persons who were treated with a regimen that combined nicotinic acid, saunas and exercise and found (not surprisingly) reduced cholesterol levels. Reduced blood pressure was also reported. More intensive tests on seven of the study subjects reportedly showed reductions in previously measured levels of various toxins, including PCBs and such pesticides as heptachlor and dieldrin.

The nicotinic acid/sauna/exercise "Purification Program" was apparently named and started by the Church of Scientology. The only explanation given for its claimed benefits is that nicotinic acid supposedly frees up toxic substances that are stored in fatty tissues; prolonged saunas and long-distance running then expel the toxins in perspiration.

Others have claimed that nicotinic acid, in doses ranging between 500 milligrams and 3 grams daily can significantly reduce the craving for alcohol and drugs among many of those addicted to these substances.

These reports are certainly intriguing; there is, however, no adequate support of these claims.

3) Prevents or cures schizophrenia and some other mental disorders—The most striking effect of severe niacin deficiency is the disease pellagra, which is characterized by dementia, diarrhea, depression and skin problems. Pellagra was the first form of "mental illness" to be directly linked to a physical cause: lack of B vitamins in general and especially lack of niacin. Since then a few researchers have persistently claimed that some forms of schizophrenia can also be treated successfully with nicotinic acid. There is, as yet, no adequate substantiation of these claims.

4) May be of benefit in diabetes—This is a relatively new claim. It is based on some work regarding a substance called the glucose tolerance factor, which is thought to potentiate the effect of insulin in glucose metabolism (see section on chromium). Glucose tolerance factor was earlier thought to have nicotinic acid as part of its structure. But, at present, it is unclear whether nicotinic acid is in fact present in glucose tolerance factor, and there is no evidence that nicotinic acid is of benefit in diabetes.

5) Relieves migraine headaches—Some doctors, and others, report anecdotal success in using niacin to abort migraine headaches when they first begin. Unfortunately, there are no controlled studies to substantiate these claims.

6) Alleviates arthritis—There is no evidence to support this claim.

7) Stimulates the sex drive—Nicotinic acid is a vasodilator, which means that it expands the blood vessels, increasing blood flow into certain parts of the body. The so-called niacin flush is often experienced by those who take large doses of this nutrient. The flush is something like a protracted blush and is usually confined to the face, neck and shoulders. A few, but only a very few, claim that this flush sometimes pervades the genital region as well, and is thus sexually stimulating or pleasurable. Nicotinic acid is not recommended for this purpose. The chances of your finding the flush sexually stimulating are extremely remote. Most people find the niacin flush highly annoying

(see Related to Negative Claims); some find it frightening. Moreover, nicotinic acid in high doses is not without potentially serious risks in some individuals (as explained in Related to Negative Claims).

8) Reduces high blood pressure—This has been reported, in passing, by some researchers and needs follow-up to confirm or refute.

Related to Negative Claims:

1) Toxic in high doses—Those who take nicotinic acid in large doses—usually 100 milligrams or more—experience what has been called the "niacin flush," a burning, itching, reddening, tingling sensation, usually in the face, neck, arms and upper chest, which may persist for half an hour or even longer, causing some people fright and others discomfort. This effect is due to nicotinic acid's ability to dilate the blood vessels. The flush is not considered dangerous, but the sort of doses that produce it (greater than 100 milligrams) can, in a few individuals, produce other unwanted side effects, including nausea, headache, cramps, diarrhea. Even fewer report altered heart rates and temporarily lowered blood pressure, which may produce a feeling of faintness. Persons suffering from cardiac arrhythmia (irregular heartbeat) should consult their physicians before taking nicotinic acid. Still larger doses of nicotinic acid (in excess of 2 grams daily) have been reported to produce skin discoloration and dryness, decreased glucose tolerance, high uric-acid levels, abnormal liver function tests, aggravation of peptic ulcers and even symptoms that resemble some of those that accompany hepatitis. There is some evidence that liver toxicity can be avoided, even at these doses, through very gradual increases in dosage, arriving at the 2-gram level only after some months. No one, however, should take these megadoses without medical supervision.

IV. RECOMMENDATIONS

A) *Suggested Intake:* The National Research Council recommends 13 to 19 milligrams of niacin for adults, 5 to 6 milligrams for infants and 9 to 13 milligrams for children one through ten. Large doses may be useful under certain circumstances, when ordered by and supervised by a physician. Very large doses of niacin have pharmacological effects that require careful monitoring by a doctor. Possible, but not proved, benefit may accrue from taking 20 to 100 milligrams of niacin daily if you are eleven years of age or older. Do not take more than this unless advised to do so by a physician. If you want to use high doses of nicotinic acid to lower your cholesterol it is imperative that you consult your doctor first.

B) *Source/Form:* Dietary sources of niacin include lean meats, fish and poultry. Vitamin B_3 as a supplement is available in the form of nicotinic acid or as nicotinamide (niacinamide). Nicotinamide, unlike nicotinic acid, does not cause the so-called niacin flush.

C) *Take With:* It is important to take B vitamins in a well-balanced combination, rather than individually. (See Part Three)

D) *Cautionary Note:* Discontinue if any signs of toxicity occur, such as nausea, headaches, cramps, diarrhea, feeling of faintness, accelerated or irregular heartbeat. Toxicity is highly unlikely if intake is limited to the above-recommended dose. Those with peptic ulcer disease, liver disease, gouty arthritis or significant heart-rhythm disturbances should only take supplementary niacin under a doctor's supervision.

VITAMIN B_6

I. OVERVIEW: Immune Booster

B_6 is required for the proper functioning of more than sixty enzymes and is essential for normal nucleic-acid and protein synthesis. It plays a role in the multiplication of all cells and the production of red blood cells and the cells of the immune system. Through its effects on various minerals and brain neurotransmitters, it influences the nervous system. Severe B_6 deficiency can result in anemia, nervous disorders and various skin problems. It has been claimed that women have special need of B_6—while on the Pill, during pregnancy and in order to alleviate some of the symptoms of premenstrual tension. Recently some very preliminary evidence has emerged that suggests a possible anti-cancer role for B_6. Even more important may be the role B_6 plays in immunity. In fact, of all the B vitamins, B_6 is most crucial for a healthy immune system.

II. CLAIMS

Positive:

1) Boosts immunity; 2) protects against cancer; 3) relieves the symptoms of premenstrual tension and cures some forms of infertility; 4) has anti-convulsant effects and protects against nervous disorders; 5) helps control diabetes; 6) protects against metabolic imbalances caused by oral contraceptives; 7) prevents skin diseases; 8) inhibits cataracts.

Negative:

1) Toxic in high doses and may cause serious nerve damage; 2) reduces the therapeutic effect of levodopa, a drug used by sufferers of Parkinson's disease.

III. EVIDENCE

Related to Positive Evidence:

1) Boosts immunity—Laboratory animals and human volunteers subjected to B_6 deficiencies experience severe immune depression. Many older people and alcoholics have low levels of B_6—and both groups are more likely to have weakened immunity. So are people suffering from diseases characterized by immune disorders, such as AIDS and many cancers.

Recently it has been shown for the first time that B_6 supplements can boost immunity in the elderly. And when lab animals with cancer are fed B_6-rich diets their immune responses increase and the growth of their tumors slows.

The time is at hand to test B_6 in people suffering from cancer and immune disorders.

2) Protects against cancer—B_6 has been found to inhibit the growth of a number of different types of cancer cells in the laboratory. Mice given B_6 (in the form of pyridoxal) and then injected with melanoma cells, of the sort that appear in a particularly lethal form of skin cancer, exhibited significantly greater resistance to this cancer than did control mice that did not receive pretreatment with B_6. The vitamin-treated mice had more than a twofold reduction in tumor growth compared to the control animals.

Similarly promising results with *human* melanoma cells treated with

B_6 in culture prompted researchers to test the effects of B_6 in a human subject with melanoma. The B_6 was administered in the form of a pyridoxal cream that was applied directly to the malignant nodules, both cutaneous and subcutaneous, four times daily for a two-week period. At the conclusion of this trial "cutaneous papules were no longer visible" and "the subcutaneous nodules were significantly reduced in size (some nodules showing more than 50 percent regression)." All of this must be accounted encouraging, especially in view of the fact that melanoma has heretofore resisted almost all form of treatment. More investigation is urgently needed in order to further assess these exciting but still very preliminary findings.

3) Relieves the symptoms of premenstrual tension and cures some forms of infertility—It has been claimed for some time that B_6 can relieve various discomforts to which some women fall prey. Various disturbances of estrogen metabolism are claimed to be corrected with supplemental B_6. Premenstrual tension, often characterized by breast tenderness, headaches, weight gain due to water retention, and irritability arising in the week to ten days prior to menstruation, is a significant problem for many women. This syndrome has been attributed to a variety of hormonal processes, some of which are known to be affected by B_6. It has been reported that twenty-one of twenty-five women given 500 milligrams of B_6 daily, in time-release tablets, in a double-blind study enjoyed significant relief from premenstrual symptoms. Treatment continued through three consecutive menstrual cycles. These researchers have also reported that women with unexplained infertility experienced "a high conception rate" after B_6 therapy was started.

Another study showed that B_6 is effective in alleviating the dizziness and nausea that usually accompany premenstrual syndrome. The impact on depression and anxiety were less, but those who got B_6 were less likely to withdraw from social activities than were control subjects who got placebos instead of B_6.

4) Has anticonvulsant effects and protects against nervous disorders— It is established that B_6 deficiency can cause convulsions and degeneration of peripheral nerves. In fact, it was through the administration of high doses of B_6 to infants suffering from convulsions that researchers demonstrated, in 1954, the first of many inborn vitamin-responsive

disorders of metabolism. B_6 supplementation dramatically abolishes seizures in most of these infants. A neurotransmitter in the brain thought to inhibit certain types of seizures depends in part for its existence upon adequate supplies of B_6. Except in these cases of in-born metabolic disorder, however, there is no evidence to support the claim that B_6 is effective against convulsive seizures in general.

Evidence is mounting that B_6 supplementation may be the best treatment for carpal tunnel syndrome, a compression of a nerve in the wrist that causes a pins-and-needles sensation and often quite a lot of pain in the hand. The old treatments—injecting the wrist with steroids, splinting the wrist and giving other anti-inflammatory drugs—haven't proved very useful in most cases. B_6, on the other hand, *has* proved quite effective in a large majority of patients getting 100 to 200 milligrams of B_6 per day. It sometimes takes three months of B_6 therapy before most symptoms disappear.

5) Helps control diabetes—There is some evidence that *some* forms of diabetes may be contributed to by B_6 deficiencies. Adequate levels of B_6 are required for the proper metabolism of the amino acid tryptophan. Abnormalities of tryptophan metabolism, which may contribute to glucose intolerance, have been reported in some diabetics, and these abnormalities have been found to be reversible with administration of supplemental B_6. Supplemental B_6 can reduce the need for insulin in some diabetics. Other research suggests that supplemental B_6 can enhance carbohydrate tolerance during pregnancy, when diabetes can pose special risks. If you have diabetes, discuss the possible benefits of B_6 supplementation with your physician and don't use it unless directed to do so by your doctor.

6) Protects against metabolic imbalances caused by oral contraceptives—Women who take oral contraceptives usually exhibit abnormalities of tryptophan metabolism of the sort discussed under diabetes. These abnormalities have been at least partially corrected by administration of supplemental B_6, with resulting improvement in carbohydrate (sugar) tolerance. Daily intake of 5 milligrams of B_6 is generally adequate to overcome this abnormality caused by oral contraceptives, making it clear that the megadoses of this vitamin that are often recommended during pregnancy by enthusiasts are not justified.

7) Prevents skin disease—Claims that large doses of B_6 can clear up acne and dry, itching skin have been made for some time, but without objective support. B_6 may help clear up some skin problems but only if there is a severe B_6 deficiency to begin with. See discussion of B_6 and melanoma.

8) Inhibits cataracts—It has been suggested that a number of B vitamins may help protect the lenses of the eyes from the clouding effects of cataracts. Research remains very preliminary and, though some positive data may turn up, this claim remains unproved at this time.

Related to Negative Claims:

1) Toxic in high doses and may cause serious nerve damage— Researchers have reported nerve damage in seven patients who had been taking 2 grams or more of B_6 daily. Four of the seven patients had been taking these doses for only two to four months.

   The first signs of neurotoxicity in most of these patients were unstable gait and numbness in the feet, followed by numbness and clumsiness in the hands. Extensive evaluations ruled out the presence of other or additional toxic substances. These patients gradually improved when B_6 was withdrawn, though some sensory deficits remained. The commonest reason given for taking these large doses was for relief of premenstrual edema (water retention). Clearly, it is unwise to megadose on B_6. (See Recommendations for more details on proper dose.)

2) Reduces the therapeutic effect of levodopa, a drug used by sufferers of Parkinson's disease—Vitamin B_6 is involved in the metabolism of L-dopa. If L-dopa is given by mouth, as is the case with patients suffering from Parkinson's disease, the L-dopa is inactivated by vitamin B_6 in the intestine and loses its effectiveness. Therefore, patients taking L-dopa should not consume supplementary B_6 at the same time (unless the L-dopa drug you are taking is Sinemet, in which case it *is* okay to take B_6 at the same time).

IV. RECOMMENDATIONS

A) *Suggested Intake:* The FDA's Recommended Daily Allowance is 2 milligrams for adults. Health-food stores typically sell B_6 in 50- to 500-milligram tablets. It is easy to see how an unwary consumer might soon be taking potentially highly dangerous doses of this nutrient—

four 500-milligram tablets and you're taking 2 grams a day, the same amount that resulted in significant nerve damage in several patients (see preceding discussion of toxicity). There is little in the data to justify dosages of B_6 in excess of 50 milligrams daily. That is more than an ample dose for adults, including women who are pregnant or on the Pill. Women who seek relief from the symptoms of premenstrual tension or those seeking to alleviate diabetes, symptoms of the carpal tunnel syndrome or any other disorder should consult their doctors before exceeding 50 milligrams of supplemental B_6 daily.

B) *Source/Form:* Dietary sources of B_6 include meats, whole grains and brewer's yeast.

C) *Take With:* Get your supplemental B_6 in a well-balanced vitamin/ mineral formula. (See Part Three for further recommendations.)

D) *Cautionary Note:* Don't take B_6 at the same time with levodopa, the anti-Parkinson's drug. (It *is* okay, though, to take with Sinemet.) Discontinue B_6 if any signs of toxicity occur, such as numbness in the hands or feet or unsteadiness in walking. Do not exceed 50 milligrams of supplemental B_6 daily.

Vitamin B_{12}

I. OVERVIEW: The Energizer

Here's a vitamin that appears to be doing a remarkable about-face. B_{12} has long been regarded by medical orthodoxy with something akin to suspicion or, in some cases, outright derision. A minority of doctors and many "alternative" practitioners have prescribed B_{12} for decades, claiming that it has remarkable rejuvenation and powerful energizing qualities, that it can pick a person up when everything else fails, that it improves memory and ability to reason and concentrate, dispels mental disturbances, prevents mental deterioration and, in general, makes one feel younger. In the face of all this, many "mainstream" doctors dismissed B_{12} as modern-day "snake oil."

Now it is beginning to look like B_{12} really does have some remarkable properties beyond those that have long been accepted. (We know, for example, that B_{12} is essential in humans for the healthy metabolism of nerve tissue. We know that deficiencies can result in nervous disorders and brain damage, as well as a form of anemia.) It is also beginning to look like more of us may have subtle deficiencies of B_{12} than was previously believed.

There is a striking new evidence that B_{12} may have important anti-cancer effects and that it may energize not only the body but the mind, alleviating a number of neuropsychiatric problems. It may also have a role in protecting us from toxins and allergens. Additional new research suggests a greater need than ever for supplementing vegetarian/macrobiotic diets with B_{12}.

II. CLAIMS

Positive:

1) Energizes the body; 2) alleviates neuropsychiatric disorders and prevents mental deterioration; 3) protects against cancer, especially smoking-induced cancer; 4) protects against toxins and allergens; 5) needed to supplement vegetarian/macrobiotic diets.

Negative:

1) Toxic and a waste of money.

III. EVIDENCE

Related to Positive Claims:

1) Energizes the body—There is no doubt that those who have clear-cut B_{12} deficiencies to begin with feel far more energetic once their problem is diagnosed and they increase their B_{12} intake. Individuals who suffer from pernicious anemia often benefit dramatically from injections of B_{12}. But the claim over the years has been that even generally healthy people can often benefit from supplemental B_{12}, especially during periods of stress, fatigue or recovery from illness. It is this claim that has most galled the medical profession, partly because most of the people for whom these benefits have been claimed are not, by the standard measures, deficient in B_{12}.

New research (see evidence related to other positive claims) suggests, however, that tests more sensitive than the standard ones often turn up subtle deficiencies. It is quite possible, therefore, than an enormous and continually growing and persistent body of anecdotal evidence in support of this particular claim has some real validity. More and more doctors seem to be coming out of the B_{12} "closet" all of the time, admitting that they have long used injections of this vitamin in their practice simply because they seem to have such favorable impact on their patients.

One doctor, writing in *Medical World News* recently, stated that he and "thousands of other physicians" have gradually come to be convinced that B_{12} can help patients recover faster from viral and bacterial diseases and sometimes from surgical procedures. B_{12} seems to accelerate a restoration of appetite and vigor.

Clearly this claim has not yet been *proved* in the most rigorous sense—and it *is* desirable that such proof be sought. But, in the meantime, it is also very clear that a growing number of doctors and patients are not about to forgo what they perceive to be the very real energizing benefits of B_{12}. In view of other recent, very promising findings related to B_{12} (see below), it appears now that there is a good chance that this claim will finally be adequately investigated.

2) Alleviates neuropsychiatric disorders and prevents mental deterioration—It is well known that B_{12} deficiencies are linked to deterioration of mental functioning, to neurologic damage and to a number of psychological disturbances. Up to 10 percent of the elderly have fairly clear-cut B_{12} deficiencies accompanied by these neuropsychiatric disorders. Now there is good evidence that B_{12} deficiencies may occur commonly in the general population, even in the absence of those manifestations long thought to be hallmarks of this deficiency (such as anemia). Newly developed and more sensitive tests have enabled researchers to make this determination.

In a series of thirty-nine patients treated for neurologic symptoms related to B_{12} deficiency, 100 percent showed improvement, sometimes dramatic improvement. The neuropsychiatric symptoms included abnormal gait, memory loss, decreased reflexes, weakness, fatigue, disorientation, psychiatric disorders and impaired touch or pain perception. Such symptoms were present in varying degrees and combinations.

3) Protects against cancer, especially smoking-induced cancer—Because smokers have been shown to have abnormally low levels of B_{12} and folic acid (another B vitamin), researchers decided to see whether supplements of these substances might offer some protection

against the ravages of smoking. Components of cigarette smoke are known to reduce levels of these vitamins in the cells that line the lungs. Since folic acid is involved in cell division, interference with its activity, researchers believed, might lead to lung or bronchial cancer. Interference with B_{12} also concerned them because of its interrelationship with folic acid.

To test their hypothesis, these researchers recently studied seventy-three men who had been smoking a pack of cigarettes a day for at least twenty years. All had potentially precancerous changes in their bronchial tissues but none had yet developed cancer. The men were divided into two groups, one receiving 10 milligrams of folic acid and 500 micrograms of B_{12} daily, the other receiving placebos. After just four months the protective effects of the B_{12}/folic acid combination were apparent. The vitamin-treated group had significantly fewer cells classified as potentially precancerous.

The researchers properly cautioned that their findings are still preliminary and that, even if borne out by follow-up studies, no smoker should assume that he/she can now evade cancer by simply taking B_{12}/folic acid while continuing to smoke.

4) Protects against toxins and allergens—Little investigation into this claim has been made, but a recent study showed that B_{12} can effectively block most of the adverse reactions to sulfites, common food (and wine) additives. Many people are allergic to sulfites, which can produce headache, congestion, drippy nose and bronchial spasms.

Eighteen sulfite-sensitive individuals were given 2,000 micrograms of B_{12} and were then given sulfites. All but one evaded any adverse reaction. Subsequent tests comparing B_{12} with placebos showed similar effectiveness for the vitamin. The B_{12} in this study was given not by injection but sublingually—via tablets that dissolve under the tongue (where the many vessels transport the vitamin quickly into the bloodstream).

Given the dramatic results that were obtained in this study, it is clear that B_{12} should be tested for other possible benefits related to food/chemical sensitivities and allergies. As for those who have known sulfite allergies, a 2,000 to 4,000 microgram dose of B_{12} once a day was found to be adequate to prevent most symptoms.

5) Needed to supplement vegetarian/macrobiotic diets—Even many of the proponents of macrobiotic diets and other schools of vegetari-

anism are now conceding the real danger of B_{12} deficiency, especially among children on these diets. Claims that miso, tempeh and other soy products are rich in B_{12} have been convincingly refuted in a number of recent studies. Meanwhile another study has found serious B_{12} deficiencies in some vegetarian children.

Tests of more that fifteen different tempehs, more than a dozen different misos and tamari and numerous brands of spirulina and sea vegetables revealed: no B_{12} at all in the tamari, only trace amounts in the tempehs, much less than was claimed by the manufacturers in the spirulinas. Only some of the sea vegetables seemed to contain significant amounts of B_{12}. Even here, however, there are problems, for there is now accumulating evidence that what is found in sea vegetables is not the real B_{12} but B_{12} analogues that don't fulfill the same biological requirements in the human body. Nor can vegetarians count on getting their B_{12} in grains and cereals, barley malt, shiitaki mushrooms and so on. Even unpasteurized miso, long thought to be a good source of B_{12}, is as devoid of B_{12} as the pasteurized version. Claims that brewer's yeast is another good source of B_{12} have now also been discredited.

So, vegetarians, be warned! Whatever the tempeh package labels may claim, you are gambling with your health and that of your children if you don't take a supplement containing adequate amounts of B_{12}. Vegetarians who regularly eat egg and dairy products, however, will, in most cases, be getting adequate amounts of B_{12} in their diet. Fish is also a good source of B_{12}.

Related to Negative Claims:
1) Toxic and a waste of money—There is no evidence that B_{12}, even in large doses, is toxic when taken orally, by which route very little is absorbed. Those who receive intravenous injections may develop skin problems that generally clear within one to two weeks.

IV. RECOMMENDATIONS

A) *Suggested Intake:* Unless you have a medical problem that can be benefited by taking higher doses of B_{12} (in which case your use of the vitamin should be under the supervision of a physician), I recommend a daily intake in the range of 5 to 50 micrograms daily. This dose range is adequate for those on vegetarian and macrobiotic diets, as well.

B) *Source/Form:* B_{12} is available from a number of dietary sources, including fish, dairy products, organ meats (especially kidney and liver), eggs, beef and pork. Spirulina, nori and other sea vegetables, tofu and other soy products, fermented or otherwise, pasteurized or not pasteurized, grains, yeast, cereals are *not* good sources of B_{12}. Vegetarians who object to taking combination vitamin/mineral preparations are nonetheless encouraged to take supplemental B_{12} alone, both for themselves and their children. Others should get their B_{12} in a well-balanced vitamin/mineral preparation. B_{12} supplements are also available in sublingual and intranasal forms. All have their merits, but the sublingual forms deliver more to the bloodstream.

BIOTIN

I. OVERVIEW: The Hair Vitamin?

Biotin is a water-soluble B vitamin which is produced in our intestines by bacteria as well as being obtained from our diets. It serves as a cofactor for carboxylase reactions that are involved in the synthesis of fatty acids, purine nucleotides (involved in nucleic acid synthesis and formation of the biological energy molecule ATP) and in the metabolism of the branched chain amino acids.

Biotin deficiency, which is not common, mainly affects the skin and hair. Symptoms include baldness, dry, flaky skin and a rash around the nose and mouth. At risk for biotin deficiency are those who eat a lot of raw egg white. Raw egg white contains the anti-vitamin avidin, which binds to biotin to prevent its absorption by the body. Also at risk are those who have poorly balanced diets and are, at the same time, on chronic oral antibiotics.

If any of you were ever on very low calorie weight-loss diets and lost more than just some pounds, now you know why. A number of people on those diets also lost their hair. It came back, usually along with the pounds, when the diets were discontinued. Baldness due to severe biotin deficiency from whatever cause is usually reversible with biotin supplementation.

II. CLAIMS

Positive:
1) Produces healthy hair and prevents graying and baldness; 2) boosts athletic performance.

Negative:
1) Toxic in high doses.

III. EVIDENCE

Related to Positive Claims:
1) Produces healthy hair and prevents graying and baldness—Many hair treatment products contain biotin, which is supposed to promote healthy hair. It is unclear what effect, if any, the biotin in these products has.

Biotin deficiency in rats does cause hair loss. The same is true in humans with severe deficiencies; supplementation in those cases *can* promote hair growth. For most people with graying hair or baldness, it appears highly unlikely that biotin supplementation will do any good, in the absence of a real deficiency—and, as pointed out earlier, few of us are deficient in this vitamin.

There *is* one hair claim, however, that seems to stand up: biotin has been used successfully in the management of the "uncombable hair syndrome," a disorder in children which causes a profusion of cowlicks—hair that stubbornly sticks up in odd directions and won't settle down. For some reason, biotin tames these cowlicks.

2) Boosts athletic performance—Claims were made several years ago that biotin levels were reduced in athletes and that supplementation could improve athletic performance. There has been no confirmation of this to date.

Biotin is important in the metabolism of the branched chain amino acids valine, isoleucine and leucine. It has been suggested that supplementation with these amino acids can improve athletic performance and that biotin supplementation is necessary for this to happen. Again, there is no evidence to support this.

Related to Negative Claims:
1) Toxic in high doses—There is no evidence that this is the case.

IV. RECOMMENDATIONS

A) *Suggested Intake:* The U.S. RDA for adults is 300 micrograms daily. Those at risk of biotin deficiency include those who eat a lot of raw egg whites (eating a lot of whole raw eggs is also risky in this respect), those with inadequate diets who are on chronic oral antibiotics and those who are on very low calorie weight-loss diets. For these, supplementation with 100 to 300 micrograms of biotin daily is advised.

B) *Source/Form:* Good sources of biotin are nuts, whole grain foods, milk, vegetables, organ meats and brewer's yeast. Biotin is available in supplement form either as an individual vitamin or in combination with other vitamins and minerals.

C) *Take With:* Best taken in a well-balanced vitamin/mineral formula.

FOLIC ACID

I. OVERVIEW: Help for Smokers?

Folic acid is the parent compound of a large group of naturally occurring, structurally related compounds collectively known as the folates. They are produced in higher plants and microorganisms and occur abundantly in fresh leafy green vegetables (folic acid was originally isolated from four tons of spinach, such was the crudity of isolation techniques more than sixty years ago), yeasts and liver.

Folic acid participates in several important metabolic processes in the body, the most important being the synthesis of DNA. Deficiency leads to an anemia which is very similar to that caused by vitamin B_{12} deficiency. This type of anemia is called megaloblastic anemia. Folic acid deficiency can exist, however, without anemia and can produce a broad spectrum of symptoms including generalized weakness, easy fatigability, irritability and cramps.

Most folic acid deficiency results from unbalanced diet. Alcoholics are good candidates for this deficiency. So are the elderly because of their frequently poor diets, malabsorption problems and drug interactions. Pregnancy puts women at risk. A deficiency in B_{12} often puts one at risk for folic acid deficiency, as well. Those with sickle cell anemia or any condition in which there is an unusually high production of red blood cells (such as hemolytic anemia) are at higher risk of folic acid deficiencies. See Recommendations for a list of drugs that can cause folic acid deficiency.

Recent findings suggest that folic acid can prevent certain types of cancer as well as birth defects.

II. CLAIMS

Positive:
1) Protects against cancer; 2) prevents birth defects and is beneficial in the treatment of mental retardation; 3) beneficial in the treatment of atherosclerosis.

Negative:
1) Toxic in large doses and can cause severe neurologic problems.

III. EVIDENCE

Related to Positive Claims
1) Protects against cancer—Studies done in the 1970s showed that potentially precancerous cervical cells could be improved if folic acid supplements were consumed in large doses. In 1986 researchers at the National Cancer Institute found depressed blood levels of folic acid in smokers with abnormal bronchial cells of a type prone to becoming cancerous. Researchers at the University of Alabama decided to study the effect of supplemental folic acid on the potentially precancerous lung lesions of smokers. They reported their results in 1988.

The researchers studied seventy-three male long-time heavy cigarette smokers with potentially precancerous bronchial changes. About half the study group received oral doses of 10 milligrams of folic acid and 500 micrograms of vitamin B_{12} daily. The others received placebo. After four months of the vitamin regimen, there was a significant decrease in the number of patients who had abnormal bronchial cells. These results are very encouraging and will be followed up with further studies. However, smokers should not use these results as an excuse not to quit.

Inadequate folic acid status may not only increase susceptibility to cancerous changes in the lungs of smokers, but may also increase the malignant potential of other types of cancer. For example, a researcher at the University of Vermont recently reported that mouse melanoma cells grown in the test tube and made folic acid deficient had a much higher rate of spreading when injected into mice than melanoma cells that had adequate amounts of folic acid. The increased cancer-spreading potential of the cells persisted even after the folic acid deficiency was corrected, suggesting that something occurred in those cells during the period of folic acid deficiency which was irreversible.

What this something was could have been breaks in the chromosomes.

There are at least fifty-one fragile sites in human chromosomes. Twenty of these sites correspond with chromosome breakpoints associated with human cancers. It was recently reported that certain cells grown in the test tube are much more likely to have chromosome breaks if they are deficient in folic acid. Oral intake of folic acid appears to prevent chromosome breakage and this may lower the risk of cancer. This exciting work is being pursued.

2) Prevents birth defects and is beneficial in the treatment of mental retardation—There is evidence that folic acid supplementation of pregnant women may prevent neural tube defects. These defects can lead to mental retardation.

Fragile-X syndrome is an inherited disorder of males and is second only to Down's syndrome as an identified cause of mental retardation. French investigators reported, in 1981, that oral supplements of folic acid improved many of the behavior abnormalities of the disorder.

One study reported in 1986 that some fragile-X syndrome patients given 10 milligrams daily of folic acid showed some improvement in behavior. A few prepubertal boys in the study showed some improvement in IQ but not the older children. Another study used 250 milligrams of folic acid daily. In that study, two subjects, ages eight and thirteen, showed IQ increases but not the older ones. Other studies find folic acid to be beneficial in some children but not usually those over the age of thirteen. It is unpredictable as to which fragile-X syndrome patient will respond to folic acid, but considering the nature of this disease it is worth a trial, and it is certainly worthwhile pursuing this line of research.

3) Beneficial in the treatment of atherosclerosis—The foremost proponent of this claim is the physician Kurt Oster. He reported that in the treatment of patients who had atherosclerotic heart disease, 80 milligrams daily of folic acid (200 times the RDA) prevented recurrence of heart attacks in twenty-five cases. He reported at the same time that this treatment alleviated angina (heart pain) and reduced nitroglycerin needs in thirty-one cases.

Another study looked at the effect of folic acid on peripheral vascular diseases. Four patients whose average age was eighty were given 7.5 milligrams of folic acid intravenously. After forty minutes these patients showed marked improvement in their visual acuity. In two patients, the improvement lasted only for a few hours, while in the other two it lasted more than twenty-four hours. Another group of seven patients whose average age was sixty-two was also given 7.5 milligrams of folic acid intravenously. These patients noted pleasant warm feelings in various parts of their bodies which lasted for two days. A final group of six diabetic patients whose average age was seventy-two years was given 5 milligrams of folic acid orally for four weeks. Four of the group noted improvement in visual acuity and improvement in skin temperature. It was postulated that folic acid had its effects by opening up blood vessels in the collateral circulation of the patients.

Unfortunately there has not been any follow-up of the above studies and so we really don't know if folic acid could be beneficial in the treatment of atherosclerosis. Such studies are warranted given the preliminary findings.

Related to Negative Claims:

1) Toxic in large doses and can precipitate severe neurologic problems—Very high doses of folic acid have been used over long periods of time without any adverse effects. However, there is one situation where folic acid supplementation, not toxic by itself, can unmask the symptoms of another nutrient deficiency. That is the case with B_{12} deficiency. Deficiency of either B_{12} or folic acid leads to the same type of anemia. But B_{12} deficiency also can lead to some very serious neurologic problems. If B_{12} deficiency anemia, such as pernicious anemia, is treated with folic acid, the anemia can improve, but the neurologic symptoms progress. Fortunately, laboratory testing is very adequate to distinguish which of the vitamins is causing the anemia.

IV. RECOMMENDATIONS

A) *Suggested Intake:* The U.S. RDA for adults is 400 micrograms daily. The list of those at risk for folic acid deficiency is quite a long one and includes alcoholics, pregnant women, the elderly, those on low-calorie diets, those with sickle cell anemia or other blood disorders in which there is an unusually high production of red blood cells, those with B_{12} deficiency, those with intestinal malabsorption problems and those taking certain medications. These medications include the anticonvulsants phenytoin (Dilantin), phenobarbitol and primidone, triamterene (found in Dyazide and Maxzide), oral contraceptives and sulfasalazine

(Azulfidine). Pregnant women should supplement with 400 to 800 micrograms daily. Supplementation with 400 micrograms daily is advised for all the others at risk. Smokers or others who wish to supplement with much higher doses should discuss this with their physicians, mentioning the studies discussed in this section.

B) *Source/Form:* Good sources of folic acid are dark green leafy vegetables (broccoli, spinach, romaine), oranges, beans, rice, brewer's yeast and liver. Folic acid is available in supplementary form either as an individual vitamin or in combination with other micronutrients. Recently, a folate form called folate triglutamate has become available. I see no advantage to this form since most of this substance gets converted to folic acid anyway, before it gets absorbed.

C) *Take With:* Best to take in a well-balanced vitamin/mineral formula.

D) *Cautionary Note:* Do not take supplementary folic acid if there is a suspicion that you have B_{12} deficiency anemia. Have this checked out with your physician. If you do have this problem then it is all right to take folic acid as soon as you receive treatment for the B_{12} deficiency.

PANTOTHENIC ACID AND PANTETHINE

I. OVERVIEW: Youth and Beauty

Pantothenic acid is part of the vitamin B complex and plays a number of essential metabolic roles in the human body, including some of those related to the production of adrenal-gland hormones and the production of energy. It has become increasingly popular as a nutritional supplement, widely used for its alleged abilities to boost energy, increase athletic performance, alleviate arthritis, restore color and luster to hair and, in general, rejuvenate. Deficiencies in humans can result in abdominal distress, vomiting, cramps, burning pain in the heels, fatigue, insomnia. Signs of reduced immunity to some infectious agents have also been noted in pantothenate deficiency.

Recently a metabolite of pantothenic acid called pantethine has come into the supplement supermarket. It has excited quite a lot of research, most of it directed toward cholesterol lowering and protection against cardiovascular disease. In addition, pantethine is showing early promise as a detoxifier of alcohol and as an immune stimulant.

CLAIMS

Positive:

1) Boosts energy and athletic ability; 2) lowers cholesterol and protects against cardiovascular disease; 3) prevents and alleviates arthritis; 4) speeds wound healing; 5) detoxifies alcohol; 6) stimulates immunity; 7) prevents hair loss and graying of hair; 8) retards aging.

III. EVIDENCE

Related to Positive Claims:

1) Boosts energy and athletic ability—This claim has been around for a long time. There's a lot of anecdotal evidence attesting to it. Scientific evidence, on the other hand, has been scarce. Some twenty-five years ago there was an animal study showing that rats given large doses of pantothenic acid survived twice as long as unsupplemented rats when forced to remain in cold water. In the last few years a couple human studies were finally conducted to investigate this intriguing claim. The results were mixed but interesting.

In one study, highly conditioned distance runners were given 1 gram of pantothenic acid daily for two weeks. Their performance on a treadmill was compared with equally well-conditioned distance runners who received only placebos during the study period. No difference in performance was noted.

More positive results were obtained in a more recent study in which well-trained distance runners were given 2 grams of pantothenic acid daily for two weeks. These athletes out-performed other, equally well-trained distance runners who received placebos for comparison purposes. Those who got the pantothenic acid used 8 percent less oxygen to perform equivalent work and had almost 17 percent less lactic acid buildup. These differences, particularly in the context of athletic competition, are quite significant if they are confirmed in subsequent studies.

2) Lowers cholesterol and protects against cardiovascular disease—This claim has been made with respect to pantethine, not pantothenic acid. Several studies have been reported recently indicating that pantethine can lower both cholesterol (an average of about 15 percent) and triglycerides (an average of 30 percent) in those with elevated cholesterol and triglyceride levels. These results have been achieved at doses in the range of 600 to 1,200 milligrams daily. There were no adverse side effects at those doses. Additional studies indicate pantethine may have effects that will help inhibit dangerous blood clots and irregular heart beats. Pantethine's ability to lower blood fats and the other findings related to possible cardiovascular protective effects deserve further work and confirmation.

3) Prevents and alleviates arthritis—The evidence related to this claim is intriguing. Nearly forty years ago, researchers noted that young rats acutely deficient in pantothenic acid suffered defects in the growth and development of bone and cartilage, defects that were reversed with pantothenate supplementation. This experimental work suggested a possible therapeutic role for pantothenic acid in the treatment of human bone and joint disorders.

Some years later other investigators reported that blood levels of pantothenic acid are significantly lower in humans with rheumatoid arthritis than in normal individuals. From that observation they conducted a clinical trial in which twenty patients with rheumatoid arthritis were injected daily with 50 milligrams of calcium pantothenate. Blood levels quickly rose to normal and relief from many rheumatoid symptoms was quickly achieved in most cases. Symptoms gradually returned, however, when pantothenate was discontinued. Interestingly, still better results were obtained among arthritic patients who were vegetarians. The best results were achieved among the vegetarians who were given a combination of pantothenic acid and royal jelly. (See analysis of royal jelly elsewhere in this book for further details.)

With the exception of a 1963 study attributing relief from symptoms of osteoarthritis in a small number of human patients to oral pantothenate supplements, there was no further work on these promising early findings until 1980 when the General Practitioner Research Group conducted a double-blind study that recorded "highly significantly effects for oral calcium pantothenate in reducing the duration of morning stiffness, degree of disability, and severity of pain" in patients suffering from rheumatoid arthritis. Control subjects (who received placebos) did *not* obtain relief in any of these particulars. The oral dose used in this study was one tablet of 500 milligrams daily for two days, followed by one tablet twice a day (for a total of 1,000 milligrams daily) for three days, followed by one tablet three times daily (1,500 milligrams daily) for four days, followed by one tablet four times a day (2,000 milligrams, which equals 2 grams daily) thereafter.

Pantothenate was not found to be effective, in this study, against forms of arthritis other than the rheumatoid variety. Clearly, as the Research Group concluded, further trials are justified and needed.

4) Speeds wound healing—Studies have appeared in recent years showing that surgical wounds in animals heal faster and more firmly with pantothenic acid supplementation. The vitamin seems to stimulate cell growth in the healing process. The definitive research into this issue has not yet been performed, but pantothenic acid looks promising in this regard.

5) Detoxifies alcohol—There is one recent study showing that pantethine speeds up the body's detoxification of acetaldehyde, lowering levels of it in the blood following alcohol consumption. This is significant because acetaldehyde appears to be a major player in the toxic process that accompanies long-term alcohol use. Given the magnitude of alcoholic abuse in this country and worldwide, this finding needs to be further investigated as soon as possible.

6) Stimulates immunity—This claim, made for pantethine, is based upon a single study which showed an immune-boosting effect in animals. More work will have to be done to determine whether similar effects can be obtained in humans. The effects noted in this study were activation of natural killer cells and macrophages.

7) Prevents hair loss and graying of hair—Perhaps because pantothenic acid deficiency in rats leads to graying of hair and loss of hair, many manufacturers have added pantothenyl alcohol (panthenol) to hair conditioners and other hair treatment products. There is anecdotal evidence that pantothenic acid can restore some color to human hair and prevent or slow its loss, but these claims have not been tested in scientific studies.

8) Retards aging—The claim is that megadoses of pantothenic acid will retard and remove age spots (pigments), "re-energize" old cells and extend lifespan. The lifespan claims are based upon a study conducted some years ago in which pantothenic-acid-supplemented mice lived 18 to 20 percent longer than unsupplemented control mice. This was a well-designed study, but it does not by itself prove that pantothenic acid can make mice, let alone humans, live longer. This research needs to be followed up.

IV. RECOMMENDATIONS

A) *Suggested Intake:* In the absence of any information indicating toxicity, daily doses of pantothenic acid up to 100 milligrams do not seem unreasonable as part of a preventive regimen for healthy people. Individuals with rheumatoid arthritis should consult their physicians, calling attention to the findings discussed above, before taking larger doses. Those interested in taking pantethine in the 600- to 1,200-milligram dose ranges discussed above should also consult their physicians for approval. Remember that those doses were designed for specific therapies, not for prevention of problems. Effective preventive doses will presumably be smaller.

B) *Source/Form:* Dietary sources include organ meats, eggs and whole-grain cereals. Supplements are widely available.

C) *Take With:* Best if incorporated into a well-balanced vitamin/mineral "insurance" formula. (See Part Three for further recommendations.)

D) *Cautionary Note:* At present there is no known toxicity. This does not mean, however, that large doses are safe. Research on this issue has been inadequate.

VITAMIN C

I. OVERVIEW: The Cancer Preventive

Vitamin C, also known as ascorbic acid, was the subject of the first controlled clinical experiment in recorded medical history. In the

1750s, a British doctor put limes, rich in vitamin C, in the rations of one group of sailors and then compared this group with a second group of sailors who got precisely the same rations except for the limes, which were withheld. The limeless group, after having been at sea a long time, showed the expected tendency to develop scurvy, a disease characterized by wounds that don't heal, gums that bleed, skin that is rough, muscles that waste away.

The sailors whose rations included limes, however, did not get the dreaded scurvy. And thus it was that British sailors became known as "limeys," for they regularly thereafter carried limes or other citrus fruits rich in vitamin C with them on long sea voyages.

Until recently most of us thought scurvy was pretty much a thing of the past, especially in developed countries. Now there is a growing recognition that this scourge continues in certain subsets of our population: some of the elderly, the alcoholics, the chronically ill. Vitamin C deficiencies that fall short of producing outright scurvy are also far more prevalent than most expected. Among the institutionalized elderly, up to 95 percent have been found to have vitamin C deficiencies. Other studies have shown that 100 percent of some populations of the institutionalized young have these deficiencies, 75 percent of cancer patients are deficient and that 20 percent of the healthy elderly are deficient. Other studies have shown deficiencies between 17 percent and 72 percent for different groups studied, including dental and orthodontic patients and even dentists themselves. Those undergoing dialysis for kidney failure, some food faddists and some vegetarians have also been shown often to be vitamin C deficient.

This is true despite the fact that there are probably more people taking vitamin C today than any other supplement. Surveys indicate that fully *half* of all adult Americans now take supplemental vitamin C. The great popularity of this substance proceeds in part from the tireless work of two-time Nobel Laureate Dr. Linus Pauling, who has persistently claimed that vitamin C is effective in preventing/alleviating colds and treating cancer.

While the best available evidence does not fully support Dr. Pauling, it *does* indicate that vitamin C can significantly reduce the severity of colds and that it can help prevent cancer but not inhibit established advanced cancer. There is also good evidence that vitamin C can be of benefit in the management of asthma, that it offers some protection against cardiovascular disease, speeds wound healing, helps prevent gum disease and helps protect us from pollutants, including those in cigarette smoke. Recently some research has indicated that vitamin C might even be useful in the treatment of certain mental disorders, lending support to a claim Dr. Pauling made some time ago.

II. CLAIMS

Positive:
1) Fights cancer; 2) boosts immunity against colds and other infections including AIDS; 3) lowers cholesterol and combats cardiovascular disease; 4) speeds wound healing; 5) helps maintain good vision; 6) helps overcome male infertility; 7) counteracts asthma; 8) protects against smoking and various pollutants; 9) prevents diabetes; 10) combats gum disease; 11) useful in the treatment of some mental disorders.

Negative:
1) May cause kidney stones and gout in susceptible individuals; 2) causes diarrhea and abdominal cramps; 3) leads to scurvy in those individuals (and their newborn babies) who abruptly discontinue megadose usage; 4) interferes with a number of laboratory tests; 5) waste of money since the body quickly excretes most supplemental vitamin C.

III. EVIDENCE

Related to Positive Claims:
1) Fights cancer—A protective role for vitamin C in cancer is inferred in part from population studies showing that those who regularly eat foods high in ascorbic acid are at lower risk of developing various malignancies, especially those of the stomach and esophagus. Some of these studies suggest that the often-noted high rate of stomach cancer in Japan may be due to diets high in cancer-causing substances and low in vitamin C. The relationship between high cancer rates and low ascorbic acid intake has been reported by numerous researchers.

One study noted an apparent protective effect of vitamin C against esophageal cancer even after "controlling for" alcohol use and smoking, that is, even after taking these additional cancer-contributing factors into account. Similar findings, again after controlling for smoking and alcohol consumption, were found with respect to cancer of the larynx.

The population studies suggesting a vitamin C protective effect against certain cancers are given further support by findings that ascorbic acid, through its antioxidant properties, can block the formation of various cancer-causing substances, principally the nitrosamines, within the body. Vitamin C, in fact, is now added to some bacon and other foods to help prevent the formation of nitrosamines even before they enter the human body. Much has been done to reduce, remove or inactivate nitrosamines in malt beverages and cured-meat products, but cigarette smoke and other tobacco products remain major sources of exposure. Some cosmetics also contain nitrosamines. Many public water systems carry significant quantities of these chemicals. Large (1 gram) doses of vitamin C have been shown to block nitrosamine formation in the human body.

Recently researchers in Great Britain demonstrated for the first time a direct link between levels of vitamin C in the stomach and the relative ability of stomach juices to promote potentially cancerous changes in the cells of the stomach. The finding was that vitamin C reduces by almost half the sort of changes in cells that typically lead to stomach cancer. The subjects in this study received 4 grams of vitamin C a day (in four 1-gram doses spread across the day) for one week.

Vitamin C appears, in addition, to have a protective effect against cervical dysplasia, a condition that predisposes women to cancer of the cervix. Detailed dietary and nutrient analyses of women studied reveals that those with cervical dysplasia are significantly deficient only in beta-carotene and vitamin C. The rate of cervical dysplasia, in fact, was seven times greater among women whose daily intake of vitamin C was less than half the RDA of 60 milligrams than among women whose intake exceeded the official RDA. This finding persisted even after controlling for age, sexual activity and some other pertinent variables. Analysis of results further revealed that women whose daily intake of ascorbic acid is below 90 milligrams (which is 150 percent of the RDA) will have a 2.5 times greater risk of developing this precancerous condition than will women whose intake exceeds 90 milligrams daily. It is estimated, on the basis of current U.S. Department of Agriculture data, that 20 to 40 percent of all women in the United States have daily vitamin C intakes *less than* 70 milligrams.

Still more recent work has again confirmed the lower levels of vitamin C in the blood of women with cervical dysplasia and cancer of the cervix. The researchers involved in this study suggest, as I do, that it is time for a clinical trial to directly test vitamin C's ability to prevent cervical cancer. All indications are that it should be effective.

Claims that large doses of vitamin C can prevent or inhibit familial polyposis (precancerous rectal growths) have not been as convincingly demonstrated; nor have claims been confirmed that ascorbic acid can lower the risk of colon cancer. In one recent study, however, those given supplements of vitamins C and E had a 10 percent lower rate of polyp recurrence than did those who only got placebos. The dose in this study was a relatively modest 400 milligrams each of vitamins C and E. Additional studies need to be done.

There is evidence, too, that vitamin C can suppress the growth of human leukemia cells in culture and that when given in combination with certain anti-cancer drugs and hormones, it can make those substances act more effectively.

What *hasn't* been proved is that vitamin C is useful in the *treatment* (as opposed to the prevention) of cancer. So far, however, on the treatment front, vitamin C has only been tested in *advanced* cancers. Dr. Pauling and his associates have reported significant extension of survival time among terminal cancer patients given 10 grams of vitamin C daily. The control subjects (against whom the vitamin-C-supplemented cancer patients were compared) in this study were "historical," meaning they were drawn from hospital records. In a better controlled "double-blind" study (where the researchers did not know until the end which patients had received vitamin C and which had received placebos instead), the Pauling findings were *not* duplicated. This follow-up study, however, was criticized by some because most of the patients involved had received chemotherapy or radiation therapy or both prior to receiving vitamin C; these other treatments may have so compromised their immune systems, it has been argued, that they could not respond to the ascorbic acid.

In the wake of that controversy, another study was launched—this time using patients who had *not* been given other therapies first. Again, however, the researchers failed to find any benefit from vitamin C. This time Dr. Pauling criticized the study for withdrawing 10-gram daily doses of vitamin C in otherwise untreatable cancer patients after only a short period of time. The patients in this study got vitamin C for a median of 2.5 months, making it impossible, Dr. Pauling said, to adequately test his thesis that megadose ascorbate can significantly extend the lives of cancer patients who have been declared terminal.

In fairness to Dr. Pauling and others who support his work, it must be said that these follow-up studies did *not* scientifically refute his claims with respect to ascorbate's ability to extend the lives of terminal cancer patients. On the other hand, they certainly gave no support to those claims, either. *Some* of the patients in the second follow-up continued to get 10 grams of vitamin C for up to fifteen months, and their cancers reportedly continued to progress at the same rate as those who received only the sugar pills (placebos).

The issue remains unresolved and needs more study.

Meanwhile, there is little doubt about vitamin C's promise as a cancer *preventive*.

2) Boosts immunity against colds and other infections, including AIDS—It was the claim that vitamin C can cure or prevent the common cold that first made it a topic of major discussion in public circles. The disease-fighting white blood cells have been shown to be particularly dependent upon vitamin C for normal functioning. Levels of the vitamin in these cells drop during colds and other infections, after surgery, during pregnancy and whenever the body is under stress due to exposure to radiation, drugs, alcohol, cigarette smoking. It's not at all irrational to assume, therefore, that high doses of vitamin C might fight infection or, even more likely, prevent infection.

A great many studies have now been done on vitamin C's effects on colds. An analysis of a dozen of these clinical studies showed a 37 percent average reduction in the *duration* of colds treated with vitamin C. Most of the studies have found that vitamin C (often in 1-gram daily doses) can reduce the severity and length of colds—but not the number of colds a person gets. One study found that even an 80-milligram daily dose can reduce the duration and severity of a cold.

In a recent test of ascorbic acid's effects on colds, college men were given either 2 grams of vitamin C daily or placebos. Then they were exposed to other students who had already come down with colds. Six of those who got vitamin C caught colds, while seven of those who got placebos became infected. The men who had taken vitamin C had cold symptoms that were judged to be two times less severe than those who had taken placebo. Coughs among the vitamin-C group were judged to be three times less severe.

Recent claims that vitamin C can be useful in the prevention or treatment of AIDS have not been substantiated.

3) Lowers cholesterol and combats cardiovascular disease—It was almost fifty years ago that Russian researchers first reported that large doses of vitamin C can retard atherosclerosis (narrowing of arteries) in rabbits. Continuing investigations have been sporadic since then. Guinea pigs with atherosclerosis resembling that which afflicts humans have typically been found to have severe vitamin C deficiencies. Vitamin C supplementation reduces cholesterol levels in these animals, usually to the normal range.

Humans with coronary artery disease have lower cellular levels of ascorbic acid than do healthy individuals. Postsurgical patients given 1 gram of ascorbic acid daily, in a double-blind study, developed significantly fewer life-threatening blood clots than did control subjects who did not get vitamin C. In one study it was demonstrated that a daily dose of 2 grams of vitamin C can inhibit blood clotting. In another study 500 milligrams given twice daily via injections did the same job.

Studies related to the claim that vitamin C can lower cholesterol levels have come in with mixed results. At this point it does not appear that vitamin C is particularly potent in this respect. Given its other possible benefits in fighting cardiovascular disease, however, continuing research appears justified.

4) Speeds wound healing—It is well established that vitamin C plays a crucial role in the body's manufacture of collagen, which is the principal protein "glue" that holds connective tissue and bone together. It seems almost certain, therefore, that vitamin C is involved in wound healing, though little research has been done related to this claim. There is evidence that large doses of vitamin C can substantially speed up the healing of burns in the cornea of the eye.

5) Helps maintain good vision—There are reports that vitamin C may help prevent cataract formation and may be useful in the treatment of glaucoma. A recent Canadian epidemiologic study suggests that supplemental vitamin C helps prevent cataracts in humans. Other studies are being conducted on this potentially fruitful area.

6) Helps overcome male infertility—Researchers have found that a common form of male infertility—caused by agglutination or clumping together of sperm cells, making it difficult or impossible for them to swim to the egg—can be reversed by the simple addition of vitamin C supplementation. Vitamin C levels were found to be a quarter to a third

below normal in thirty-five young infertile males studied. Improvement was noted within a few days of beginning supplementation with 1 gram daily of vitamin C. Within a week, blood levels of vitamin C were normal and so were the sperm. More than a dozen of the men's wives were reported pregnant soon after the vitamin C was administered; other pregnancies were expected to follow shortly. There is some evidence that vitamin C enhances the body's utilization of various minerals—especially zinc, magnesium, copper and potassium—that are vital to normal sperm functioning.

7) Counteracts asthma—Evidence has mounted over the years that shows reduced levels of vitamin C in most asthmatics; supplementation with vitamin C can reduce some of the airway spasms that characterize this disease. One study showed that a 500-milligram dose of vitamin C taken an hour and a half before vigorous exercise lessens bronchial spasms in some patients. Another study found that 1 gram of vitamin C daily reduces airway reactivity to harmful stimulants in asthmatics.

8) Protects against smoking and various pollutants—Smokers have been found, in many studies, to have lower levels of vitamin C both in their blood and in their white blood cells. These levels are reduced by 25 percent in those who smoke fewer than twenty cigarettes per day; they are diminished up to 40 percent in those who smoke more than twenty cigarettes per day. One study has shown that vitamin C supplements can restore ascorbic acid levels to normal in smokers. Vitamin C's role as an antioxidant in the lungs lends support to the idea that ascorbate can provide some protection against various airborne pollutants.

Vitamin C can also neutralize chloramines, chemicals that are, increasingly, being added to public water systems to purify it in place of chlorine. Chlorine has been found to combine with other substances to produce carcinogens. Unfortunately, chloramines are also showing some evidence of toxicity. So far this toxicity has clearly been demonstrated only in some fish and in humans who are on dialysis due to kidney failure. It seems likely, however, that any exposure to chloramines entails some toxicity.

9) Prevents diabetes—Blood and cell levels of vitamin C are low in many diabetics. There is, as yet, no evidence that supplemental vitamin C can prevent diabetes, but a recent study does show that vitamin C

supplements may help diabetics overcome several problems they frequently encounter: gum disease, slow wound healing and rapidly aging skin. These benefits are suggested by results that have been obtained in animal experiments with doses that would translate, in humans, to about 3 grams of vitamin C daily. This work needs to be followed up in humans, and those diabetics wishing to use large doses of vitamin C should do so only with the knowledge and consent of their physicians.

10) Combats gum disease—Periodontal (gum) disease is a feature of scurvy; following from that observation researchers have been investigating the relationship between vitamin C and this disease. It is now known that even subtle deficiencies in ascorbic acid can increase susceptibility to gum disorder. Recent experiments have shown that animals deficient in vitamin C are at much greater risk of getting periodontal disease. The vitamin deficiency weakens immune defenses and makes the surfaces of the gums more permeable, letting more bacteria and toxic substances into the tissues of the gums. Supplemental vitamin C, on the other hand, decreases the permeability of the gum surfaces, protecting the inner tissues.

12) Useful in the treatment of some mental disorders—More than twenty years ago Linus Pauling proposed a role for vitamin C in the treatment of schizophrenia. The American Psychiatric Association Task Force dismissed that proposal out of hand. Three psychiatrists later examined the claim again and rejected it in a more reasoned fashion, stating that it was an interesting theory worthy of some further consideration but that no proof existed then for its validity. They did nothing, however, to test the hypothesis themselves. Now another group of researchers has found that vitamin C can enhance the effectiveness of an antipsychotic drug, which may make it possible to reduce the dosages of the drug and thereby the unwanted side effects. The researchers favorably cited the earlier work of Pauling and believe that their findings reopen the issue of a possible role for ascorbic acid in the management of some mental disorders.

Vitamin C alone was shown in these experiments to have a small but still statistically significant effect, reducing psychotic-like behavior. When combined with the anti-psychotic drug haloperidol, there was a very dramatic decrease in the psychotic-like behavior. Vitamin C's antioxidant effects may be protecting the drug, so that less of it gets degraded before it arrives at its target tissues. It is also possible that vitamin C works directly to block dopamine receptors in the brain. This exciting research is currently being followed up. It is hoped that we will soon learn whether vitamin C can boost the effects of other drugs used in the management of mental disturbances and whether it can by itself, perhaps at higher doses, favorably affect these disorders.

A double-blind, placebo-controlled clinical study has shown that vitamin C can be helpful in the management of manic-depressive illness, especially in combination with some other therapies (see discussion of vanadium under Minerals). The favorable effect seems to be on the depressive aspect of the illness. Dramatic results were additionally reported anecdotally in some individuals whose disease had been particularly severe and persistent. One woman using the vitamin C/low-vanadium regimen avoided a depressive episode for the first time in the ten years she had been under treatment for her disease. Another woman whose long-term illness had resisted all other treatments emerged from her depression and remained free of it for the two months she used the supplements. Within a few days of withdrawal of the supplements she slipped back into severe depression. When the supplements were given to her again she once more quickly shook off the depression. The regimen appears to work by regulating defects in water and electrolyte metabolism.

These very promising results also need further investigation. They may herald an exciting new era for vitamin C.

Negative:

1) May cause kidney stones and gout in susceptible individuals—Most people taking vitamin C—even large doses of it—need not worry about kidney stones or gout. A few people who are prone to stone formation and gout (mostly for reasons that have nothing to do with vitamin C) may, however, become more susceptible if they take large doses of ascorbic acid. Individuals with histories of gout, kidney stone formation or kidney disease should not use vitamin C supplements without the consent of their physicians.

2) Causes diarrhea and abdominal cramps—Individual tolerance to vitamin C is highly variable. Some individuals get diarrhea and cramping on 500 milligrams daily while others tolerate several grams daily

for years without difficulty. If these problems arise, cut back on intake until symptoms clear.

3) Leads to scurvy in those individuals (and their newborn babies) who abruptly discontinue megadose usage—There have been a few cases of scurvy when large doses of vitamin C are *abruptly* discontinued. Large doses apparently condition accelerated metabolism and excretion of vitamin C, so that even if normal amounts of the vitamin are found in diet after discontinuing supplementation some hazard of scurvy remains. Unfortunately there is nothing in the research literature yet to tell us what dosage or dosage period poses a risk in the event of sudden discontinuance of the vitamin. If you have been taking 500 milligrams or more of vitamin C daily for at least a few weeks and then wish to discontinue supplementation, I believe it would be wiser to taper off *gradually* over a period of several days.

Pregnant women who are using large doses of vitamin C should be aware that their unborn babies may develop "rebound scurvy" after birth unless they, too, are given vitamin C supplementation. Pregnant women should consult their doctors before taking any supplements, especially megadose supplements.

4) Interferes with a number of laboratory tests—Large doses of vitamin C may make it difficult to determine if there is hidden blood in the feces; they may also interfere with tests to monitor sugar levels in the blood of diabetics. Any time you have laboratory tests tell your physician what drugs, vitamins, minerals and other supplements you are taking.

5) A waste of money since the body quickly excretes most of the vitamin C obtained through supplements—This oft-heard criticism of vitamin C supplementation is inaccurate and unwarranted. What we know is that about 200 milligrams of vitamin C daily will *maintain* ascorbic tissue saturation in humans. But the argument that supplementation beyond those 200 milligrams is just going to go down the drain, so to speak, is too simplistic and fails to account for many of the recent reports finding significant effects only at higher levels of supplementation. Blockage of carcinogenic nitrosamines (see previous discussion), for example, takes place for the most part in the gastrointestinal tract. Vitamin C's activity in this area is not necessarily reflected in or dependent upon tissue stores of vitamin C or amounts being excreted in the urine.

IV. RECOMMENDATIONS

A) *Suggested Intake:* The National Research Council has recommended 60 milligrams of vitamin C daily for adults. The new guidelines recommend smokers increase their intake to 100 milligrams daily. Many nutritional researchers now regard that as too little for optimal health, though few agree with Linus Pauling that the daily dose should be between 2,000 and 9,000 milligrams (2 to 9 grams). Need for ascorbic acid varies considerably from one individual to another. Exposure to infection, tobacco smoke, environmental pollutants, various drugs, surgery, burns, trauma, alcohol and other "stresses" may increase need for vitamin C. So may pregnancy (but consult your doctor first) and advancing age. Though many people tolerate very high doses of ascorbic acid for prolonged periods, the assumption should not be made that these doses are *always* safe. The best available data suggest that adults and children over ten years of age may benefit from a daily intake of 250 milligrams to 1,000 milligrams (1 gram) of vitamin C daily. Children under ten years of age may benefit from 50 milligrams to 100 milligrams daily. Vitamin C will be best utilized by the body if taken in divided doses, preferably with each meal, or, in any case, at least three hours apart. Since there is some negative evidence regarding doses of 1,500 milligrams daily for periods greater than two months, doses higher than 1,000 milligrams daily are not recommended. This evidence suggests that a high ascorbic acid intake is antagonistic to the copper status of men. However, no adverse effects of the reduced copper status of men were noted in this study. (See section on copper.)

B) *Source/Form:* Fresh fruits and vegetables are the best natural sources of vitamin C. Some of the research cited above indicates that many Americans get quantities of vitamin C in their diets insufficient to significantly protect against various disorders and pollutants. Hence the plethora of vitamin C supplements currently on the market. Many manufacturers hype their individual products as somehow different and better than all others; some declare that their product is "natural" rather than synthetic, that their product is "derived from" rose hips, acerola and other "rich" sources of ascorbic acid. Some vitamin C products come mixed with bioflavonoids (see discussion of these later in this book) and other substances that are supposed to "potentiate" vitamin C. Do not be misled by these claims. There is no meaningful difference between "natural" and "synthetic" vitamin C; nor do bioflavonoids add anything of demonstrated value to vitamin C. (One study—see bioflavonoid analysis—has, in fact, shown that *synthetic* vitamin C is more readily absorbed by the body than *natural* vitamin C both alone and in combination with the bioflavonoid rutin.) Recently, ascorbyl palmitate has been touted as the "best" form of vitamin C. This is a synthetic substance made by combining vitamin C with palmitic acid (a saturated fatty acid derived from fat and used as a food additive). There is no evidence that this is a better form of vitamin C. For those who find vitamin C hard on their stomachs, palm-derived ascorbate *may* be easier to tolerate. One of the best ways to get your vitamin C is in the pure granular form. Note that chewable varieties may be hard on the enamel of your teeth.

C) *Take With:* Best if incorporated into a well-balanced vitamin/mineral preparation. (See Part Three for more specific recommendations.)

D) *Cautionary Note:* Avoid taking vitamin C with *inorganic* selenium; take with selenium derived from yeast (see analysis of selenium later in this book for more details). Do not take at the same time with aspirin, as this may increase the bleeding and intestinal irritation associated with aspirin. Discontinue vitamin C if you have a tendency to develop kidney stones or gout. Suspend use temporarily, according to your doctor's instructions, if you are scheduled for glucose tests or "occult blood" tests (hidden blood in feces), as vitamin C intake can interfere with the accuracy of these tests. If you have been taking vitamin C for long periods of time and want to quit taking it, taper off slowly over a period of days. Scurvy has been reported in a few cases where individuals who were taking large doses abruptly discontinued supplementation.

Vitamin D

I. OVERVIEW: New Roles in the Treatment and Prevention of Cancer

Vitamin D is the only vitamin whose biologically active form is a hormone. It can be produced in the skin from the energy of the ultraviolet rays of the sun but is also obtained from diet. It is *not,* however, very abundant in the food chain. It is mainly found in fatty fish, liver, egg yolks and, to some extent, milk fat.

There are two major forms of vitamin D: vitamin D_2 or ergocalciferol and vitamin D_3 or cholecalciferol. These are also the major food forms of vitamin D. Vitamin D_2 is the form most commonly used for food fortification and in vitamin formulations.

The classic vitamin D deficiency disease is rickets, a disease of growing children characterized by defective mineralization of the bones. Rickets is now rare in the Western world owing to food fortification with vitamin D, particularly of milk. Vitamin D plays a central role in the regulation of calcium metabolism. It promotes calcium absorption from the gut among other things.

Recently there has been an explosion of information regarding other roles for the vitamin—roles that include control of cellular proliferation and differentiation, which could have enormous impact on the prevention and treatment of cancer; immunomodulation, which could be important in protection against and treatment of infectious diseases; and maintenance of cell membrane fluidity, which could have significance for all biological processes, including aging.

New and exciting studies suggest that vitamin D does indeed protect against colorectal and breast cancers and that it may be beneficial in the treatment of certain cancers. There is speculation that chronic vitamin D deficiency finally shows up as cancer of the breast and colon.

The elderly are at risk for vitamin D deficiency for several reasons. Many have inadequate exposure to sunlight, consume low amounts of vitamin D-containing foods and take drugs which interfere with uptake and/or metabolism of the vitamin, such as cholestyramine (used to control cholesterol and certain cases of diarrhea), mineral oil and the anticonvulsants diphenylhydantoin (Dilantin) and phenobarbitol.

Others at risk for deficiency of the vitamin include alcoholics, those who do not drink milk and who do not receive much sunlight, those with malabsorption problems and those who live in regions where they receive little natural light. It is important to note that as more and more of us use sunscreens and decrease our exposure to the sun, as we should, then dietary and supplementary sources of vitamin D will become increasingly more important as the principal source of the vitamin.

II. CLAIMS

Positive:

1) Protects against cancer; 2) beneficial in the treatment of cancer; 3) enhances immunity; 4) beneficial in the treatment of psoriasis; 5) protects against osteoporosis.

Negative:

1) Toxic.

III. EVIDENCE

Related to Positive Claims:

1) Protects against cancer—The claim that vitamin D protects against cancer was made in 1985 and the evidence that this indeed may be the case is gaining momentum. Investigation of an epidemiologic map of the United States with regard to mortality rates from cancer of the colon and breast reveals the rates are highest in populations exposed to the least amount of natural sunlight.

Vitamin D is formed in the skin by the action of ultraviolet light from the sun. The active form of vitamin D, calcitriol, is necessary for the transport of calcium from the gut into the body. Thus, differences in vitamin D production and calcium absorption could be responsible for the above phenomenon.

In 1985, researchers at the University of California, San Diego, published the results of their analysis of the relationship between dietary vitamin D and calcium intake and the incidence of colorectal cancer in a group of men who were the subjects of the Western Electric Health Study. The Western Electric Health Study was a nineteen-year, prospective, epidemiologic study which followed about 2,000 men who were selected in 1957 from workers at the Western Electric Company's Hawthorne Works in Chicago. These men completed detailed twenty-eight day dietary histories during the period 1957–1959. The men who developed colorectal cancer differed from those who did not in only two major respects—their consumption of foods containing vitamin D and calcium was much lower.

The highest incidence of both colorectal and breast cancer is in areas where people are exposed to the least amount of natural light. An increasing number of researchers now believe that it is vitamin D as well as calcium deficiency which is responsible for this. This is not only true in the United States; the worldwide pattern is the same.

Aggravating this situation is acid rain. Cedric Garland, a researcher involved in the above study, believes that the pollutants, especially sulfur dioxide, which contribute to acid rain, absorb from the sun the ultraviolet light that is responsible for the induction of vitamin D in the skin.

Interestingly, a country which is an exception to the link between low sunlight exposure and high incidence of colorectal and breast cancer is Japan. Even though people living in Japan are exposed to the low amount of sunlight which is associated with these cancers in other areas, the incidence is very low in that country. This is undoubtedly because the Japanese eat a large quantity of fatty fish, which *is* rich in vitamin D.

The active form of vitamin D does have anti-cancer activity. It has recently been found to inhibit cells from human colon cancer metastasis in the test tube. It also inhibits the growth of human malignant melanoma cells in the test tube.

A couple of hundred years ago the high sulfur coals from Newcastle burned in London and regurgitated sulfur dioxide into the skies to block out the sunlight. Rickets was the legacy of these burning coals from Newcastle. Are cancers of the colon and breast the rickets of modern times?

2) Beneficial in the *treatment* of cancer—Vitamin D in its active form, calcitriol, has been found to have anti-cancer activity *in vitro* (in the test tube). Calcitriol inhibits the growth of human leukemia cells, breast cancer cells, malignant melanoma cells, lymphoma cells and colon cancer cells. It also inhibits chemical carcinogenesis in mouse skin.

Retinoblastoma is the most common intraocular tumor of childhood. In 1966 it was suggested that retinoblastomas might be sensitive to treatment by vitamin D. Recently it has been reported that calcitriol inhibits the growth of mouse retinoblastoma both *in vitro* and in mice, and that ergocalciferol, or vitamin D_2 (one of the forms of dietary vitamin D), also inhibits the growth of the tumor in mice. The finding that a dietary form of vitamin D can inhibit tumor growth is of enormous importance. Vitamin D_2 could be effective in the treatment of human retinoblastomas and probably other cancers, as well.

3) Enhances immunity—Years ago, before the age of antibiotics, those with tuberculosis who could afford it would go to a sanitarium somewhere in the mountains where there was plenty of fresh air, sunlight, good food and relaxation. Thomas Mann's *Magic Mountain* was such a place. This therapy actually cured many. What we are now coming to understand is that the cure had something to do with the sunlight: the sunlight and its ability to produce vitamin D in the skin.

It turns out that vitamin D probably boosts resistance to tuberculosis. Two independent groups of researchers recently reported that the active form of vitamin D, calcitriol, stimulated human macrophages, the white blood cells most active in fighting tuberculosis, to slow down or stop the proliferation of the bacterium that causes the disease. This work was done *in vitro* (in the test tube). Thus, vitamin D, or its active form, is an immunomodulator. There has been an increase in tuberculosis in the U.S. over the past few years which is related to the AIDS epidemic. Worldwide, 8 to 10 million people contract this disease annually. There aren't too many magic mountains on this planet anymore, but we do have plenty of vitamin D. This immunomodulator begs to be studied in other diseases of immunity such as AIDS.

4) Beneficial in the treatment of psoriasis—Psoriasis is a skin disorder caused by overactive growth of certain skin cells, resulting in reddish, scaly patches over various parts of the body. Recently, a Boston University School of Medicine researcher reported on the use of the active form of vitamin D in the treatment of the disorder. It appears to benefit some patients. These patients had normal levels of vitamin D. Vitamin D itself was not studied, but it is interesting to note that sunlight itself is often helpful for psoriasis.

5) Protects against osteoporosis—To date, the best regimen to prevent osteoporosis in postmenopausal women includes estrogen, calcium and the hormone progesterone. Research suggests that the addition of fluoride may be useful (see fluoride under Minerals), and preliminary work suggests that manganese, boron and vitamin K may offer some additional protection as well.

There are still no convincing studies that indicate vitamin D would be helpful in protecting against osteoporosis except in the care of steroid (cortisone)-induced osteoporosis. Vitamin D might help prevent osteoporosis in those regularly taking cortisone. Calcitriol may hold more promise in the prevention and treatment of osteoporosis. Studies are in progress.

On the other hand, several reports have indicated an increased incidence of osteomalacia in the elderly. Osteomalacia is a disorder of bone characterized by decreased mineralization and caused by vitamin D deficiency. It is the adult equivalent of rickets. Osteomalacia might increase the risk of hip fracture in such patients. Since many elderly are deficient in vitamin D, it would seem prudent for the elderly to take supplementary vitamin D to prevent osteomalacia, if not osteoporosis. This could significantly reduce their incidence of hip fractures.

Related to Negative Claims:

1) Toxic—High doses of vitamin D can be toxic. The major effects of vitamin D toxicity are hypercalcemia (high levels of blood calcium) and soft tissue calcification. Symptoms of hypercalcemia include anorexia, nausea, vomiting, constipation, tiredness, drowsiness and, when more severe—confusion, high blood pressure, kidney failure and coma. Doses of less than 1,000 IUs of the vitamin daily are highly unlikely to cause any adverse effects.

IV. RECOMMENDATIONS

A) *Suggested Intake:* The U.S. RDA is 400 IUs daily. See the Overview for those at risk for vitamin D deficiency. For these, supplementation with from 200 to 400 IUs of the vitamin is desirable.

B) *Source/Form:* Very few foods are natural sources of the vitamin. These are fatty fish, liver and egg yolks. Remember that egg yolks and liver are also sources of lots of cholesterol. One quart of milk, which is fortified with D, has 400 IUs of the vitamin. Vitamin D is available in supplementary form as D_2 (ergocalciferol) either individually or in combination with other micronutrients.

C) *Take With:* If used in supplementary form, it's usually best to take in a well-balanced vitamin/mineral formula.

D) *Cautionary Note:* High doses of vitamin D may cause hypercalcemia (see negative claims). Doses less than 1,000 IUs daily are highly unlikely to have adverse effects. If you do have elevated levels of calcium in your blood, do not take supplementary vitamin D except under your physician's advice and supervision. To use calcitriol, the hormonal form of D, you must be under a physician's supervision.

VITAMIN E

I. OVERVIEW: The Nerve Protector

The discovery of vitamin E dates back to the early part of this century. Its important role in the reproduction of some animal species gave it the name tocopherol, which in Greek means "to carry and bear babies." It turns out that vitamin E does not play this role in humans. For a long time many scientists scoffed at the idea that it plays *any* role in humans. Now the best evidence suggests that vitamin E is probably essential for the survival of all oxygen-breathing forms of life.

Vitamin E is an important antioxidant. In fact, it is the oldest recognized biologic antioxidant. But it may have a function even more basic, for it appears that vitamin E is of great importance in the production of energy. In these two capacities, vitamin E is of the utmost importance in maintaining good health at the most basic level.

The claims for vitamin E over the years have been numerous and, not infrequently, off the mark. Meanwhile some very important *real* benefits of vitamin E have been, until recently, largely overlooked.

Most of the claims in the recent past have focused on heart disease and other cardiovascular disorders. It turns out that there is actually much better evidence for an active role on the part of vitamin E in nerve disorders and immunity.

We are gradually coming to better understand the roles vitamin E plays in human health. We may even soon know the optimal amounts of this substance we should take in order to ensure maximum health and life span. The quest for these answers continues to some extent, unfortunately, to be impeded by a polarity of opinions. The more hidebound of the nutritional conservatives, relying upon anecdotes and poorly designed studies of the sort they would normally deride, insist that vitamin E is to blame for a galaxy of ills, ranging from nausea and fatigue to vaginal bleeding, blood clots, breast tumors and aggravation of diabetes. At the other extreme, some nutritional true-believers, showing they can be equally cavalier about the data, ascribe to vitamin E a plethora of miracles, including beautification of the skin, enlargement of the male sex organ, enhancement of athletic prowess and, incidentally, the cure for cancer.

The truth is quite interesting enough without all the embroidery. Vitamin E is no panacea but it *is* being employed in medicine for a slowly but steadily expanding range of ailments.

Vitamin E deficiencies may be more commonplace than previously believed. One study of affluent elderly Americans revealed that 45 percent of them were getting under three-quarters of the RDA for this crucial vitamin.

II. CLAIMS

Positive:

1) Protects against neurologic disorders; 2) boosts the immune system; 3) protects against cardiovascular disease; 4) protects against air pollution and other toxic substances; 5) prevents cancer; 6) prevents diseases of the breast; 7) reduces the symptoms of premenstrual syndrome (PMS); 8) fights skin problems and baldness; 9) relieves muscular cramps; 10) prevents spontaneous abortion; 11) increases sexual and athletic prowess; 12) extends life span.

Negative:

1) Toxic in high doses; 2) may cause bleeding and delay wound healing; 3) may elevate blood pressure; 4) may cause or contribute to dangerous blood clots; 5) may result in serious lipid and hormonal disturbances.

III. EVIDENCE

Related to Positive Claims:

1) Protects against neurological disorders—It has been established that vitamin E plays a crucial role in normal neurologic functions in humans, as well as in many other animals. Various neurologic disorders arise in humans deficient in vitamin E and may be slowed or even reversed with prompt vitamin E therapy. Among those who may have the kind of vitamin E deficiencies that can contribute to nerve damage are people with chronic disorders of fat absorption, chronic liver disease and cystic fibrosis. Patients and physicians alike need to be especially alert to the possibility of underlying vitamin E deficiencies whenever malabsorption/maldigestion disorders arise. Increasingly, those at risk of neurologic disease will be given vitamin E as a *preven-*

tive and protective measure. These individuals may require very high doses of supplemental vitamin E—under their doctors' supervision.

Here, for those of you who may already have been diagnosed as having disorders you think might fall into these categories, are the names of some of the malabsorptive disease states associated with vitamin E deficiencies: biliary atresia, intrahepatic cholestasis syndromes, primary biliary cirrhosis, abetalipoproteinemia, short bowel syndrome, bacterial overgrowth and, as previously mentioned, cystic fibrosis; also Whipple's syndrome, sprue and non-tropical sprue, sclerodermal bowel disease, chronic pancreatitis and gluten enteropathies.

The vitamin E therapies for each of the above conditions vary and each requires individual medical management—so be sure to consult your physician if you even think you may have one of these disorders before self-dosing with vitamin E. The younger the age at which you start vitamin E therapy for these disorders the better the outcome.

Some of the neurologic symptoms of these diseases include muscle weakness, abnormal eye movements, loss of reflexes, restriction of field of vision, unsteady gait, loss of muscle mass. The commonest non-neurologic symptom is a diarrhea in which one excretes a lot of fat.

There is a chance that vitamin E may also be able to play a role in slowing or even stopping the progression of Parkinson's disease, which currently afflicts more than 1 million Americans. A long-term study is currently underway to see whether vitamin E, in combination with the drug Deprenyl, can alleviate the symptoms of this disease.

Also under investigation is a possible role for vitamin E in the management of epilepsy. Several studies have shown that epileptic children have abnormally low levels of vitamin E. Improved seizure control in children given vitamin E supplementation was recently reported.

Vitamin E has proved beneficial in another neurologic disorder called tardive dyskinesia. This disorder is a side effect of long-term use of neuroleptic drugs (major tranquilizers typically used to curb psychotic behavior). In a double-blind, placebo-controlled pilot study using 400 to 1,200 IUs of vitamin E daily there was a 43 percent reduction of involuntary movements among those receiving the vitamin.

2) Boosts the immune system—There has been an explosion of interest recently in vitamin E as a potential immune stimulant. Numerous studies have shown that the immune systems of various animals tend to

sag when vitamin E intake is low. High vitamin E levels, on the other hand, correlate with optimum immunity. In one experiment, aging mice were given vitamin E seventeen times greater than that normally found in their diet. This regimen restored declining immunity to levels found in much younger mice.

In humans, increased cancer risk has been associated with low blood levels of vitamin E. In one study, those with the highest levels of vitamin E in their blood were found to be 2.5 times less likely to get lung cancer than those with the lowest blood levels of the vitamin.

There are a number of ways in which vitamin E is likely to have immune-protective and immune-stimulating effects. As an antioxidant it protects against the free radicals that are known to play a role in the cancer process. There is evidence that it also blocks some of the chemicals called prostaglandins, which dampen immune responses. In addition, vitamin E protects cell membranes, making it more difficult for viruses and some other pathogens to attack them.

3) Protects against cardiovascular disease—For a long time, this was the claim most widely made for vitamin E. It was reported in the late 1940s that large doses of vitamin E can alleviate the symptoms of angina pectoris, the intense chest pain caused by insufficient oxygenation of heart muscle. From there the claims expanded to include benefits in a number of other cardiovascular disorders.

One claim that has been validated relates to a condition called intermittent claudication, which is characterized by pain in the calves of the legs and is caused by narrowing of the leg arteries. Supplementation with vitamin E in doses of 300 to 800 IUs daily for periods of at least three months resulted in clinical improvement in a number of patients with this disease. The patients who got vitamin E in this study required far fewer amputations than did those who got other substances or placebos. The vitamin E-treated patients were better able than the others to walk without pain, and blood flow through the arteries of their legs was much improved in most cases, although it sometimes took as many as twenty-five months of supplementation before this improvement was apparent.

There have been claims that vitamin E can lower cholesterol and other blood lipids. Results on this issue are mixed. One recent double-bind, placebo-controlled study found that 500 IUs of vitamin E daily can elevate the so-called good cholesterol, HDL, by about 14 percent. HDL helps transport the dangerous forms of cholesterol out of the body. Other cholesterol abnormalities were partially corrected in another study in which women with precancerous breast lesions were treated with vitamin E.

Several studies indicate that vitamin E can help protect against potentially life-threatening blood clots. And vitamin E deficiencies have been linked to increased stickiness of blood platelets, predisposing to clots.

4) Protects against air pollution and other toxic substances—Vitamin E has a protective effect, in animal experiments, against ozone and nitrogen dioxide, both major constituents of smog. Animals given vitamin E and then exposed to various levels of ozone live longer than animals who are not given vitamin E. The formation of cancer-causing nitrosamines can also be blocked by vitamin E. There are also preliminary findings that vitamin E may confer some protection against the toxins in cigarette smoke.

5) Prevents cancer—Vitamin E increases the ability of the mineral selenium (see discussion under Minerals) to inhibit breast cancers in some experimental animals. There is evidence that vitamin E can inhibit a precancerous breast condition in humans (see following section). Low blood levels of vitamin E (as well as beta-carotene) have been linked to an increased risk of lung cancer. That vitamin E might be a tumor preventive in humans has been suggested by researchers who showed that the vitamin could completely prevent tumor development in hamsters exposed to a potent cancer-causing substance. Hamsters not given vitamin E and exposed to the same carcinogen all developed tumors.

Vitamin E has also been shown to protect against the adverse side effects of radiation therapy and to reduce the toxicity of some cancer chemotherapies in additional animal studies.

6) Prevents disease of the breast—One form of breast disease (fibrocystic) can be treated with vitamin E, especially in combination with other therapies. This disorder, also known as mammary dysplasia, is a potentially precancerous condition. Some researchers have reported that 600 milligrams of vitamin E daily provide a safe and effective treatment for this disorder, leading to relief in 70 percent of those

treated. These studies have a strong subjective component in that they have relied for signs of "clinical response" upon patient reports of reduced discomfort. Objective regression of the disease has also been seen, however, in ten of twenty-eight patients in a double-blind study in which patients got 600 IUs daily.

7) Reduces the symptoms of premenstrual syndrome (PMS)—All major categories of PMS symptoms are improved with supplementation of 400 IUs of vitamin E daily, according to researchers who conducted a double-blind, placebo-controlled study of this issue. This study confirmed earlier results reported by the same research group. This work awaits confirmation by other researchers.

8) Fights skin problems and baldness—Vitamin E has no demonstrated effect on hair loss and baldness. Claims of favorable effects on skin remain purely anecdotal. So do claims that vitamin E promotes healing of burns and cuts and minimizes scar tissue.

9) Relieves muscular cramps—Remarkable relief from persistent nocturnal leg and foot cramps was reported in 82 percent of 125 patients, many of whom obtained nearly complete relief with less than 300 IUs of vitamin E daily. Others have reported similar benefits. Further research is indicated.

10) Prevents spontaneous abortion—There is no evidence that this is true in women with other than severe vitamin E deficiencies.

11) Increases sexual and athletic prowess—Claims that vitamin E increases sex drive in both men and women and that it enlarges the male sex organ abound. Unfortunately, there is no evidence to support these claims. Similarly, many have claimed that vitamin E supplements can increase stamina, muscle strength and athletic performance, supposedly by increasing blood flow into the muscles and by improving the "oxygen quality" of each cell of the body. There have, in fact, been a few *uncontrolled* reports attesting to such effects. Again, it is unfortunate that these reports have not been substantiated by more objective, double-blind trials like those that failed to find any objective effect of vitamin E on athletic performance. It may turn out (see Overview) that vitamin E plays a hitherto largely unsuspected role of great importance

in energy production, in which case those *deficient* in vitamin E might indeed experience a greater sense of energy with supplementation. Frank vitamin E deficiency, however, is rare.

12) Extends life span—One researcher has found that although giving mice vitamin E lengthens their mean life span it does not extend maximum life span. The question of how much vitamin E is the correct amount for optimal human health and longevity is a very important one for which there is not yet an answer. The assumption that *more* vitamin E is likely to be better than less is a naive and dangerous one. Vitamin E has proved time and again just how complex and sometimes unpredictable it is. It may be that we will determine what is optimum for vitamin E only after we have done so for a number of the other major antioxidant nutrients.

Related to Negative Claims:

1) Toxic in high doses—Many researchers regard vitamin E as nontoxic in doses up to 600 IUs per day. Avoid higher doses unless taking them under a doctor's supervision.

2) May cause bleeding and delay wound healing—Persons who are taking anti-coagulation drugs should be followed closely by their physicians and especially when they take vitamin E supplements. This applies as well to persons who have reduced coagulation factors. These include those who have vitamin K deficiencies. Even moderate coagulation-factor deficiency may predispose one to potentially dangerous bleeding if vitamin E is taken in doses greater than 400 IUs daily. Vitamin E has not been found, however, to interfere with coagulation factors in *normal* individuals. As for delayed wound healing, this has been noted in a study with animals and was attributed to an inhibitory effect of vitamin E on the synthesis of collagen, the protein that helps bind tissue together. Delayed wound healing has been reported anecdotally in humans. There is no evidence that this presents a problem for normal individuals.

3) May elevate blood pressure—Again, this adverse effect has not been reliably observed in normal individuals. It has been reported anecdotally in persons with preexisting hypertension or predisposition to hypertension. Vitamin E has also been reported to be dangerous in high doses in persons suffering from rheumatic heart disease. Some who

advocate megadoses of vitamin E caution users to begin with small doses and gradually increase them in order to avoid hypertension. Hypertensives are advised to consult their physicians before taking vitamin E supplements.

4) May cause or contribute to dangerous blood clots—This has been reported anecdotally by one researcher in patients who report daily intake of vitamin E in the range of 800 to 1,200 IUs. Though these and some of the other adverse effects reported by that researcher have not been observed by most other researchers, it would be unwise to conclude that doses above 600 to 800 IUs of vitamin E daily are entirely safe. The popularity of doses in that range is of relatively recent origin, and study of long-range effects of these doses has, necessarily, only now begun. It is possible that while certain smaller doses of vitamin E may have beneficial effects in specific disorders, some larger doses may have adverse effects in those *same* disorders.

5) May result in serious lipid and hormonal disturbances—Again, this is the contention of a single investigator, based on uncontrolled observations. A recent, better documented report indicates that supplementary vitamin E does *not* alter lipid patterns in *normal* adults. More research is needed. At present, however, adverse side effects have not been reported when daily doses of vitamin E do not exceed 600 IUs.

IV. RECOMMENDATIONS

A) *Suggested Intake:* Many people are now taking 600 to 1,200 IUs of vitamin E daily. No adverse effects have been reported for normal people (not taking anti-coagulant medications) using up to 1,600 IUs daily. I see no reason, however, for adults to take more than 400 IUs daily. The benefits of vitamin E—and there are many—can be obtained with daily doses between 30 and 400 IUs. Infants under the age of one should not be given more than 50 IUs daily. Children between age one and ten should not take more than 200 IUs daily. People who use fish oils or eat a diet rich in polyunsaturated fatty acids should take at least 30 IUs of vitamin E daily in order to protect against rancidification of the oils they are consuming.

B) *Source/Form:* Most of us apparently get about 15 IUs of vitamin E in our daily diets, from such sources as whole-grain cereals, eggs, vegetable oils, enriched flour, leafy greens and many other vegetables. Real deficiencies are rare. If you buy vitamin E supplements you will note that some manufacturers stress the "natural" origins of their products. In fact, however, there is no evidence that natural vitamin E is any better or more active than synthetic versions. Acceptable supplementary forms of vitamin E include d-alpha-tocopheryl acetate, d-alpha-tocopheryl succinate, dl-alpha-tocopheryl acetate and dl-alpha-tocopheryl succinate.

C) *Take With:* Best if incorporated into a well-balanced vitamin/mineral preparation. (See Part Three for further recommendations.) Because of widely reported synergistic effects, a daily 50- to 200-microgram dose of *organic* selenium should be accompanied in adults by 30 to 400 IUs of vitamin E daily. Children under seven should not take more than 100 micrograms of selenium with their vitamin E. Infants should not take more than 50 micrograms of selenium daily.

D) *Cautionary Note:* Don't take vitamin E at the same time that you take inorganic iron or the contraceptive pill, if possible, both of which may interfere with vitamin E activity. Take vitamin E several hours before or after you take the birth-control bill or iron supplements. This should not pose any problem as far as the Pill is concerned, but iron may be troublesome since you are likely to get it in a multivitamin/mineral preparation that also contains vitamin E. Fortunately, most forms of iron used in these preparations, such as ferrous fumarate, are thought to be compatible with the vitamin E forms used. If you take extra iron, however, that is, iron beyond that which you get in your multivitamin/mineral formulation, you'll derive the most benefit if you take this separately and, if at all possible, on an empty stomach. (See discussion of iron for more details.) Don't take vitamin E if you are on anti-coagulant drugs, such as warfarin, or if you have a known vitamin K deficiency (which results in diminished blood-clotting ability) unless your physician approves and carefully monitors your condition. Discontinue vitamin E supplementation if any signs of toxicity occur, such as fatigue, nausea, muscle weakness, stomach upset, skin disorders. Also discontinue if cuts or burns take unusually long to heal or if you experience unexplained bleeding. If you are diagnosed as having blood clots of any kind, alert your physician to the fact that you are taking vitamin E and do not continue without his or her permission.

VITAMIN K

I. OVERVIEW: The Natural Band-Aid

Though not widely known, vitamin K is a very real vitamin and is essential to human health. It is most recognized for its role in preventing bleeding. In fact, K is from the German "Koagulation."

Vitamin K is the generic term for several different forms of the vitamin. The most important naturally occurring forms are vitamin K_1, or phylloquinone (aka phytonadione), and vitamin K_2, which refers to a family of substances called menaquinones. Vitamin K_3, or menadione, is a synthetic substance.

Vitamin K has several known biological roles, the most important being in the synthesis of several factors involved in blood clotting. It also plays a significant role in the mineralization of bone and thus in the maintenance of normal bone and fracture healing. Preliminary studies suggest that vitamin K may be beneficial in the prevention and treatment of postmenopausal osteoporosis. Recently there has been some excitement regarding a possible role in the treatment and prevention of human cancer.

Vitamin K deficiency is uncommon because of the widespread distribution of the vitamin in the food chain and because bacteria in the human gut synthesize a major portion of our vitamin K requirement. Deficiency, however, can occur. Those at risk include individuals with malabsorption problems, those who require nourishment through their veins, those on prolonged oral antibiotic therapy, those on very low calorie diets and those taking certain drugs, such as cholestyramine (lowers cholesterol levels), mineral oil, the anticonvulsants Dilantin and phenobarbitol and some cephalosporin antibiotics. Symptoms of vitamin K deficiency are easy bruising and black-and-blue marks on the skin. (Of course, there can be other causes for such symptoms, as well.)

II. CLAIMS

Positive:
1) Beneficial in the treatment of cancer; 2) protects against osteoporosis.

Negative:
1) Toxic.

III. EVIDENCE

Related to Positive Claims:

1) Beneficial in the treatment of cancer—Vitamin K, especially menadione (vitamin K_3), has been found to inhibit a variety of human tumors *in vitro*. The tumor types include breast, ovary, colon, stomach, kidney and lung. The activity of the vitamin is comparable to that of some highly toxic chemotherapeutic agents. Currently, some human trials are in progress using vitamin K alone or in combination with other agents in the treatment of human cancers. The results of these studies are eagerly awaited.

This is another case of a nutrient that may become an important player in the fight against cancer. (See vitamins A, B_6, C, D, folic acid, B_{12} and the minerals calcium and selenium for others.)

2) Protects against osteoporosis—A Japanese study reported that in three postmenopausal women with osteoporosis the loss of calcium was found to be reduced 18 to 50 percent by daily treatment with vitamin K. In a more recent study from London, it was reported that sixteen elderly patients with osteoporosis and fractures had significantly lower blood levels of vitamin K when compared with normal controls.

Vitamin K is known to play a significant part in the calcification of bone. The above studies suggest that vitamin K may play an important role in the prevention of osteoporosis and fractures. Studies should be performed to test this. It is of interest to note that women are commonly treated with antibiotics for bladder infections. This could put them at risk for vitamin K deficiency.

Related to Negative Claims:

1) Toxic—High doses, greater than 500 micrograms daily, have been reported to cause some allergic-type reactions, such as skin rashes, itching and flushing. Liver problems have been reported but are not very common. Very rarely, those who receive vitamin K by intramuscular injection may develop a scleroderma-like patch (hard skin) at the site of the injection after several months.

IV. RECOMMENDATIONS

A) *Suggested Intake:* The RDA for vitamin K for men is 80 micrograms daily and for women, 65 micrograms daily. The vitamin is widely present throughout the food chain, and deficiency is rare. For those at risk for K deficiency (see Overview), supplementation with 50 to 100 micrograms daily is both safe and desirable.

B) *Source/Form:* Vitamin K is widely available throughout the food chain. Vegetables and dairy products are excellent sources. In fact, foods containing the lactobacillus bacteria, such as yogurt and kefir, are particularly good since these foods add to the intestine a bacterium that produces the vitamin. Vitamin K_1 is available in some micronutrient supplements. Most supplements do not contain the vitamin. Vitamin K_3, or menadione, is also available, but this form is usually used by physicians to treat frank vitamin K deficiencies.

C) *Take With:* Some well-balanced vitamin and mineral supplements contain vitamin K in a dose of 50 to 100 micrograms daily.

D) *Cautionary Note:* Those who have frank vitamin K deficiency should be treated by a physician. Those who take the blood thinner coumadin should not take supplementary vitamin K unless approved by a physician. There is no reason at this time to supplement with more than 100 micrograms daily except in the case of frank vitamin K deficiency.

FIVE

Minerals

Carbohydrates, proteins, lipids (fats, fatty acids, cholesterol) and vitamins are all organic substances. What this means is that they are all compounds of the chemical element carbon. We require, in addition to these nutrients, certain chemical elements in their *inorganic* forms, i.e., *not* bound to carbon. These chemical elements in their non-organic forms are classified as the dietary minerals. These nutrients participate in a multitude of biochemical and physiologic processes necessary for the maintenance of health.

These substances are often grouped in two categories: those that are required in our diets in amounts greater than 100 milligrams per day and those that are required in amounts much less than 100 milligrams daily. The term "mineral" is applied to the former group, while "trace element" is applied to the latter.

Minerals include compounds of the elements calcium, magnesium, phosphorus, sodium, potassium, sulfur and chlorine. Trace elements that are required for human health are iron, iodine, copper, manganese, zinc, molybdenum, selenium and chromium. There are trace elements that appear to be important for other warm-blooded animals. These are fluorine, tin, boron, vanadium, silicon, nickel, arsenic, cadmium and lead. Whether these elements play roles in human nutrition remains to be determined. Recent evidence suggests that boron protects against osteoporosis.

Mineral-insufficiency and trace-element-insufficiency states are actually more likely to occur than are vitamin-insufficiency states. Those at increased risk of such insufficiencies include people who eat low-calorie diets, the elderly, pregnant women, people on certain drugs (such as diuretics), vegetarians and those living where the soil is deficient in certain minerals. Vitamins are usually present in foods in similar amounts throughout the world, but this is not true of the minerals and trace elements. Because of differing geologic conditions, minerals and trace elements may be scarce in the soils of certain regions and rich in those of other regions. The soil of South Dakota, for example, is very rich in selenium, while the soil in certain parts of China and New Zealand is very poor in this element. Thus, you can live in some areas, eat a perfectly "balanced" diet and still develop mineral deficiencies or trace-element deficiencies that can only be averted through dietary change or supplementation.

There is increasing evidence that those whose nutritional status is suboptimal in certain trace elements, such as selenium, for example, may be at greater risk for certain forms of cancer and heart disease. Suboptimal intake can be due to factors other than soil depletion. These factors are as diverse as the effects of acid rain and the overrefining, overprocessing of foods.

Our vulnerability to even minute dietary imbalances in minerals can be appreciated by comparing, to begin with, our daily mineral intake (about 1.5 grams) with our total intake of carbohydrates, proteins and lipids (about 500 grams). Thus our mineral intake represents only about 0.3 percent of our total intake of nutrients, yet they are so potent and so important that without them we wouldn't be able to utilize the other 99.7 percent of foodstuffs and would quickly perish. Our total daily intake of zinc accounts for only 0.003 percent of our total nutrient intake. So it becomes easier to see how even what would seem to be a tiny decrease in zinc intake can have enormous negative impact on health, especially if that decrease persists.

There has been a strong tendency on the part of some dietetic and other medical professionals to discourage people from taking more than the RDAs (Recommended Daily Allowances) of minerals and vitamins, which can be obtained, they say, in the typical American diet. Unfortunately, numerous studies have shown, repeatedly, that many, possibly *most,* Americans are *not* getting the RDAs for the minerals in their daily diets. Supplementation, therefore, seems advisable, particularly since, except in a few medical conditions I identify in the following pages, such supplementation poses no peril.

Evidence is accumulating from recent studies that mineral/trace-element supplementation may help prevent various forms of cancer, heart disease and some other degenerative processes. More of these studies need to be done. The impact prudent supplementation may have on medicine may turn out to be enormous.

Finally, for the purists, it is herewith noted that although the trace elements are classified as inorganic nutrients, some of the dietary *delivery forms* of the inorganic elements are structures in which the element is bound to a carbon-containing molecule. This is true of selenium and chromium.

BORON

I. OVERVIEW: The Bones Like It

Boron has begun attracting attention, mainly due to a recent study which indicates that it may be beneficial in the prevention of postmenopausal osteoporosis. Boron is a trace mineral mostly found in foods of plant origin. It appears to be essential for plant growth and development. Although it is thought to be important for the growth and development of animals, its essentiality in animals and humans has still to be proven. On the other hand, its health-promoting effects in humans are becoming increasingly apparent.

II. CLAIMS

Positive:
1) Prevents osteoporosis in postmenopausal women; 2) beneficial in the treatment of arthritis; 3) builds muscle.

III. EVIDENCE

Related to Positive Claims:

1) Prevents osteoporosis in postmenopausal women—Researchers recently reported on the effects of dietary boron in twelve postmenopausal women between the ages of forty-eight and eighty-two. They followed these women closely for twenty-four weeks. During the first seventeen weeks, the women were given a low-boron diet (not much different from what many people consume). During the next seven weeks, the diet was supplemented with 3 milligrams daily of boron in the form of sodium borate capsules.

About eight days after receiving boron supplementation, the women markedly reduced their excretion of both calcium and magnesium. They also were found to have significant increases (about twofold) in the production of an active form of estrogen and also testosterone.

This work suggests that supplementation of a low-boron diet with boron causes changes in postmenopausal women consistent with the prevention of calcium loss and bone demineralization. Follow-up research is currently in progress.

The finding that supplementary boron reduces magnesium excretion is also of potential great interest. Suboptimal magnesium appears quite common, particularly in those taking diuretics and digitalis. Low magnesium status may be an important factor in ischemic heart disease and other forms of cardiovascular disease. The magnesium-sparing effect of boron could have enormous significance in these matters.

2) Beneficial in the treatment of arthritis—This claim has been around for a longer time. It has to do with the finding that chicks fed diets low in magnesium and boron developed rickets-like lesions. Chicks fed diets deficient only in boron did not.

There is no evidence this claim is true.

3) Builds muscle—Some athletes, especially body builders, are constantly watchful for substances that are neither drugs nor steroids that can help build their muscles. Boron supplements are now available and are claimed to double testosterone in a short time, contributing to muscle growth.

The claim goes back to the study mentioned above which showed a twofold increase in testosterone *in postmenopausal women* after eight days of boron supplementation. No one knows yet what effect, if any, boron might have on *male* testosterone levels, but there is certainly no validity in extrapolating results from a study of postmenopausal women and applying them to male athletes. Since women have very low levels of testosterone to begin with, a twofold increase in those women translates to an insignificant drop in the bucket in males—and even that minuscule increase may not occur in boron-supplemented males.

IV. RECOMMENDATIONS

A) *Suggested Intake:* The study reported in this section suggests an intake of about 3 milligrams daily to prevent osteoporosis.

B) *Source/Form:* Foods rich in boron are fruits and vegetables. Foods poor in boron are meat and fowl. Boron supplements are now available. The most common form is sodium borate. If you eat a good mixed diet, including fruits and vegetables, you will get 1.5 to 3 milligrams of boron in your food daily.

C) *Take With:* Best if taken with a well-balanced vitamin and mineral supplement including manganese, calcium and riboflavin. See Part Three for specific recommendations.

CALCIUM

I. OVERVIEW: Your Mother Was Right

Mothers have been telling us from time immemorial to drink our milk. That isn't news. But in 1984 a panel of medical experts brought together by the National Institutes of Health set off what the media called "the calcium craze" by announcing that most women in the United States aren't getting enough calcium in their diets. They recommended that women consume 1,000 to 1,500 milligrams per day in an effort to stem a widespread form of bone degeneration known as osteoporosis, an affliction of 20 million Americans.

Other recent research lent further fuel to the "craze," suggesting that calcium might be useful in preventing high blood pressure and even some forms of cancer. Additional research suggests a possible role in lowering cholesterol. The calcium craze, the biggest brouhaha in the supplement supermarket since Linus Pauling declared that vitamin C could prevent the common cold, reached such a pitch that *Newsweek* made the mineral calcium its cover story and the national TV talk shows buzzed for weeks with the wonders of this substance.

Plenty of people were quick to jump on the calcium bandwagon. Today you can find dozens of calcium supplements on the market, whereas not many years ago you'd find only one. Sales have quadrupled to about $200 million per year since the NIH-convened panel issued its recommendations. Savvy food packagers are even adding calcium to such things as orange juice and diet soda.

Has all of this been justified? As the calcium dust begins to settle, along with the "craze," the mineral continues to look promising. It is certainly no panacea, however, and has no doubt been oversold in some respects. The recent calcium craze has, if nothing else, alerted us to the fact that most Americans are getting only a third to a half of the calcium they need for the maintenance of good health.

Calcium is essential for human life. Apart from being a major constituent of bones and teeth, calcium is crucial for nerve conduction, muscle contraction, heartbeat, blood coagulation, the production of energy and maintenance of immune function, among other things. Severe calcium deficiency may lead to abnormal heartbeat, dementia, muscle spasms and convulsions.

Increasing complexity characterizes the evolution of life. The complex functions of human cells require messengers to mediate and coordinate their responses. There is perhaps no more sensitive a regulator of cellular activity than the calcium ion. It is so sensitive that even a slight change in its concentration can cause a biologic event, such as a heartbeat, to occur—or not occur. The highly sensitive command mechanism itself requires very fine regulations, for if the concentration of calcium ions in cells exceeds certain levels, even slightly, those cells can be destroyed via the generation of toxic oxygen forms. Magnesium appears to be the prime regulator of calcium flow within cells. It is this delicate collaboration that may well be the major determinant of the rate at which the cellular flame burns.

There are many groups at risk of marginal calcium deficiency. The elderly, in particular, are vulnerable. As we age we have increasing difficulty in absorbing calcium from our intestines. Add to this the fact that as we age we also have a tendency to reduce our dietary intake of calcium. To compensate for this lack, the body begins taking calcium from our bones, thinning them and making them brittle in the process. Postmenopausal women are often deficient in calcium, as are many aging men. Others at special risk include: users of antacids containing aluminum, consumers of alcohol, users of cortisone, inactive people, people on low-calorie diets, high-protein diets and high-fiber diets, people who are intolerant of lactose (milk sugar) and pregnant women.

"Eating" our bones for calcium, rather than getting it from our diets, can have devastating clinical consequences. There is evidence that calcium supplementation is beneficial in decreasing the incidence of bone fractures in postmenopausal women and appears to be indicated, along with other factors, for the prevention of postmenopausal osteoporosis; supplementation is likely to be warranted in general for the maintenance of optimal health and longevity. Calcium appears to have a bright and exciting future in preventive medicine.

II. CLAIMS

Positive:

1) Beneficial in prevention and treatment of osteoporosis ("brittle bones"); 2) prevents cancer; 3) useful in the treatment of high blood pressure; 4) lowers cholesterol and helps prevent cardiovascular disease; 5) helps alleviate cramps in the legs; 6) useful in treating and preventing arthritis; 7) helps keep the skin healthy.

Negative:

1) Forms kidney stones; 2) causes tissue calcification; 3) produces magnesium deficiency and the premenstrual syndrome in women.

III. EVIDENCE

Related to Positive Claims:

1) Beneficial in prevention and treatment of osteoporosis—This degenerative bone disorder is a particularly serious problem, especially among women over the age of forty-five. Osteoporosis leads to, among other things, more than one million hip fractures each year. The complications of those fractures kill approximately forty thousand women annually; they lead to permanent crippling in many others. One of the unfortunate results of all the hype surrounding the "calcium craze" has been the mistaken idea that osteoporosis is wholly the product of calcium deficiency. It's a lot more complicated than that. Osteoporosis

is the result not only of nutritional inadequacies but also of inherited and hormonal factors, lifestyle and so on.

Unfortunately, once bone loss has occurred it cannot be restored. *Prevention* is the key in osteoporosis—and there, it appears, consuming extra calcium may be beneficial. It is now known that the dietary intake of calcium, as well as absorption of calcium from the intestines, decreases with age. It has been reported but not confirmed that the incidence of fractures in postmenopausal women can be significantly reduced by giving long-term calcium supplementation. The experts convened by the NIH recommend that premenopausal women consume 1,000 milligrams of calcium daily and that postmenopausal women (not on estrogen replacement therapy) consume up to 1,500 milligrams daily.

Most researchers now believe that calcium alone will not stop the progression of osteoporosis unless it is used in conjunction with estrogen therapy. There is some evidence that, with calcium supplementation, estrogen can be used in lower doses without sacrifice of effectiveness. Despite the inconclusiveness of the data with respect to calcium and osteoporosis, most experts nonetheless agree that it is a good idea for most Americans to increase their calcium intake. Better safe than sorry.

2) Prevents cancer—This new claim for calcium relates to colon cancer. In a nineteen-year study of middle-aged white males in Chicago, the risk of developing colorectal cancer was found to be related to the amount of vitamin D and calcium these men got in their diets. The lower the amounts the greater the incidence of colorectal cancer. Epidemiologic studies in four Scandinavian countries suggested the same thing. It has been found that men who have the lowest intake of calcium (the amount one would obtain from drinking 1½ glasses of milk daily) are at three times greater risk of developing these cancers than are those men (in the Chicago study) who were taking in the most calcium daily (an amount obtainable by drinking 4½ glasses of milk daily).

The calcium-colorectal-cancer link has now been more directly investigated. Individuals from families in which colorectal cancers are common were given 1,250 milligrams of supplemental calcium carbonate per day. After two to three months of this supplementation, abnormally high rates of cell division in their colons slowed to rates considered normal. This suggests that supplemental calcium may, indeed, exert a strong preventive effect in these high-risk individuals. Other studies indicate that at least part of calcium's protective effects may be due to its ability to detoxify potentially carcinogenic bile acids in the gut.

It appears that an exciting new role for calcium supplementation may be at hand.

3) Useful in the treatment of high blood pressure—There have been research reports that individuals with hypertension consume far less calcium than do those who have normal blood pressure. In addition, other researchers have reported successfully lowering blood pressure in some individuals by giving them supplemental calcium. This was recently confirmed in a well-designed double-blind, placebo-controlled study. The reduction in blood pressure (achieved with daily doses of 1,500 milligrams of calcium for twelve weeks) was modest but significant. It appears likely that some hypertensive individuals will benefit more than others from calcium supplementation.

4) Lowers cholesterol and helps prevent cardiovascular disease—To the extent that calcium protects against hypertension it also reduces some of the risks of cardiovascular disease. Claims that calcium may help protect against this disease by also lowering cholesterol are less known but actually date back several decades. Studies to date have yielded mixed results. More investigation is required to determine whether this claim has any validity.

5) Natural tranquilizer—Reports that calcium supplements (or a glass of milk) are good for sleep or to calm the nerves persist but remain anecdotal.

6) Helps alleviate cramps in the legs—Obstetricians occasionally prescribe extra calcium to pregnant women who complain of leg cramps. Reports of beneficial effect remain purely anecdotal.

7) Useful in treating and preventing arthritis—There is no evidence that supplementary calcium is beneficial in the treatment or prevention of any form of arthritis.

8) Helps keep the skin healthy—There is an antioxidant enzyme in the skin that is calcium-sensitive. It is possible—but not proved—that calcium deficiencies could accelerate skin aging.

Related to Negative Claims:

1) Forms kidney stones—It is true that the majority of kidney stones are formed from calcium. However, the process is still poorly understood, and there is no evidence that stone formation is related to calcium intake.

2) Causes tissue calcification—There are some who believe that calcification of soft tissue, a phenomenon that is extremely complex and that is part of the wear and tear of the aging process, is related to dietary intake of calcium. The only situation where this may be true is in the context of a frank magnesium deficiency. There is no evidence that dietary calcium is associated with tissue calcification. In fact, this process is common in the elderly consuming *inadequate* calcium.

3) Produces magnesium deficiency and the premenstrual syndrome in women—Guy Abraham is the leading proponent of this claim, arguing that the diet is already too rich in calcium. He believes that because calcium is antagonistic to magnesium a deficiency of the latter can occur, causing the premenstrual syndrome in women. This syndrome is characterized by both physical and sometimes psychologic distress prior to the commencement of menstruation. Abraham seeks to support part of his thesis by the finding that osteoporosis (discussed above) is not more common in underdeveloped countries where calcium intake is relatively low. The problems with this argument are as follows: Dietary surveys have documented declining calcium intake in Americans, and particularly in aging American women; there is evidence (cited above) that calcium supplements help prevent fractures in postmenopausal women; and, finally, the fact that there isn't more osteoporosis in underdeveloped nations than has been reported probably has more to do with low protein intake than with anything else. Protein, the consumption of which is high in the United States and most developed countries, may accelerate the loss of calcium.

There is no evidence that supplementary calcium causes magnesium deficiency or that it is related to the premenstrual syndrome.

IV. RECOMMENDATIONS

A) *Suggested Intake:* The National Research Council recommends 1,200 milligrams daily of calcium for males and females from age eleven to twenty-four and 800 milligrams daily after age twenty-four. Intake of 1200 milligrams daily is advised for pregnant and nursing women. Unfortunately, few American women consume this amount. On the basis of carefully conducted studies, the best informed researchers now recommend 1,500 milligrams daily in postmenopausal women and 1,000 milligrams (1 gram) daily for premenopausal women. I recommend that men also take 1 gram of calcium daily. The elderly, people consuming low-calorie, high-protein, high-fiber diets, consumers of alcohol and users of aluminum-containing antacids should, in particular, ensure that they get the above-recommended quantities. Supplementation of up to 2,500 milligrams (2.5 grams) daily is safe.

B) *Source/Form:* The best natural sources of calcium are milk, cheese, ice cream, yogurt, buttermilk and other dairy products. Other sources include salmon, green leafy vegetables, and tofu. One glass of milk contains 300 milligrams of calcium; a slice of Swiss cheese, 270 milligrams; four ounces of tofu, 154 milligrams; one cup of yogurt, 415 milligrams; one cup cooked broccoli, 178 milligrams. (The fat content of dairy products is unrelated to calcium content.) There are several calcium supplements on the market. Bone meal contains absorbable forms of calcium but may be contaminated with lead. Calcium chloride is irritating to the gastrointestinal tract. Calcium carbonate is the most concentrated form as well as the cheapest. It also has the advantage of being an antacid. Calcium glubionate is available as an elixir but is much more expensive. Both calcium carbonate and magnesium carbonate are found in dolomite, a popular food supplement. Although it is important to balance calcium with magnesium—this has always been the big selling point for dolomite—magnesium carbonate is not a very "available" form of magnesium, meaning it is not easily absorbed in this form by the body. Calcium gluconate, calcium lactate and calcium citrate are more soluble forms of calcium but are less concentrated in calcium. Absorbability of calcium supplements varies considerably. If the calcium supplement you are using won't completely disintegrate in half an hour (or less) when placed in room-temperature vinegar (stir every five minutes) then switch to another brand. This test more or less duplicates what happens in your stomach. Those who use calcium carbonate should take their supplements with meals because this form of calcium needs a lot of acid for absorption. Eating stimulates acid production. This is particularly important for people over sixty, since we produce less acid as we age.

C) *Take With:* Best incorporated into a well-balanced vitamin/mineral "insurance" formula. (See Part Three for more specific details and recommendations.) Contrary to popular belief and the claims of many manufacturers, neither zinc nor magnesium interferes with the absorption of calcium.

D) *Cautionary Note:* Patients with unusually high calcium concentrations in their blood should not take calcium supplements. Conditions that cause this include overactive parathyroid gland and cancer. Patients who are taking high doses of vitamin D (not recommended unless prescribed by a physician for a specific medical problem) require medical surveillance when taking calcium supplements. Those who form kidney stones should not take calcium supplements except under a physician's supervision.

CHROMIUM

I. OVERVIEW: The Sugar Regulator

It wasn't until the 1950s that chromium's potential importance in diet began to be recognized. Prior to that time chromium was widely regarded as another of the toxic trace metals. In the mid-fifties, it was reported that glucose intolerance in rats could be corrected by feeding them brewer's yeast. (Glucose intolerance is a decreased ability to remove sugar from the blood for cellular nourishment; it is a characteristic of diabetes.) A painstaking search for the factor in brewer's yeast responsible for this effect finally revealed trivalent chromium in the form of a substance named glucose tolerance factor (GTF). It was theorized that GTF potentiates the activity of insulin, required in sugar metabolism.

Chromium-deficient animals, in addition to having glucose intolerance, suffer from impaired growth, elevated blood cholesterol, fatty deposits in arteries, decreased life span, and decreased sperm count and fertility. It is now established that chromium is an essential trace element in many animals, including humans. It has been reported that chromium supplements can correct impaired glucose tolerance in malnourished children. In another report, diabetic symptoms, including glucose intolerance, weight loss and nerve disorders, were reversed in a woman given intravenous chromium. She was a hospitalized patient who had been receiving all of her nutrition intravenously for several years when these diabetic symptoms arose. Insulin itself had no effect.

There is evidence that marginal chromium deficiency is common in the United States, possibly due to high consumption of refined foods. Researchers have found a dramatic decline in the concentration of chromium in a variety of human tissues with increasing age. At the same time it is known that human aging is associated with a progressive impairment in glucose tolerance, possibly linked to an age-related decrease in tissue sensitivity to insulin. Since the supply of insulin itself remains fairly steady as we age, it appears that impaired glucose tolerance itself could be responsible for many of the pathologic changes that occur as we age. Diabetics, in many ways, appear to be the victims of an accelerated aging phenomenon associated with such diverse problems as hardening of the arteries and increased susceptibility to infection.

Another recent study yielded results suggesting that many Americans, of all ages, get amounts of chromium in their daily diets that are below the minimum safe and adequate allowance.

Glucose, like oxygen, has two sides, good and bad. We obviously can't live without it, but in some instances it seems we can't live with it—at least not in good health. It can react with many different types of biologic molecules, including hemoglobin, proteins in membranes, even conceivably the nucleic acids DNA and RNA. These reactions damage the tissues. Chromium may help restore some of the body's sensitivity to insulin and thus make better use of glucose.

Factors that appear to contribute to a depletion of body chromium stores include aging, pregnancy, high consumption of refined foods and, possibly, strenuous exercise. It has been shown that running significantly increases the urinary excretion of chromium. Although it is still unclear if urinary excretion of chromium is a valid indicator of the nutritional status of chromium, it is a factor that could lead to further chromium deficiency in an individual whose chromium concentrations are already marginal.

Chromium supplementation is expected to assume an important place in preventive medicine. I anticipate much further research with this element and its role in optimal health.

II. CLAIMS

Positive:

1) Useful in the treatment and prevention of diabetes; 2) protective against cardiovascular disease and high blood pressure; 3) useful in treating hypoglycemia.

Negative:

1) Toxic and carcinogenic.

III. EVIDENCE

Related to Positive Claims:

1) Useful in the treatment and prevention of diabetes—There is no direct evidence that chromium prevents diabetes, although there is evidence that it can increase glucose tolerance. The best double-blind, placebo-controlled studies have so far not revealed any favorable role for chromium in the treatment of established diabetes. It will be of interest to see if higher doses of GTF chromium have any effect on glucose metabolism in diabetics.

The most promising studies are those involving elderly subjects. One of these showed that impaired glucose tolerance often improved when diet was supplemented with a yeast rich in GTF. Another demonstrated a beneficial effect on glucose tolerance in ten out of twelve elderly subjects given chromium-enriched yeast. No such effect was seen in a group of control patients who did not receive chromium supplementation. Another recent study demonstrated improved glucose tolerance in elderly people given 200 micrograms of chromium trichloride daily.

Chromium supplementation may have beneficial effects in younger people, as well. Recently researchers found that supplementation with 200 micrograms daily of inorganic chromium (chromium trichloride) improved glucose tolerance in otherwise healthy, non-diabetic subjects.

Overall, research in this area is promising, but further clinical trials will have to be conducted before it can justifiably be claimed that chromium prevents or improves diabetic conditions.

2) Protective against cardiovascular disease and high blood pressure—The evidence here is contradictory. Some studies have shown favorable effects and others have not. One group reported that patients with coronary artery disease have significantly lower serum chromium levels than do healthy individuals. Other investigators report that supplemental chromium significantly increases the level of high-density lipoproteins (HDLs) in humans. HDLs are considered *protective* against cardiovascular disease. The study was double-blind and placebo-controlled. The dose was 200 micrograms daily of chromium trichloride. Another study, however, did not find any favorable effects on blood cholesterol levels.

Recently my colleagues and I found that 200 micrograms of chromium picolinate daily can significantly reduce cholesterol, increase HDL and decrease amounts of the proteins that carry the harmful forms of cholesterol. This was a placebo-controlled, double-blind study.

There is no evidence, meanwhile, that chromium is useful in treatment or prevention of high blood pressure.

3) Useful in treating hypoglycemia—A recent study showed that hypoglycemic individuals respond favorably (with increases of blood sugar) to supplementation with 200 micrograms of chromium daily.

Related to Negative Claims:

1) Toxic and carcinogenic—Hexavalent chromium is toxic, but *trivalent* chromium, the dietary form of this essential trace element, has very low toxicity. Long-term exposure to the dangerous hexavalent form may lead to skin problems, perforation of the nasal septum and lung cancer. The trivalent form is not associated with any type of cancer.

IV. RECOMMENDATIONS

A) *Suggested Intake:* The optimal amount of chromium intake is not known. The National Research Council tentatively recommends as a safe and adequate daily allowance for adults 50 to 200 *micrograms* (not milligrams). The chromium intake of a typical U.S. diet is below 50 micrograms daily. Only about 1 to 2 percent of this amount is actually absorbed. There is increasing evidence that marginal chromium deficiency is commonplace. Deficiency is most likely among the aged, pregnant women and persons who indulge in regular, strenuous exercise (such as runners). Healthy young people, as well as the aged, however, have exhibited improved glucose tolerance when taking chromium supplements. I recommend supplementation with 50 to 200 micrograms of chromium daily.

B) *Source/Form:* Good food sources of chromium include whole-grain cereals, condiments (black pepper, thyme), meat products and cheeses. Fruits are low in chromium. So are most refined foods. Brewer's yeast is a good source of chromium. Chromium-enriched yeast, which has a higher chromium content than brewer's yeast, is now being produced. GTF chromium (found in brewer's yeast and the specially prepared yeast described previously) is far better absorbed by the body than other forms studied. Less than 1 percent of chromium in the form of chromium trichloride is absorbed, whereas 10 to 25 percent of the chromium in the form of GTF is absorbed. About 10 percent of the chromium in brewer's yeast is in the form of GTF. Chromium-rich yeast and inorganic chromium are currently available. Chromium picolinate has also recently become available. I recommend organic forms of chromium, such as chromium-rich yeast and chromium picolinate.

C) *Take With:* Best if taken with a well-balanced vitamin/mineral "insurance" formula. (See Part Three for specific recommendations.)

D) *Cautionary Note:* The chemical structure of GTF is not known; thus, to determine its activity, a biologic and not a chemical assay is performed. Specifically, fat cells are used in this procedure. There are some yeast products on the market that claim to have most of the chromium in the form of GTF. If a chemical analysis was used to determine this, the claim is necessarily *invalid.* In short, there are some yeast products on the market that are questionable.

COPPER

I. OVERVIEW: The Fire Extinguisher

Copper is an essential trace mineral for humans. It plays a singular role in respiration. The protein hemoglobin carries most of the oxygen in the blood and relies upon copper as well as iron for its synthesis and function. Copper is also involved in the production of collagen, the protein responsible for functional integrity of bone, cartilage, skin and tendon; elastin, the protein that is mainly responsible for the elastic properties of the blood vessels, lungs and skin; the neuro-transmitter noradrenalin, a key molecule in the working of the nervous system; and melanin formation (pigment found in the skin and hair). Copper helps protect against the ravages of oxidant damage through the enzyme copper-zinc superoxide dismutase, as well as the protein ceruloplasmin. By oxidizing iron, ceruloplasmin inhibits free-radical formation from reduced iron. It is, in fact, one of the most important blood antioxidants. It prevents peroxidation (rancidity) of polyunsaturated fatty acids and maintains the integrity of cell membranes.

It has been reported that copper deficiency can produce emphysema (destruction of the elastic recoil properties of the lungs, resulting in diminished oxygen transfer from the air into the blood) in pigs. Copper deficiency may be at the base of this because ceruloplasmin appears to be necessary to maintain a protein (called alpha$_1$-antitrypsin) that seems to help prevent the sort of lung damage seen in emphysema. Thus, ceruloplasmin could be an important lung defense in people chronically exposed to oxidants (such as cigarette smoke and air pollution).

Finally, ceruloplasmin is one of the "acute-phase reactants." This means that the amount of ceruloplasmin available increases in direct proportion to such pathologic "insults" to the body as infection, trauma, vascular insufficiency. Production of oxygen radicals and inflammation attend these insults. Ceruloplasmin acts as something of a fire extinguisher—an emergency antioxidant. Copper-zinc superoxide dismutase is a human enzyme that protects against superoxide-induced cellular damage. It has antioxidant and anti-inflammatory properties and loses its potency when copper is removed from its structure. (See anti-inflammatory discussion below for further details.)

Probably the most important factor in protecting against free-radical generation and damage is the high degree of structural organization of the cell that has evolved over billions of years. One may expect that in the final reaction of respiration, free-oxygen radicals would be generated. This does not occur to any significant extent as long as the structural integrity of the membrane where the reaction takes place remains intact. Copper is an essential factor in preserving the integrity of this membrane.

Human copper deficiency has been demonstrated. The relatively recent clinical practice of feeding patients through their veins has resulted in dramatic demonstrations of the need for trace elements in human nutrition. Copper deficiency is the second commonest trace-metal deficiency that occurs during intravenous feeding. (Zinc is the commonest.) Symptoms of copper deficiency include an anemia that is responsive to iron, lowered white-blood-cell count and loss of bone density (osteoporosis). Copper deficiency has been noted in patients taking zinc supplements (150 milligrams daily of elemental zinc) for periods greater than a year. (Zinc is antagonistic to copper.) Signs in this context are anemia and decrease in high-density lipoproteins, which are known to be protective against coronary heart disease.

On the darker side, copper has been called a "culpable heavy metal" that can cause certain types of schizophrenia and heart disease. Indeed, in a *rare* genetic disorder of copper metabolism called Wilson's disease, excessive copper accumulates in the liver and brain, severely damaging both organs. However, there is no reliable evidence to link excessive copper to any form of schizophrenia or heart disease.

Recent studies have shown a wide variation in dietary copper intake. Many individuals may be consuming suboptimal amounts—not low enough to cause overt deficiency symptoms but possibly low enough to affect life span. Apart from its role as an antioxidant and *possible* protector against some forms of cancer and heart disease, copper's folk-remedy reputation as an anti-arthritic agent may turn out to have some scientific validity. Other risk factors for copper deficiency include diets rich in fructose (sugars in fruit, honey and cornstarch) regular consumption of antacids and prolonged megadoses of vitamin C.

II. CLAIMS

Positive:
1) Anti-cancer substance; 2) protective against cardiovascular disease; 3) anti-inflammatory and useful against some forms of arthritis; 4) immune booster.

Negative:
1) Promotes oxidation; 2) causes cancer; 3) contributes to schizophrenia; 4) toxic.

III. EVIDENCE

Related to Positive Claims:

1) Anti-cancer substance—Several reports suggest that copper may protect against cancer. One group observed that supplementary copper (copper acetate) in the diets of rats protected them against chemical-caused cancers. Another noted that several copper-containing compounds prevented the malignant transformation of chick-embryo cells by the cancer-causing (to chicks) Rous sarcoma virus. This is of interest because there is increasing evidence that RNA viruses similar to the Rous sarcoma virus may have some role in human cancers.

There are other studies demonstrating that high levels of copper salts added to the diets of animals provided protection against carcinogenesis. One found that a copper-salicylate derivative inhibited tumor promotion in mice. The speculation is that these compounds protect against cancer by acting as scavengers of free radicals thought to be involved in the promotion of cancer.

There is no direct evidence of a cancer-protective role for supplemental copper in human nutrition as yet. But in view of the fact that substances such as ceruloplasmin and superoxide dismutase are important protectors against oxidant damage, and that free-radical mechanisms appear important in the promotion of cancer, further research on the possible anti-carcinogenic role of copper is warranted.

2) Protective against cardiovascular disease—It has been reported that copper deficiency in young men (produced by taking 160 milligrams daily of zinc, a copper antagonist, for a protracted period) contributed to a significant lowering of the level of high-density lipoprotein (HDL). HDL is believed to be protective against coronary heart disease. Others have demonstrated an increase in cholesterol levels in rats fed diets elevated in zinc and low in copper, concluding that an imbalance in the zinc-to-copper ratio increases the risk of coronary heart disease by lowering the amount of protective HDL. In another study, twenty-four male subjects fed a copper-deficient diet were found to have significant increases in LDL cholesterol and total cholesterol and significant decreases in HDL cholesterol after eleven weeks. These significant studies deserve further investigation and indicate that the intake of zinc to copper should be carefully balanced at a ratio of about 10:1—milligram to milligram. (See Recommendations later in this discussion of copper.)

3) Anti-inflammatory and useful against some forms of arthritis—The use of copper bracelets in the folk-remedy treatment of arthritis has persisted despite the skepticism of most doctors. It turns out there might be something to it, after all. Researchers have discovered a) that the clinical condition of those suffering from arthritis (mainly osteoarthritis, or degenerative joint disease) who habitually wore the copper bracelets became significantly worse after discontinuing their use; b) the worsening effects were not seen in those subjects who had worn placebo bracelets (made of a different but similar-appearing metal); and c) there was evidence that copper from the bracelets, when dissolved in sweat, could be absorbed through the skin.

A number of studies have shown that victims of rheumatoid arthritis (there are five million such individuals in the United States alone) have increased blood levels of both copper and ceruloplasmin (discussed in the Overview). The copper content of the synovial fluid of the joints is also significantly elevated in these individuals. For a while researchers thought these higher levels meant that copper was one of the *causes* of arthritis. Now just the opposite is believed—that copper is a protector and that the higher levels are indicative of the body's rallying copper in an attempt to fight off the disease. Copper seems to play an important role in the body's response to inflammatory disease. Ceruloplasmin, to which copper is bound, is a scavenger of the sort of toxic oxygen radicals that are liberated in various disease processes, such as arthritis.

This possibility—that elevation of copper-related ceruloplasmin is a protective response—has stimulated the development of a number of copper-containing complexes designed to treat rheumatoid arthritis. Copper complexes of aspirin, tryptophan and even penicillamine have been found to have anti-inflammatory activity in animals.

Some very promising studies using copper superoxide dismutase as an antioxidant and anti-inflammatory agent are being carried out. That superoxide dismutase (SOD) is essential to protect against oxidant and probably also inflammatory damage is established. Taking SOD by mouth, however, does not make sense (see analysis of SOD later in this book). SOD is an enzyme that gets digested in the gut and thus in the oral form never reaches the target cells and joints. *Injections* of copper-zinc SOD (known as Orgotein) directly into arthritic joints, however, have shown *some* effectiveness in trials of patients with osteoarthritis and rheumatoid arthritis.

Others have packaged bovine copper SOD in liposomes (artificial membrane-like structures) and, by injecting these subcutaneously, have had some success in the treatment of such serious diseases as rheumatoid arthritis, systemic lupus erythematosus, Crohn's disease, scleroderma, dermatomyositis and severe radiation-induced necrosis (wasting of tissue). Some aspects of these conditions are similar to some of the arthritic conditions.

Clearly, extensive clinical trials are needed to further define the potentially important role of copper and copper SOD in these diseases.

4) Immune booster—Data on the role of copper in the immune system are very sparse. In spontaneous and controlled experiments with *Salmonella typhimurium* infection in rats, copper deficiency results in high mortality. Copper deficiency has also been shown to result in decreased antibody response in mice. Thus, copper does appear to affect the immune system, but its role needs clarification. There is no human work in this area, as yet.

Related to Negative Claims:

1) Promotes oxidation—Up until now I have been talking about the role of copper tightly bound to substances such as copper-zinc SOD and ceruloplasmin. Copper in this form has antioxidant properties. Copper may, however, exist in a form where it is *not* bound—copper ions. These ions can be powerful generators of oxygen radicals and thus promoters of oxidation. In fact, it has been suggested that the copper contraceptive loop (IUD) kills sperm by its generation of oxygen radicals. The role free copper ions play in generating oxygen radicals is unknown.

2) Causes cancer—Researchers examined copper and zinc levels in malignant and normal tissue and found significantly elevated levels of copper in the cancer of the large bowel, bladder and female reproductive organs but not in cancer of the breast, kidney and testis. There was no difference in zinc levels between malignant and normal tissue. These researchers hypothesize that copper-ion generation of free radicals may be involved in carcinogenesis.

Elevated copper levels in the blood have been found in many different types of cancer, including Hodgkin's disease, lymphoma, multiple myeloma, leukemia, lung cancer, breast cancer and cancer of the digestive system. It is quite possible, however, that these elevated levels are the consequence and not the cause of the disease process.

Other investigators have correlated per capita intake of copper with cancer mortality rates in twenty-seven countries and found direct associations for leukemia and cancer of the intestine, breast and skin. They proposed that copper is involved in carcinogenesis, not by a direct mechanism but by antagonizing selenium, thereby diminishing selenium's protective effects against cancer. (See analysis of selenium later in this book.)

At present there is no convincing evidence suggesting that dietary copper causes or contributes in any way to any form of cancer.

3) Contributes to schizophrenia—Although several researchers have reported elevated serum copper in some schizophrenic patients, these elevations are most likely nonspecific. There is no evidence of a cause-and-effect relationship. A recent study showed no elevation of copper in the cerebrospinal fluid of a range of schizophrenic patients. There is no evidence that copper is the cause of any form of mental disease.

4) Toxic—Although copper is toxic to aquatic species and sheep, it is relatively non-toxic in humans. No adverse effects in humans would be expected from a copper intake of up to 35 milligrams daily for an adult.

IV. RECOMMENDATIONS

A) *Suggested Intake:* The National Research Council lists the estimated safe and adequate daily intake of copper for adults as 1.5 to 3 milligrams; children eleven years and older as 1.5 to 2.5 milligrams; 1 to 2 milligrams for children between seven and ten; 1 to 1.5 milligrams for children between four and six; .7 to 1 milligram for children between one and three and .4 to .7 milligram for infants. These amounts appear to be sufficient to prevent copper *deficiency*. The *optimal* copper intake for maximal longevity with minimal disease, however, has not yet been defined. As previously noted, there are studies showing that many people have much lower intakes than those recommended. This is particularly true of the elderly population. Substances that interfere with copper absorption and utilization include phytates (found in cereals, vegetables), fiber, zinc, molybdenum, cadmium, vitamin C and diets high in fructose (sugars in fruit, honey and cornstarch). One report showed that young men taking 500 milligrams of vitamin C three times a day for two months developed decreased serum copper and ceruloplasmin, which increased when they stopped taking this vitamin.

Copper supplementation is prudent. Since I advocate taking 15 to 30 milligrams of zinc daily, I recommend taking 1.5 to 3 milligrams of copper daily (adult dose) to maintain the zinc-to-copper ratio of about 10:1 discussed earlier. This puts my recommendation, for all age groups, in the same range as that recommended by the National Research Council. Consult your physician before taking higher doses. If a physician recommends higher amounts of zinc than 30 milligrams daily, adjust the copper intake accordingly. Remember: You want to take about ten times as much zinc as copper (weight of elemental zinc to elemental copper).

B) *Source/Form:* The best natural sources of copper include animal livers, crustaceans, shellfish, nuts, fruits, oysters, kidneys and dried legumes. Cow's milk is poor in copper. There are several copper supplements on the market; they all have similar bioavailability and include copper gluconate and copper sulfate.

C) *Take With:* Best incorporated into a well-balanced vitamin/mineral "insurance" formula; see Part Three. Because of the antagonisms reported to exist, I suggest that a daily dose of 1.5 to 3 milligrams of copper be accompanied by 15 to 30 milligrams of zinc, 50 to 200 *micrograms* of selenium and 50 to 100 *micrograms* of molybdenum.

D) *Cautionary Note:* Copper supplements should not be used by patients with hepatolenticular degeneration (Wilson's disease).

FLUORINE

I. OVERVIEW: Anti-Aging Agent for the Bones

Fluorine or, more specifically, its electrically charged form, fluoride, is known to be beneficial to human health. It has yet to be established, however, that this element is nutritionally essential. Fluoride is found naturally in soils, water, plants, and animal tissue and hence in our foodstuffs. This natural occurrence, coupled with its health-promoting effects, make the element a prime candidate for inclusion on the list of essential trace elements, and it is expected that one day it will be included.

When and if fluoride does get voted in as an essential nutrient, it will differ from all the other nutrients in one major way: the most important source of the element is water rather than food. It has been recognized for some time that children who drink water rich in fluoride have a lower incidence of dental caries ("cavities") than those who drink water which is fluoride-poor. This beneficial action of fluoride became the basis for fluoridation of many water supplies in the United States beginning in the 1940s, occasioning some heated debates.

Fluoride used in water fluoridation was initially associated with the fluorides used to kill insects, mice and rats. These insecticides and rodenticides, however, used poisonous organic fluorides, not inorganic fluorides, which are significantly less toxic, and which are the forms used for water fluoridation. At one point, it was thought by a few that fluoridation of the U.S. water supply was a plot by the Russians to take over the country. That speculation was, of course, utter nonsense. Later on, a couple of researchers claimed that fluoridation of water causes cancer. There is absolutely *no* evidence that this is true.

Fluorides not only significantly decrease the frequency of dental caries, they may also prevent and treat osteoporosis and protect against degenerative disease of the cardiovascular system. Other health benefits for fluoride are expected to be discovered as we move away from thinking about the element as foe and toward embracing it more as friend.

It is interesting that those drinking fluoride-rich water have a lower incidence of calcified aortas when compared to those living in low-fluoride areas. Soft-tissue calcification is very common with aging, leading, in addition to calcified aortas, to calcified heart valves, calcification in the tendons and other musculoskeletal structures, and, in a contributing role, to "hardening" of all of the arteries. Fluoride could play a major role in preventing these very common and potentially deadly processes.

II. CLAIMS

Positive:
1) Protects against dental caries; 2) protects against osteoporosis and useful in the treatment of osteoporosis.

Negative:
1) Toxic; 2) causes cancer.

III. EVIDENCE

Related to Positive Claims:
1) Protects against dental caries—It was known as early as 1892 that fluoride protects against dental caries. The association between fluoride in water and dental health came about as a result of researchers trying to find out what caused brownish staining on otherwise healthy teeth. It turned out that the brown staining was due to the consumption of water containing high amounts of fluoride.

In the 1930s and 1940s, it was determined that when the natural fluoride concentration of water was about 1 milligram per liter (or 1 part per million), caries were reduced 50–60 percent (provided fluoride ingestion began before eruption of the permanent molars). And at this concentration there was no staining of teeth.

Soon several communities voted to supplement their drinking waters with fluoride to bring them to 1 milligram per liter. Communities whose water supply contained a fluoride concentration of 1.5 milligrams per liter or higher decided to reduce it to about 1 milligram per liter. Most public water suppliers of the 100 largest cities in the United States are now fluoridated as are about 60 percent of all the nation's water systems. There are still a large number of areas in the United States, however, where water fluoride levels are less than 1 milligram per liter.

Perhaps the most dramatic study on the dental health of America's youth was that reported by the American Institute of Dental Research in 1988. The study included 40,000 youngsters coast to coast, and it was found that dental cavities have declined by 36 percent among children ages five to seventeen, and that almost 50 percent of these children had no tooth decay at all. The sample population was selected to represent the approximately forty-three million school-age children in the nation.

Dental decay, the most common degenerative disease of children and a problem that has plagued people throughout history, appears to be steadily declining as the use of fluoride in the nation's drinking water increases. Also significant is the increased use of fluoride-containing toothpastes, gels and mouthwashes.

There are a few ways in which fluoride is thought to work to prevent caries. During tooth development, ingested fluoride gets incorporated into tooth structure before eruption, creating a tougher tooth. After the tooth has erupted, fluoride that washes over it gets incorporated into the enamel. There is evidence that fluoride, particularly if applied topically (for example, in gel form), reduces the number of those bacterial organisms in the mouth which are linked to cavities.

In order to maintain the reduction of caries, approximately 1 milligram per liter of fluoride-containing water should be consumed over a lifetime. Fluoride-containing toothpastes, gels, and mouthwashes may also prevent cavity formation in erupted teeth.

2) Protects against osteoporosis and useful in the treatment of osteoporosis—Fluoride is the most important trace element affecting the formation of skeletal and dental tissues. Fluoride is the only non-hormonal agent known to stimulate new bone formation. In addition to stimulating new bone growth, which is its major effect on bones, it is incorporated in bone crystal making bone stronger. Fluoride works in conjunction with calcium in this respect.

Several epidemiologic studies show that people living in regions where they drink water with high-fluoride content have substantially less osteoporosis and a lower incidence of collapsed vertebrae than those living in areas where the fluoride content of water is low. Strong support for the possible role of fluoride in preventing osteoporosis was presented by a group of researchers from Harvard's School of Public Health some years ago. They reported on the prevalence of osteoporosis in people living in areas of North Dakota where the fluoride content of the water supply was high as well as where it was low. Evidence of osteoporosis, reduced bone density and collapsed vertebrae was substantially higher in the low-fluoride area, especially in women. Their results indicated that fluoride, at a concentration between 4 to 6 milligrams per liter in the water supply, significantly decreased the prevalence of osteoporosis. A few other studies have noted decreased prevalence of osteoporosis in women from fluoridated areas (where there was at least 1 milligram of fluoride per liter of water) compared to women in low-fluoride areas. It is clear that fluoride can prevent osteoporosis, but it is still not clear what the optimal and safe intake should be over a long period of time.

Sodium fluoride was introduced in 1961 for the curative treatment of osteoporosis with vertebral fractures. Since that time several studies were conducted relative to this issue, but it wasn't until 1988 that French researchers produced the first adequately controlled prospective study of the safety and effectiveness of combined fluoride-calcium therapy in the treatment of this disorder. Their results showed that when sodium fluoride was given at a dose of 25 milligrams twice daily (50 milligrams a day) and calcium 1 gram daily for two years to patients who had at least one vertebral crush injury secondary to osteoporosis, there was a significantly lower rate of new vertebral fractures when compared to the group that did not receive fluoride. The major side effects from the fluoride treatment were pain in the ankles and feet and irritation of the stomach.

Sodium fluoride therapy for osteoporosis is, as of this writing, not approved by the U.S. FDA. However, there are two ongoing fluoride-osteoporosis studies, one at the Mayo Clinic and the other at the Henry Ford Hospital in Detroit. FDA approval will be contingent on the outcome of these studies.

Continued research on high-dose fluoride in the treatment of osteoporosis is urgently needed in order to define the most effective, as well as safest, long-term regimen. One of the most common degenerative diseases of adults is alveolar bone loss. Alveolar bone is mainly responsible for holding teeth in our mouths. It would be extremely interesting and important to study the role of high-dose fluoride in the treatment of alveolar bone loss. If this loss can be prevented, then very few of us, provided we otherwise maintain good dental/gum hygiene, will ever need false teeth.

Related to Negative Claims:

1) Toxic—Fluoride, in high doses, *is* toxic. If you consume between 2.5 to 5 grams of fluoride in one shot you will get very sick and, in fact, probably die. Fortunately, the amounts required for improved health fall *far* below that range. The amounts included in drinking water rarely, if ever, cause tooth staining or other problems.

At high doses of fluoride, skeletal fluorosis can occur. Skeletal fluorosis is abnormal hardening of bones and is associated with arthritic pain, weakness, joint stiffness and occasionally nerve damage and paralysis. Intakes of 20–80 milligrams daily of fluoride for ten to twenty years are considered necessary for significant fluorosis to occur. This is equivalent to intakes of 72–285 milligrams daily of sodium fluoride. No evidence of skeletal fluorosis nor any other signs or symptoms of fluoride toxicity have been noted in about seven million adult U.S. residents who lived for several generations in areas where the natural fluoride concentration in the drinking water was 2 to 10 milligrams per liter.

High doses of sodium fluoride (40–70 milligrams daily) used *therapeutically* even for long periods of time are unlikely to cause skeletal fluorosis. However, those who do take these doses may suffer from gastrointestinal symptoms, such as heartburn, and from pains in the feet and ankles. New forms of sodium fluoride are being developed to minimize the gastrointestinal symptoms.

2) Causes cancer—There is *no* evidence that fluoride ingestion causes any type of cancer.

IV. RECOMMENDATIONS

A) *Suggested Intake:* About 60 percent of the water supplies of the United States are fluoridated. Fluoride in the drinking water at a concentration of 1 milligram per liter appears to confer optimal protection against dental cavities and may also confer protection against osteoporosis. The best method of providing fluoride is to add it to the local water supply.

Table 1 contains the recommendations by the Committee on Nutrition of the American Academy of Pediatrics for fluoride supplementation in communities that have insufficient fluoride in the water supply.

Adults should also use 1 milligram of fluoride daily (about 3.6 milligrams of sodium fluoride daily). It is important to note that many people, even in areas where the water *is* fluoridated, use other water sources, such as distilled water and water prepared by reverse osmosis,

TABLE 1[a]   FLUORIDE SUPPLEMENTATION SCHEDULE FOR INFANTS AND CHILDREN (DAILY)[b]

Fluoride concentration in local water supply (milligrams per liter)			
Age	*< 0.3*	*0.3 to 0.7*	*> 0.7*
0–2[c] years	0.25 mg	0	0
2–3 years	0.50 mg	0.25 mg	0
3–16 years	1.00 mg	0.50 mg	0

[a] Table from *Pediatrics*, vol 77, p 758, 1986.
[b] Values are milligrams of fluoride supplement per day.
[c] Supplementation should begin in the first two weeks after birth.

which are fluoride-poor. For protection against dental caries and osteoporosis, supplementation with 1 milligram of fluoride daily is desirable. For protection against caries, those over six years of age may use a mouthwash containing about 4 milligrams of fluoride (per rinse) every day. This exposes the teeth to about 1 milligram of fluoride daily and should not be swallowed. Alternatively, a toothpaste or gel containing about 4 milligrams of fluoride per daily application can be used.

Intakes from food and water of up to 10 milligrams of fluoride daily can be considered safe for adults.

B) *Source/Form:* The major source of fluoride is from drinking water. In the United States, the typical daily intake of fluoride from drinking water is from 1–2 milligrams and from foods, 0.2 to 0.6 milligrams. Foods high in fluoride include seafood, animal meat (especially if the bones are included in the preparation), and tea. One cup of tea can have from 1–4 milligrams of fluoride. Foods poor in fluoride include fruits, cereals, milk and other dairy products.

Sodium fluoride tablets are available but require prescription by a doctor or dentist. Likewise, fluoride is available by prescription as a 0.4 percent stannous fluoride gel which is useful for the treatment of sensitive teeth and gums. Sodium fluoride-containing mouthwashes and toothpastes are widely available without prescription but should not be used by anyone under six years of age unless recommended by a dentist and then only under strict supervision since fluoride in these products could cause some side effects if swallowed. The fluoride found in some toothpastes is usually in the form of sodium monofluonophosphate.

C) *Take With:* All those who take oral fluoride supplements should make sure that their calcium intake is adequate (see Calcium). Those who take fluoride therapeutically for the treatment of osteoporosis, for example, should take 1 gram daily of supplementary calcium unless contraindicated.

D) *Cautionary Note:* The use of fluoride for therapeutic purposes must be supervised by a physician or dentist. If a mouthwash or fluoride-containing toothpaste is inadvertently swallowed, then drink a glassful of milk or take some calcium-containing supplement (e.g.,

Tums). Calcium is an antidote for fluoride toxicity. Children under six years of age are at greatest risk for dental staining from regularly drinking fluoride-rich water if their calcium intakes are low.

GERMANIUM

I. OVERVIEW: "Cure For Everything?"

If you happened to be at the checkout counter of your local super-market during the last week of 1987, you likely saw a well-known tabloid displaying a remarkable headline that shouted: "New miracle pill cures *everything*." The miracle pill referred to contained the element germanium. A list of diseases that the pill was reputed to cure included cancer, immune disorders, viral diseases, arthritis, high blood pressure, allergies and more. One physician was quoted as saying about the substance, "It's simply the most important healing substance on the planet." Another researcher said, "It is a landmark development in the field of nutritional medicine."

Since the article appeared, germanium sales soared. In a way, germanium's dramatic entrance onto this scene is reminiscent of another "miraculous" substance which made its entrance ten years before. I refer to "pangamic acid," which, interestingly enough, supposedly cured almost all of the same diseases and was speculated to work in an identical manner. Unfortunately, pangamic acid didn't even remotely live up to any of its many promises. Let us hope that germanium turns out to have some real merit.

Germanium is relatively abundant in the earth's crust, and its position in the periodic table of the elements *is* in the region of the biologically active trace elements. However, there is no evidence that germanium itself has *any* nutritional, biochemical or biological role in humans. In fact, the *only* biological role presently known for germanium is that germanium supplementation can delay boron deficiency signs in tomatoes and sunflowers.

The idea that germanium can be beneficial in human health was introduced by the Japanese metallurgist and coal engineer Dr. Kazuhiko Asai, who describes the work at his clinic in his book *Miracle Cure: Organic Germanium*. Asai discusses work with a synthetic organic compound of germanium, not found naturally. This substance is known as Ge-132, or, popularly, organic germanium. The researcher expresses a deep religious connection to the compound and states, "I believe that my life is inextricably linked with germanium and that my germanium compound was divinely conferred on mankind through an actual being, that being happened to be I."

Despite the fact that this kind of talk no doubt makes a lot of us wince, there have been some recent studies suggesting that organic germanium compounds, including Asai's, *may* have some immune-enhancing, anti-cancer and anti-viral qualities.

II. CLAIMS

Positive:

1) Useful in the treatment of AIDS Related Complex (ARC) and AIDS;
2) stimulates the immune system; 3) useful in the treatment of cancer;
4) useful in the treatment of chronic Epstein-Barr Virus syndrome.

III. EVIDENCE

Related to Positive Claims:

1) Useful in the treatment of ARC and AIDS—Some who are infected with the AIDS virus, HIV, including those with ARC ("pre-AIDS") and AIDS itself are using Asai's organic germanium compound, and some are claiming that it is helpful. Russian scientists reported, at a recent international AIDS conference (1989) that some synthetic organic germanium compounds *do* inhibit the reproduction of HIV in the test tube. Researchers are studying the effect of organic germanium in the treatment of ARC and AIDS patients. Although Asai's compound has not shown any significant toxic effects to date, we do not know at this time if it has any beneficial effects in these disorders.

2) Stimulates the immune system—There are a few papers demonstrating that organic germanium compounds have immune-enhancing properties. It has been reported that two new organic germanium compounds (different from Ge-132), PCAGeS and PCAGeO, inhibited the growth of certain mouse cancers when the tumor-containing mice were given oral preparations of these compounds. Macrophage activity (type of immune cell that kills cancer cells) was enhanced by these compounds.

It has also been reported that serum from mice treated orally with

Ge-132 exhibited anti-cancer activity against some cancers in mice. The authors think that Ge-132 induces the activity of certain immune-enhancing substances called lymphokines, an example of which is gamma interferon.

Further research is anticipated.

3) Useful in the treatment of cancer—Ge-132 and other organic germanium compounds appear to inhibit the growth of some mouse cancers by an immune-stimulating effect. (See previous section.) Human studies are urgently needed.

4) Useful in the treatment of Chronic Epstein-Barr Virus syndrome—Chronic Epstein-Barr Virus syndrome is a chronic fatigue disorder which may occasionally be associated with reactivation of Epstein-Barr virus (a member of the herpes family) in someone who has previously been infected with the virus (frequent cause of "mono" or infectious mononucleosis). Although Chronic Fatigue Syndrome is a real entity, it may actually have many causes. Likewise, there exists a long laundry list of treatments, *some* of which work—*sometimes.*

One of the most recent additions to this therapeutic laundry list is Ge-132, and there are some clinical anecdotes suggesting that it may be of some benefit in this disorder, probably via immune-enhancing effects. More study is warranted.

IV. RECOMMENDATIONS

Asai's organic germanium, Ge-132, is now available in health food stores in capsules of 25 milligrams. A granular form is also available. Apparently the pure substance has low toxicity even if taken up to 10 grams daily for several months. Studies regarding its immune-enhancing, anti-cancer and anti-viral activities seem promising and should be continued. However, we need some good human studies to see what this and related substances can really do. In the meantime, those who are taking this substance should inform their physicians that they are doing so. The physician will thus be in a position to assess any health benefits that may occur. I would not recommend that anyone take this substance unless participating in a research study with medical supervision. A small percentage of those taking Ge-132 have been reported to develop reversible skin eruptions and stool softening. Some germanium supplements have been associated with more serious side effects such as kidney failure. It is thought the toxic substance in these supplements was not Ge-132 but another germanium compound or an unknown contaminant.

IODINE

I. OVERVIEW: Your Friend in Fallout

Iodine is present in low amounts in the earth's crust and thus in its soils. It is plentiful in the oceans and is found in sea animals and sea plants, such as the brown seaweed kelp.

Iodine was first discovered in 1812 in kelp. Elemental iodine was extracted from the seaweed and was named iodine because of its color, which means violet in Greek. Iodine occurs naturally as iodide or iodate salts. It is a crucial part of the thyroid hormones, which, in turn, play a vital role in the production of energy. Iodine deficiency is still the major cause of hypothyroidism in the world. Deficiency of thyroid hormones really slows you down. Symptoms include chronic fatigue, apathy, dry skin, intolerance to cold, weight gain and enlargement of the thyroid (goiter).

Iodine deficiency, of course, can cause the same symptoms. Hypothyroidism due to endemic goiter was fairly common in the United States during the early years of the century, but the introduction of iodized table salt has made this disorder uncommon. However, endemic goiter is still occasionally observed in the United States, and at the global level the disorder continues to be a major public health problem, particularly in Africa, Asia and South America.

II. CLAIMS

Positive:
1) Protects against toxic effects from radioactive materials; 2) relieves pain and soreness associated with fibrocystic breasts; 3) good for loosening up clogged mucus in the breathing tubes; 4) good antiseptic.

Negative:
1) Toxic.

III. EVIDENCE

Related to Positive Claims:

1) Protects against toxic effects from radioactive materials—Many of you will undoubtedly remember that following the Chernobyl nuclear plant meltdown, there was a rush to purchase potassium iodide tablets to protect against radioactive fallout. Did this make any sense whatsoever? It actually did. Radioactive iodides are released into the environment following a nuclear power plant accident. The radioiodides could enter the body and accumulate in an unprotected thyroid gland where they would remain for varying periods of time. Radioiodides can cause thyroid cancer.

Iodide is the most effective blocker of radioiodide uptake by the thyroid. In fact, thyroid radioiodide uptake can be reduced to less than 1 percent by the daily oral intake of 130 milligrams of potassium iodide, which is equivalent to 100 milligrams of iodide. Blockade with a single 130-milligram dose of potassium iodide lasts between twenty-four and forty-eight hours. A daily dose of 130 milligrams of potassium iodide, if started before any exposure to radioiodide or even right after initial exposure and continued for no more than seven to fourteen days (unless exposure continues), should be effective in preventing radio-iodide toxicity to the thyroid gland. Significant adverse side effects are unlikely at this dose for this time period. (See discussion on toxicity in this section.) The major source of radioiodide following a nuclear power-plant explosion is cow's milk.

Interestingly, iodine-rich seaweed contains other substances that provide protection against some other forms of radiation, as well. (See discussion of Alginates elsewhere.)

2) Relieves pain and soreness associated with fibrocystic breasts—Fibrocystic breasts are a very common condition in premenopausal women, as well as in postmenopausal women taking supplementary estrogens. Fibrocystic breasts are still referred to as fibrocystic disease in many medical textbooks and by many physicians. However, fibrocystic breasts are not diseased breasts, but they frequently are associated with pain and soreness. There are a number of theories on the cause of fibrocystic breasts and a number of therapies, all of which are not without controversy. Some researchers believe that fibrocystic breasts are the result of iodine deficiency.

A Canadian physician reported in 1988 that a majority of women with fibrocystic breasts experienced complete relief from their symptoms after being treated with elemental iodine for four months. When treatment was discontinued the symptoms returned. Other researchers have reported positive results with other iodine-containing compounds. More research is needed to substantiate this claim.

3) Good for loosening up clogged mucus in the breathing tubes—A cough that doesn't quit is often associated with some mucus getting lodged in the breathing tubes causing continuous irritation. Some iodine-containing compounds, such as SSKI (super saturated potassium iodide) and Organidin, are sometimes helpful in breaking up the mucus. These so-called mucolytic agents are drugs that require a physician's prescription.

4) Good antiseptic—Iodine is the most effective substance for purifying backcountry water. The form of iodine that is best for this purpose is called tetraglycine hydroperiodide, and tablets containing the substance are widely available for hikers and campers. Elemental iodine also has excellent antiseptic properties but it is rather toxic. Fatalities have been reported in those ingesting less than 2 grams of the element. Hikers and campers should stay away from using elemental iodine for water purification.

Povidone iodine, an organic form of iodine sold as Betadine, is an excellent topical antiseptic agent. Some, however, are allergic to this substance.

Related to Negative Claims:

1) Toxic—High doses of iodine may aggravate or precipitate acne. Rarely does the amount of iodine consumed in the diet or from the typical vitamin/mineral supplement affect acne, but it may in certain very sensitive individuals.

Iodine is essential for the synthesis of the thyroid hormones, and its deficiency leads to hypothyroidism. However, a large dose of iodide can lead to a temporary block of hormone synthesis and produce temporary hypothyroidism. The gland quickly adapts to this situation. However, consumption of large doses of iodide over an extended period of time occasionally, but not commonly, produces hypothyroidism. By high dose I refer to pharmacologic and not nutritional doses, that is, several milligrams daily.

Hyperthyroidism may also be induced by the administration of high doses of iodide. This is quite rare but has been reported.

Although iodide-induced thyroid disorders do occur, as discussed above, they are rare. In Japan there are a number of people who consume up to 20 milligrams of iodine, mainly from high seaweed diets, who have very low incidences of goiter, hypothyroidism, or hyperthyroidism.

Perhaps the most common adverse side effect from the consumption of high doses (greater than 50 milligrams daily) of iodide is a condition known as iodide mumps or sialadenitis. This refers to inflammation of the salivary glands, especially the parotid and submaxillary glands, and is easily reversed after stopping iodide.

There are those who are allergic to certain iodine dyes used in some X-ray procedures. These substances are different from the nutritional forms of iodide.

IV. RECOMMENDATIONS

A) *Suggested Intake:* The RDA of 150 micrograms of iodide daily appears to be adequate. Foods rich in iodine include seaweeds such as kelp, fish, shrimp, lobster, clams, oysters, some other animals (thyroid gland) and iodized salt. Those restricting their salt intake and at the same time not eating any of the above foods are vulnerable to iodine deficiency.

Cruciferous foods such as cabbage, brussels sprouts, broccoli, cauliflower, rutabaga and others may confer protection against certain types of cancer and so it is good to include them in our diets. However, these vegetables contain goitrogens, substances which may cause goiters and hypothyroidism. They do so by antagonizing iodine. A well-known newspaper columnist recently cautioned that those who have a tendency toward hypothyroidism or who have the disorder should stay away from these vegetables. Not good advice. It is easy to treat hypothyroidism, and the goitrogenic effects of these excellent foods can be neutralized by increasing iodine intake. It is not easy to treat cancer.

B) *Source/Form:* Naturally occurring iodine exists as iodide or iodate salts or as the thyroid hormones. Seafoods, which include sea animals and sea vegetables (seaweed), are the best natural source of iodine. Iodized salt is, of course, also a good source of iodine. However, many have to restrict their salt intake. Potassium iodide is available as a nutritional supplement, either by itself or in combination with other vitamins and minerals. Those who restrict their salt intake, those who eat large amounts of cruciferous vegetables, and those who do not eat seafoods should seriously consider taking supplementary potassium iodide at 150 micrograms daily (of iodide).

IRON

I. OVERVIEW: Biologic Gold

Iron has journeyed together with copper and oxygen for a very long time. It is thought that some of the earliest proteins formed on this planet some three billion years ago contained iron and that soon afterward copper-containing proteins evolved. Iron and copper appear to have participated very closely together in the evolution of aerobic life.

There is a remarkable parallel in the history of human civilization. Iron and copper are the backbone of civilized life. One of the greatest achievements in human history was the ability to work copper by heating it with fire and to create from this marriage the very tools, vessels, utensils and ornaments that have themselves catalyzed the cultural evolution of man. This period became known as the Bronze Age and was succeeded by the Iron Age, when man learned how to work iron to produce steel.

The alchemists were concerned with another metal, gold. These medieval philosophers-scientists-magicians sought to change base metals into gold. They saw in this a way of converting the corruptible to the incorruptible, a means of extracting the permanent, the eternal, from mutable, everyday life. But, in fact, gold is worthless compared with iron, for nature, the greatest alchemist of them all, has transformed iron into life.

Respiration is the process of burning foodstuffs (carbohydrates, fats, proteins) to produce biologic energy without which life could not be sustained. Iron is involved in the entire process of respiration. It is the backbone of the energy-producing process. Hemoglobin is the protein that carries most of the oxygen in the red blood cells; its function and synthesis depend profoundly on iron. The basic reaction that produces energy in the metabolic furnaces of the cells—the mitochondria—is the combination of oxygen with hydrogen to form water. This reaction occurs by means of a flow of electrons, derived from the oxidation of foodstuffs, across electron-carrier proteins called cytochromes and via the final combination of these electrons with oxygen, catalyzed by an enzyme called cytochrome oxidase, to produce water. The cytochromes and cytochrome oxidase do not work without iron, which, in turn, depends in some particulars upon a collaboration with copper.

Apart from its fundamental role in biologic energy production, iron is involved in the production of carnitine (see analysis of carnitine later in this book), a small molecule that is necessary for the oxidation of fatty acids. Iron plays roles in the production of collagen and elastin, two major components necessary for the integrity of connective tissue, in the maintenance of the immune system, in the production and regulation of several brain neurotransmitters and in the protection against oxidant damage.

That iron is a trace mineral essential for human health is firmly established. The condition most commonly associated with iron deficiency—iron-deficiency anemia—was described by Egyptian physicians at the very beginning of the Iron Age, 1500 B.C. Of course they did not know that they were diagnosing an iron-deficiency anemia, but the symptoms they described, such as pallor and difficulty in breathing, were almost certainly due to this disorder. Iron was identified as having an important role in human health in the middle of the seventeenth century when Thomas Sydenham recommended iron supplementation as a specific remedy for chlorosis, or green sickness (iron-deficiency anemia). Iron deficiency is frequently seen in infants, adolescents and pregnant women. Iron supplementation is particularly recommended for these groups. It should be noted that iron deficiency can also occur *without* anemia, producing such symptoms as fatigue, behavioral problems (decreased alertness and attention span), muscle weakness and increased susceptibility to infections. Iron-deficiency anemia remains the most prevalent nutritional disease in the world, affecting at least one billion people.

As with copper, iron has a dark side. Biologically, it exists in two states: ferrous and ferric. Free iron (not bound to protein structure) in the ferrous state is a powerful generator of destructive oxygen radicals. Free iron is terribly toxic to living cells. There are rare pathologic conditions characterized by an excessive amount of free iron in the body. Hemochromatosis is a genetic disorder wherein there are excess deposits of iron in the liver, heart, pancreas, skin and other organs, all of which are subject to serious damage from the toxic oxygen radicals generated by free iron. Fortunately, iron is usually bound very tightly to biologic structures; thus most of us are exposed to very little free iron.

Iron is enormously important in human health.

II. CLAIMS

Positive:

1) Prevents and cures iron-deficiency anemia; 2) anti-carcinogenic; 3) stimulates immunity; 4) boosts physical performance; 5) prevents learning disorders in children.

Negative:

1) Promotes oxidation; 2) depresses immunity; 3) toxic after prolonged use; 4) destroys vitamin E.

III. EVIDENCE

Related to Positive Claims:

1) Prevents and cures iron-deficiency anemia—Clearly, iron is necessary to prevent iron-deficiency anemia; it is *the* treatment for that disorder.

It should be understood that anemia is not a disease. It is a sign of the presence of disease process. Anemia (literally, without blood) refers to a significant decrease in the number of red blood cells. The adult body normally has about twenty-five trillion red blood cells (more in men than in women). Hemoglobin, the protein pigment that gives blood its color (red if oxygenated, blue if not) comprises about 30 percent of the red blood cell. This protein is responsible for carrying oxygen in the blood to the tissue. When the red-blood-cell count falls, so does the hemoglobin content and the oxygen-carrying capacity of the blood. Decreased oxygenation of tissues leads to decreased energy production with all its attendant symptoms of fatigue, muscle weakness and the like. Significant anemia occurs when the red-blood-cell count falls below about fifteen trillion (in adults).

Anemia occurs in three situations: decreased production of red blood cells, abnormal red-blood-cell destruction, or bleeding. Abnormalities in the production of red blood cells occur either because of a defect in the synthesis of the major protein of the cell, hemoglobin, or because of a defect in the synthesis of DNA. A defect in the synthesis of hemoglobin produces a small, pale-appearing cell. This is the case with iron deficiency. When DNA synthesis is interfered with, the cell is usually very large and not pale in appearance. This is what occurs with pernicious anemia, which is thought to be an autoimmune disorder affecting the stomach and producing a vitamin B_{12} deficiency. The treatment of *pernicious* anemia is with B_{12}.

2) Anti-carcinogenic—Iron deficiency has been associated with the Plummer-Vinson syndrome. In this condition, there is difficulty swallowing solid food because of a thin, web-like membrane that grows across the upper passageway of the esophagus (gullet). People with this problem are at increased risk of cancer of the esophagus and stomach. This syndrome has been fairly common in Sweden, but iron supplementation has now practically eliminated it.

In experimental research, iron deficiency has been found to accelerate chemical tumor induction in rats, though the significance, if any, of this for humans remains to be demonstrated.

Evidence of an anti-cancer role for iron remains meager. Long-term iron deficiency appears to increase the risk of cancer of the esophagus and stomach in patients with Plummer-Vinson syndrome. On the flip side of the coin, there is no evidence that long-term oral use of iron is associated with a decreased incidence of cancer.

3) Stimulates immunity—Resistance to infection depends mainly on the function of the white blood cells, particularly the lymphocytes and the neutrophils. Candida, a pathogenic yeast infection of the skin and mucous membranes, and herpes simplex infections are more common in patients who are iron deficient. Immune responses to skin tests, total lymphocyte numbers and some other indicators of healthy immunity have been shown to decrease in patients with iron deficiency.

There is little, if any, effect of iron deficiency on the production of immunoglobulins (B-lymphocyte function). That iron deficiency affects the T-lymphocyte arm of the immune system may have something to do with an enzyme called ribonucleotide reductase. This iron-requiring enzyme is essential for the synthesis of DNA. Decreased activity of this enzyme, due to iron deficiency, could lead to diminished T-cell production and thus impair cell-mediated immune response.

Iron deficiency is also known to impair intracellular killing of bacteria. Certain white blood cells (neutrophils) have iron-requiring proteins that, by generating toxic oxygen radicals, kill bacteria. This is one of the beneficial roles of oxygen radicals. These proteins are lactoferrin and cytochrome b. Another enzyme that requires iron is myeloperoxidase; it kills bacteria by generating iodine. Lactoferrin is also present in human milk and is thought to confer resistance to infection in nursing infants. Iron deficiencies can interfere with all of these important enzymes.

In summary, it appears that iron plays an important role in cellular immunity and in protection against some infections. Too much iron, on the other hand, may increase susceptibility to certain rare infections.

4) Boosts physical performance—Muscle weakness and decreased exercise tolerance, two rather non-specific symptoms, are frequently associated with iron-deficiency anemia. Remarkably, the degree of disability to perform muscular work is often much greater than would be expected from the degree of anemia present. In fact, these symptoms can occur when there is iron deficiency but no anemia and can be resolved when the iron deficiency is corrected.

From my own clinical experience, I have observed that not only does skeletal-muscle weakness appear out of proportion to the degree of anemia, but cardiac-muscle performance does as well, suggesting that iron deficiency has other effects that are in addition to and perhaps independent of the anemia. Frequently, patients with preexisting coronary heart disease develop symptoms of heart failure (shortness of breath, edema) when they develop an iron deficiency (usually from internal bleeding or frequent blood drawing) that is similarly out of proportion with the degree of their anemia.

Iron plays several roles in biologic energy production: the transfer of oxygen to tissues by hemoglobin and myoglobin; the transfer of electrons, by means of the cytochromes and cytochrome oxidase in the metabolic furnaces of the cells, to oxygen; the activation of enzymes that oxidize foodstuffs to produce energy; the transport of fatty acids into the metabolic furnaces via involvement with carnitine (fatty acids are the major source of energy in muscle, and carnitine, discussed later in this book, requires iron for its synthesis).

The decrease in oxygen transport to muscle seen in iron-deficiency anemia results in decreased muscular activity since oxygen is necessary for energy production. But it has been demonstrated that iron-deficient animals still often exhibit muscle weakness even when there is no apparent anemia.

It can be concluded that muscular performance (skeletal and car-diac) depends upon adequate availability of iron. Even iron deficien-cies that do not produce anemia can affect this performance. Iron deficiency without anemia is not uncommon among distance runners (in women more often than men). This is frequently the cause of fatigue among these athletes. More research is needed and justified to help fully clarify the role of iron—and perhaps carnitine—in muscular performance.

5) Prevents learning disorders in children—Iron-deficiency anemia has been implicated in emotional, social and learning difficulties in infants, adolescents and adults. Iron-deficient infants are often irritable and lack interest in their surroundings. Researchers have reported abnormal reactivity in infants with iron-deficiency anemia and demon-strated improvement after treatment with iron supplements. Other in-vestigators have clearly showed differences in behavior between iron-deficient and iron-sufficient infants. The anemic infants were less responsive, more tense, less active and more fearful than the non-anemic infants. However, one week of oral-iron treatment used in a study of these iron-deficient infants proved insufficient to change this behavior. Others also report behavioral differences between iron-sufficient and iron-deficient infants. In one study, two weeks of oral-iron therapy succeeded in removing these differences. This study was particularly interesting because the same behavioral abnormalities were found in infants with iron-deficiency anemia and in infants with iron deficiency but no anemia, indicating that the abnormalities are not simply a matter of decreased oxygen to the brain.

There is mounting evidence that iron deficiency affects infant be-havior. And since iron deficiency is a significant problem in infants, particularly disadvantaged infants, it is imperative that the nature of the relation between iron deficiency and behavioral problems of infants be studied and corrected. Some of the behavioral alterations observed in iron deficiency may be related to the synthesis or action of such brain molecules as serotonin, dopamine and noradrenalin, all of which are thought to play crucial roles in behavior.

Related to Negative Claims:

1) Promotes oxidation—It has been argued that iron can generate free radicals that can cause genetic mutations, atherosclerotic plaques and

cancer. Some hypothesize that iron in the membranes of the joints of patients with rheumatoid arthritis contributes to this disease by its generation of free radicals and subsequent lipid peroxidation. Others postulate that the greater incidence of coronary heart disease in men, compared to women, in affluent societies is due to higher levels of stored iron in men.

That iron can generate free radicals is well known. *Unbound* iron in the ferrous (or "plus two") state is a potent generator of hydroxyl radicals, which can be very destructive to cells. However, unbound iron occurs only under certain conditions. Patients with hemochromatosis, a genetic disorder of excessive iron accumulation, can have a significant quantity of unbound iron in their cells, and this may give rise to extensive damage to liver, heart, pancreas and skin. These genetic disorders, however, are rare. And there is no convincing evidence at present that iron is active in either rheumatoid arthritis or atherosclerotic disease. Most iron we come in contact with is tightly bound to protein and does not generate dangerous free radicals.

2) Depresses immunity—Though iron deficiency is usually associated with decreased resistance to infection, there are a few reports contending just the opposite, that iron deficiency decreases *susceptibility* to infection. However, except under rare circumstances, there is little reason to expect iron to depress immunity. People on long-term iron supplementation are *not* noted for problems with infection. Some pathogens, especially bacteria, require iron for growth. Thus some have thought that iron-deficient individuals would actually be *less* susceptible, but this has never been demonstrated.

3) Toxic after prolonged use—Prolonged administration of iron supplements very rarely causes iron overload. It is possible that in those situations where iron overload does occur, the individual has the predisposition for excessive iron absorption called hemochromatosis. Iron supplements are widely used in the United States, and reports of toxicity from iron overload are very rare.

4) Destroys vitamin E—We've known about an iron/vitamin E connection for some time. Ferric chloride, a form of iron, converts vitamin E to an inactive substance. Ferric chloride has also been shown to make rats infertile, apparently by inactivating vitamin E; fertility was restored

by the addition of more vitamin E to the diet. A number of additional reports also document an antagonism between *inorganic* iron and vitamin E.

IV. RECOMMENDATIONS

A) *Suggested Intake*: Iron requirements and Recommended Dietary Allowances are shown in Table 2. The average American diet contains 6 milligrams of iron per 1,000 kilocalories. Groups at risk for iron

TABLE 2   IRON REQUIREMENTS AND RECOMMENDED DIETARY ALLOWANCES

Age (Years)	Iron Requirement[a] (Milligrams/Day)	RDA[b] (Milligrams/Day)
Infants and Children		
0–6 mos.	0.5–1.5	6
6 mos.–1	0.5–1.5	10
1–3	0.4–1	10
4–6	0.4–1	10
7–10	0.4– 1	10
Males		
11–18	1–2	12
19–50	0.65–1.3	10
51+	0.65–1.3	10
Females		
11–18	1–2. 7	15
19–50	0.7–2.3	15
51+	0.6–0.9	10
Pregnant	1.65–3.5	30
Lactating		15

[a] Iron requirements refer to amount of absorbed iron needed. Estimates taken from Beutler, *Modern Nutrition in Health and Disease*, eds. Goodhart and Shils, Lea and Febiger, Philadelphia, 1980.
[b] Recommended Dietary Allowance (RDA), National Research Council, *Recommended Dietary Allowances*, 1989.
    The values refer to daily food intake. The assumption is made that 10 percent of the iron gets absorbed. Since it is unlikely that a pregnant woman can get 30 milligrams of dietary iron daily, supplemental iron is recommended.

deficiency include infants, adolescents, premenopausal women (especially those on low-calorie diets), pregnant and lactating women, vegetarians, endurance athletes (especially women) and the elderly with poor dietary habits over long periods of time. Iron supplementation is commonly recommended by pediatricians for infants and children at a dose of 10 to 12 milligrams daily (elemental iron). Pregnant and lactating women usually are prescribed 30 to 60 milligrams of iron daily. It is wise for adults on low-calorie diets to take 10 to 15 milligrams of supplemental iron daily. Adult men who eat well-balanced diets of 2,000 calories or more do not need iron supplements. Elderly persons who feel weak and tired most of the time should see their doctors before starting on iron, since they may be anemic from internal bleeding. Iron itself will do nothing to combat bleeding. In general, I see no reason for adults to consume more than 15 milligrams of iron daily (except during pregnancy or in the event of iron-deficiency anemia, which should be treated by a physician).

B) *Source/Form:* The best dietary sources of iron are meat (especially organ meats, such as liver), poultry, fish and ground-up soybean hulls. Foods with low iron availability include eggs, spinach and many green vegetables. The most bioavailable form of iron, that is, the type that can be most easily absorbed by the body, is heme iron found in red meats. Red meats, moreover, have a factor that increases the availability of nonheme iron.

There are several iron supplements on the market; these include ferrous sulfate, ferrous fumarate and ferrous gluconate. They all have similar bioavailability. Carbonyl iron is now on the market. It is *more* bioavailable and has fewer side effects than the other forms but requires adequate stomach acid for absorption. Thus it is best taken with food (which stimulates acid secretion). It should not be taken with antacids. Ferrous sulfate is the cheapest. Time-release or enteric-coated products are *not* reliably absorbed; moreover, they usually cost more. Absorption is best if taken between meals—unless you are taking the carbonyl form, as noted above. Calcium decreases iron availability, while vitamin C increases it.

C) *Take With:* (See Part Three for recommendations.)

D) *Cautionary Note:* Iron supplements may cause abdominal pain, diarrhea or constipation and they may color the stool a very dark brown to black. If such symptoms arise and persist, cut back on the amount of supplementation, and in any event, do not exceed the amounts recommended above. Do not take iron supplements at all if you have been diagnosed as having idiopathic hemochromatosis (a tendency toward excessive absorption of iron). Persons with anemia should use supplemental iron according to the prescriptions of their physicians. A complete blood count, including hemoglobin and hematocrit determination, will tell you if you are anemic. To determine if you are iron deficient, the tests used are: serum iron (low in iron deficiency), serum transferrin (normal or elevated in iron deficiency) and serum ferritin (low in iron deficiency).

MAGNESIUM

I. OVERVIEW: One for the Heart

The primordial oceans on this plant were rich in magnesium and potassium. Sodium rules the seas today, but the waters within our cells remain true to the "primordial soup" from which all life arose, rich in magnesium and potassium. Optimal health depends upon the maintenance of this condition. Magnesium is not a trace mineral but a major entity in our bodies. Most of it is in our bones and in the waters within the cells. Magnesium is absolutely essential for life. It is necessary for every major biologic process, including the metabolism of glucose, production of cellular energy, and the synthesis of nucleic acids and protein.

It is also important for the electrical stability of cells, the maintenance of membrane integrity, muscle contraction, nerve conduction and the regulation of vascular tone. It is intimately interlocked, biologically, with calcium. In some reactions, such as the synthesis of nucleic acids and protein, calcium and magnesium are antagonistic. Magnesium is necessary for these processes, while calcium inhibits them. Magnesium and calcium collaborate, however, in the production of the crystal of biologic energy, adenosine triphosphate. Magnesium appears to regulate the gate through which calcium enters into cells to switch on such vital functions as the heartbeat.

Magnesium deficiency is characterized by loss of appetite, nausea, vomiting, diarrhea, confusion, tremors, loss of coordination and, occasionally, fatal convulsions. Magnesium deficiency is sometimes associated with concurrent deficiencies of calcium and potassium.

It is becoming increasingly evident that marginal magnesium deficiency is very common. Particularly vulnerable groups include the elderly, those on low-calorie diets, diabetics, those taking diuretics and digitalis preparations, consumers of alcohol, pregnant women, and people who exercise regularly and strenuously. The adequacy of our dietary magnesium has been questioned. It is now recognized that even marginal magnesium deficiency can predispose one to life-threatening cardiac dysrhythmias (disruption of normal heart rhythm). Although it has not been proved, magnesium supplementation may protect against the plague of Western civilization—ischemic heart disease (oxygen starvation of heart muscle caused by spasms or narrowing and clogging of the arteries leading to the heart).

Magnesium supplementation appears poised to play a key role in preventive medicine.

II. CLAIMS

Positive:
1) Protective against cardiovascular disease and helpful in the treatment of high blood pressure; 2) beneficial in the treatment of the premenstrual syndrome; 3) helps prevent kidney stones and gallstones; 4) useful in the treatment of prostate problems; 5) useful in the treatment of polio and the postpolio syndrome; 6) aids in fighting depression; 7) effective in the treatment of convulsions in pregnant women and prevents premature labor; 8) beneficial in the treatment of neuromuscular and nervous disorders; 9) effective in the treatment of diarrhea, vomiting and indigestion.

Negative:
1) Toxic.

III. EVIDENCE

Related to Positive Claims:
1) Protective against cardiovascular disease and helpful in the treatment of high blood pressure—Epidemiologic studies suggest that the death rate from ischemic heart disease is increased in areas with soft, as opposed to hard, water. Hard water contains both magnesium and calcium. However, it is the view of some researchers that magnesium

is the more important factor in the protection against ischemic heart disease. They have presented evidence that Western diet is deficient in magnesium and propose that this may underlie the very high incidence of cardiovascular disease in Western nations, especially among men. Findings have conflicted to some extent, but the foregoing hypothesis certainly warrants further investigation, particularly in view of recent findings that magnesium does indeed play an extremely important role in the maintenance of the electrical and physical integrity of heart muscle.

One of the causes of ischemic heart disease, wherein the coronary arteries fail to provide all of the oxygen that the heart demands, is spasm in the smooth muscles of the artery walls. It seems reasonable to postulate that inadequate magnesium may make the coronary arteries more susceptible to muscle spasm. Too little magnesium may mean too much calcium, and the toxic effects of calcium ions could potentiate spasm. The same applies to the muscular activity of the heart itself. Calcium is crucial for this activity, but if too much ionic calcium enters the heart cells (because the "gatekeeper," magnesium, is in short supply) then the effect can be disruptive, introducing toxic, killing forms of oxygen. This may be at the very root of heart-tissue death and thus of myocardial infarction (heart attack). A magnesium-calcium imbalance may not only predispose to cardiovascular disease but may also make repair very difficult. Once calcium has the upper hand its natural antagonism to magnesium makes it all the more difficult for the latter to promote the nucleic acid and protein syntheses that are at the literal heart, in this case, of the mending process.

More research will have to be done before it can legitimately be claimed that magnesium supplementation is of benefit in ischemic heart disease. But we do know that magnesium deficiency predisposes humans to potentially fatal disruptions of normal cardiac rhythm (cardiac dysrhythmia). Investigators have successfully treated ventricular dysrhythmias with magnesium. These disorders had not been improved by conventional drug therapy. Remarkably, the levels of magnesium in the blood of these patients were normal. That *cellular* magnesium deficiency can exist in the context of normal blood magnesium levels, however, has been demonstrated by researchers who report successful treatment (with magnesium) of cardiac-dysrhythmia patients taking diuretics and digitalis. Cellular (lymphocyte) levels of magnesium were depleted in these patients even though their blood levels were normal. The cellular measure is a far more accurate gauge and should be employed more often, especially when dealing with patients on diuretics and digitalis, both of which are known to diminish magnesium levels.

The most recent studies have shown that those with acute heart attacks have a much higher survival rate or fewer life-threatening dysrhythmias if given magnesium right after the attack.

Patients with essential hypertension have better control of their blood pressure when given magnesium supplementation. These patients were also taking diuretics. Follow-up studies have yielded conflicting results on the blood pressure issue. More research is needed.

2) Beneficial in the treatment of the premenstrual syndrome—This syndrome refers to cyclic symptoms experienced by women during their reproductive years; these symptoms may include anxiety, irritability, mood swings, breast tenderness, fatigue, dizziness, headache, etc. Some believe that magnesium, zinc and some vitamin deficiencies play a central role in this syndrome, reasoning that refined sugars and high dairy-product intake decrease magnesium absorption and that the resulting deficiency leads to a decreased synthesis of the brain neurotransmitter dopamine, which, in turn, causes an imbalance in other brain chemicals. This and other disruptions are thought to cause the symptoms of premenstrual syndrome. It has been reported in one trial that vitamin and mineral supplementation, including magnesium, provided some measurable relief for some women with this syndrome. The trial was not placebo-controlled.

There are insufficient data at present to substantiate or refute this claim. More research will have to be done.

3) Helps prevent kidney stones and gallstones—A few studies report the beneficial effect of magnesium supplementation in the prevention of recurrent calcium-oxalate stones. One study used 200 milligrams daily of magnesium oxide plus 10 milligrams daily of vitamin B_6. In a second study, magnesium was used alone—in the amount of 300 milligrams of magnesium oxide daily. Magnesium hydroxide was used in a more recent study. The current evidence suggests that magnesium supplementation is effective in preventing calcium oxalate stones in people who have this recurrent problem. (It is presently estimated that about one million Americans now living will die from causes related to

kidney stones, the causes of which remain obscure.) Gallstones, in contrast to kidney stones, only rarely contain calcium; there is no evidence that magnesium either prevents or is useful in the treatment of gallstones.

4) Useful in the treatment of prostate problems—There is no evidence to support this claim.

5) Useful in the treatment of polio and the postpolio syndrome—There is no evidence to support this claim.

6) Aids in fighting depression—Depression is one of the most complex human phenomena. It is characterized by sleep disturbances, loss of interest in the world, guilty feelings, loss of energy, inability to concentrate, decreased appetite for food (and often for all of life), diminished psychomotor activity and occasionally by suicidal thoughts. Depression is not uncommon, especially in the elderly, and is one of the most difficult challenges faced by the physician. We still know very little about the bases of depression. There is no evidence as yet that magnesium can play any useful role in the treatment of depression. Almost no research has been done in this context, but we do know that magnesium is involved in the synthesis of some of the brain neurotransmitters. We also know that marginal magnesium deficiency increases with age. The preliminary data on magnesium in the treatment of premenstrual syndrome (see discussion above) at least suggest that supplementary magnesium might have some favorable effect on some of the neurotransmitters. Here is an area that that needs more research.

7) Effective in the treatment of convulsions in pregnant women and prevents premature labor—A very threatening syndrome that occasionally occurs during pregnancy is called preeclampsia/eclampsia. Preeclampsia is characterized by high blood pressure, swelling of the body (sometimes the entire body) and the finding of protein in the urine. Preeclampsia can develop into the far more serious eclampsia, in which convulsions, coma and even death can occur. Intravenous magnesium (magnesium sulfate) has been used successfully for many years in the treatment of this syndrome. The mechanism by which magnesium works in this case is unknown. It is possible, however, that women who develop this disorder have a marginal magnesium defi-

ciency. If there is not enough magnesium in the body to regulate the flow of calcium into the cells, an excess of calcium may cause constriction of the smooth muscles in blood vessels and in the uterus, accounting for at least part of the syndrome. A recent report showed intravenous magnesium sulfate to be beneficial in the inhibition of premature labor. Prematurity is the single greatest cause of disease and death in the newborn. Magnesium may, in this instance, be helping to maintain the muscle of the uterus in a relaxed condition until the fetus is clearly called for.

8) Beneficial in the treatment of neuromuscular and nervous disorders—It is true that in clear-cut cases of magnesium deficiency, muscle weakness, tremors and various movement disorders may arise that can be resolved with supplemental magnesium. There is no evidence, however, that magnesium supplements can be of benefit in these disorders in individuals not suffering from severe magnesium deficiency. On the other hand, respiratory muscle weakness—something the elderly are at particular risk for—can be aggravated by magnesium deficiency.

9) Effective in the treatment of diarrhea, vomiting and indigestion— Loss of appetite, nausea, vomiting and diarrhea are, in fact, among the early symptoms of magnesium deficiency. However, these symptoms are so general that they could be—and usually are—related to a multitude of other factors. Most of the magnesium products on the market do not have an anti-diarrhea effect but actually *cause* diarrhea. Such products as Phillips' Milk of Magnesia and Haley's M-O, both of which contain magnesium hydroxide, are sold as laxatives in the treatment of constipation. Some of the magnesium-containing antacids on the market, though they help with indigestion, also can cause diarrhea.

Related to Negative Claims:
1) Toxic—There are two situations in which increasing magnesium intake is not desirable. Magnesium should not be administered to patients with severely decreased renal (kidney) function and in those with high-grade atrioventricular blocks or bifascicular blocks. Magnesium, in these instances, could slow down the heart rate and lead to depression of neuromuscular function and even to respiratory depres-

sion. Paradoxically, many of the cardiac patients with these blocks may be suffering from marginal magnesium deficiency, in part because they often use diuretics and the heart drug digitalis. If such patients are fitted with artificial pacemakers, magnesium supplementation will not present the same risks—but all such patients should consult with their physicians before taking any magnesium supplements. They should also be careful about using over-the-counter magnesium-containing antacids and laxatives.

Except in the conditions described above, there is no evidence that magnesium supplements are harmful to people. Diarrhea may be avoided by taking magnesium in the form of magnesium gluconate.

IV. RECOMMENDATIONS

A) *Suggested Intake:* The National Research Council recommends a daily allowance of 350 milligrams of magnesium for men and 280 milligrams for women. Additional allowances of 40 and 60 to 75 milligrams daily are recommended for pregnant and lactating (nursing) women, respectively. The magnesium content of the average American diet is estimated at 120 milligrams per 1,000 kilocalories. Dietary intake of magnesium may be inadequate in large segments of the population. It is prudent to take supplementary magnesium. I recommend a supplementary intake of 200 to 400 milligrams daily. Those who may, in particular, benefit from such supplementation include the elderly, those on low-calorie diets, diabetics, people taking diuretics and digitalis preparations (though the latter should consult their physicians before taking any supplements), consumers of alcohol, pregnant women, and those who indulge in regular and strenuous exercise.

B) *Source/Form:* Foods rich in magnesium include meats, seafoods, green vegetables and dairy products. Supplementary forms include magnesium oxide, magnesium carbonate, magnesium hydroxide, magnesium gluconate, magnesium aspartate and magnesium orotate. Magnesium oxide and magnesium hydroxide often cause diarrhea, unless taken in a multimineral vitamin combination that includes calcium carbonate (or various other calcium forms often used in these preparations). The calcium carbonate (which, by itself, is constipating) may counteract the diarrhea. Magnesium carbonate is not recommended because it is not easily absorbed. Magnesium gluconate is less likely to cause diarrhea. The oxide and hydroxide forms should be taken with meals to stimulate acid secretion sufficient to ensure adequate absorption. The gluconate, aspartate and orotate forms need not be taken with meals.

C) *Take With:* Best if incorporated into a well-balanced vitamin/mineral preparation. (See Part Three for more specific recommendations.)

D) *Cautionary Note:* People with renal failure and high-grade atrioventricular blocks should not take supplementary magnesium. (See Evidence section, Related to Negative Claims, for details.) Patients with high-grade heart blocks may take supplementary magnesium if they have artificial pacemakers, though they should first consult with their physicians and follow their instructions. Note that the conventional test for magnesium deficiency—a measure of blood levels of this mineral—*does not* necessarily reflect actual body stores of magnesium. The best test—not commonly available—analyzes magnesium levels in *lymphocytes* (white blood cells).

MANGANESE

I. OVERVIEW: An Elemental Enigma

Oxygen was absent from the atmosphere when the earth was newly born about four and a half billion years ago and did not appear until about two and a half billion years later. At that time the blue-green "algae" (a type of bacteria) came into being and were able to split water into oxygen by using the energy of the sun. It was manganese that made this possible. Today, one of manganese's principal roles is that of antioxidant and, as such, may help protect humans from toxic oxygen forms.

Manganese, for the most part, however, remains an enigma with respect to its possible roles in human biology. Manganese-deficiency states are known in animals (these include defective growth and neurologic disorders) but have not been documented in man. There is one report of what may be such a deficiency in man. In this instance, manganese deficiency developed in a patient who was maintained for four months on a manganese-deficient diet and who simultaneously was given manganese-containing antacids. The signs and symptoms included: decrease in serum cholesterol, impaired blood clotting, reddening of his black hair and beard, slowed growth of hair and nails, and scaly dermatitis. It is suggested that in humans this element functions in both glycoprotein synthesis (some of the clotting factors are protein with carbohydrates attached to them) and cholesterol synthesis.

A fascinating pathologic state in humans is manganese intoxication, an understanding of which may eventually yield important clues regarding the role of manganese in the human body. Dietary manganese has low toxicity, but mine workers exposed to high concentrations of manganese dust develop what is known in the mining villages of northern Chile, where this disorder is most common, as "locura manganica," or manganese madness. The early stage of this disorder is marked by unaccountable laughter, heightened sexuality, impulsiveness, inability to fall asleep, delusions and hallucinations. This manic state is followed by a state of deep depression, which is distinguished by slow speech, impotence and inability to stay awake. In the final stage of the disease process, symptoms similar to those of Parkinson's disease are observed. Parkinson's is a degenerative disease of the brain resulting from the loss of dopamine-containing cells. The treatment is a drug called L-dopa, which the brain can convert to dopamine. L-dopa is also the treatment of the chronic stage of manganese poisoning.

Although to this date we do not know the unique functions of manganese in human biology, what we do know suggests that it is essential. It is conceivable that this element is so important that nature has invented ways to ensure that manganese-deficiency states do not occur or almost never occur. Such mechanisms may include the ability of magnesium to substitute for manganese in many biochemical reactions, thus sparing manganese when its stores are low. With regard to the aging process, manganese's probable role as an antioxidant is interesting. In this regard, it is noteworthy that all tumors examined to date have diminished amounts of the manganese-containing superoxide-dismutase enzyme. This provides a hint, but certainly not proof, that manganese deficiency may play a role in degenerative processes in humans. Manganese has a fascinating past; I suspect it has a promising future.

II. CLAIMS

Positive:

1) Important for the normal functioning of the brain and effective in the treatment of schizophrenia and some nervous disorders; 2) necessary for reproduction; 3) needed for normal bone structure and helpful in the treatment of osteoarthritis; 4) necessary for normal glucose metabolism and beneficial in the treatment of diabetes mellitus; 5) miscellaneous.

Negative:

1) Toxic.

III. EVIDENCE

Related to Positive Claims:

1) Important for the normal functioning of the brain and effective in the treatment of schizophrenia and some nervous disorders—Manganese appears to be involved in the synthesis of the neurotransmitter dopamine in the brain, although more research will have to be done before this role is convincingly established. There are anecdotal reports of the effectiveness of manganese in the treatment of schizophrenia. One researcher has been arguing for years that copper contributes to certain types of schizophrenia. He believes that manganese, as well as zinc, decreases dietary copper absorption (see analysis of copper elsewhere in this book) and in so doing aids in the treatment of schizophrenia. There are no controlled studies to substantiate any of this. There is no proof that copper plays a role in any form of schizophrenia and no evidence that manganese lowers copper levels in humans, although zinc certainly can do this. (See discussions of zinc elsewhere in this book.) There are also reports that manganese can be useful in the treatment of tardive dyskinesia, a neurologic disorder caused by neuroleptic drugs (major tranquilizers). These reports are anecdotal.

2) Necessary for reproduction—Manganese-deficient animals sometimes exhibit reproductive difficulties; this may be due to the requirement for manganese in the synthesis of cholesterol, which is itself the precursor of the sex steroids. Manganese may have this function in humans, but this has not been demonstrated to date.

3) Needed for normal bone structure and helpful in the treatment of osteoarthritis—Skeletal abnormalities have been observed in manganese-deficient animals and have been linked to a reduction in the synthesis of mucopolysaccharides, which make up the matrix of the cartilage at the ends of bones (within which bone formation takes place). Manganese is involved in this synthesis in animals and may play a similar, though yet unestablished, role in humans.

One researcher proposed some years ago that manganese should be useful in the treatment of osteoarthritis, a degenerative joint disease characterized by a loss of joint cartilage and hypertrophy (overgrowth) of bone. He reasoned that if manganese were involved in mucopolysaccharide formation, then manganese may function to repair worn-out cartilage. More recently it has been reported that the blood level of manganese was significantly lower in a group of women with osteoporosis than in a similar group of women who do not have osteoporosis. Further investigation is definitely warranted.

4) Necessary for normal glucose metabolism and beneficial in the treatment of diabetes mellitus—Manganese deficiency in animals does lead to decreased glucose tolerance (the ability to metabolize this sugar); however, there is no evidence that this is true in humans, and there are no studies showing manganese to be useful in the treatment of any form of human diabetes.

5) Miscellaneous—There is no evidence whatever for claims that manganese is important for the formation of thyroid hormone, that it promotes maternal instincts, that it is useful in the treatment of multiple sclerosis and myasthenia gravis, or that it helps overcome dizziness and eliminate stress, fatigue, absentmindedness and irritability.

Related to Negative Claims:

1) Toxic—The toxicity of dietary manganese is low. Inhaled manganese dust can, as explained in the Overview, cause serious neurologic disease. A matter of concern is the recent practice of adding manganese as an anti-knock agent in automobile fuel (to replace lead). The use of these manganese compounds has not yet caused dangerous levels of manganese air pollution, but this could change. The situation should be carefully monitored and studied. "Manganese madness" is a very serious matter.

IV. RECOMMENDATIONS

A) *Suggested Intake:* Optimal manganese intake is unknown. The National Research Council lists the estimated safe and adequate daily dietary intake of manganese for adults at 2 to 5 milligrams. Up to 10 milligrams daily are considered safe. High dietary or supplemental intake of magnesium, calcium, iron or phosphate may decrease the absorption of manganese. So may antacids, laxatives that contain magnesium, fiber (e.g., bran), phytates in vegetables, tannins in tea and oxalic acid in spinach. Given the low toxicity of manganese and the potentially important role that it plays in human health, I believe it is prudent to incorporate 5 milligrams daily (adults) in one's supplement program. Doses higher than 10 milligrams daily are not recommended.

B) *Source/Form:* The best dietary sources of manganese include whole grains and nuts. Fruits and green vegetables contain moderate amounts, content depending upon the soil in which the crops were grown. The more alkaline the soil the less manganese there will be in the food. Manganese is concentrated in the bran of grains, which is removed during processing. Organ meats, shellfish and milk are additional good sources of this element. The most common supplementary forms of manganese are manganese sulfate and manganese gluconate. They both deliver about the same amount of manganese to the body; the sulfate is usually less expensive.

C) *Take With:* Best incorporated into a well-balanced vitamin/mineral "insurance" formula; see Part Three.

D) *Note:* There is no routine test presently available to assess individual manganese status. Promising tests, which may become available in the future, include whole-blood analysis and mitochondrial manganese superoxide-dismutase levels. Manganese can be assessed in the serum using atomic absorption spectrophotometry.

MOLYBDENUM

I. OVERVIEW: Detoxicant

Compounds of molybdenum are among the scarcer constituents of the earth's crust. This scarcity has been associated with one of the world's highest incidences of esophageal cancer—in an area of China. The discrepancy between its rarity in the earth and its abundance in living things has been used in support of a postulate that life on this planet was seeded by microorganisms sent by some form of intelligent life on another planet rich in this element.

Molybdenum is a trace mineral that is found in all tissues of the human body and is required for the activity of several enzymes. Only recently has a human deficiency state for molybdenum been described. A patient fed intravenously who became intolerant of the sulfur-containing amino acids and developed a fast heartbeat, increased rate of breathing, visual problems and who finally became comatose was found to have high blood sulfite levels. After molybdenum (as ammonium molybdate) was added to the intravenous feeding solution, the patient improved and the sulfite level returned to normal. At least from this isolated case it appears that the deleterious effects of molybdenum deficiency are due to the accumulation of sulfite, which is toxic to the nervous system. There have been no other reports of molybdenum deficiency.

Sulfiting agents are extensively used for the preservation of foods and drugs. These are not harmless substances and can cause nausea, diarrhea, acute asthma attacks, loss of consciousness and even death in certain individuals. Bisulfite, itself, can destroy vitamin B_1. Ideally, less toxic substances should be substituted. These substances are probably detoxified in the body by means of the molybdenum-activated enzyme sulfite oxidase. Thus, in this capacity, molybdenum is a detoxifier of potentially hazardous substances we all come in contact with almost daily.

Molybdenum may also play a useful antioxidant role. Uric acid has been shown to be a powerful antioxidant and a scavenger of singlet oxygen and hydroxyl radicals. Toxicity of oxygen radicals is thought to be a major factor in degenerative diseases and aging. Uric acid is produced by the molybdenum-activated enzyme xanthine oxidase. Most clinicians see uric acid as, at best, a useless and, at worst, a very destructive molecule in that it can cause gouty arthritis. Biologic phenomena, however, often have two sides, as is the case here. Conceivably, an optimal uric-acid level (maybe just short of the point where it begins to cause problems) is essential for optimal health and to slow down the wear and tear of aging. If this is true, then molybdenum does indeed enter the realm of useful antioxidants.

All signs point toward the essentiality of molybdenum for optimal health and life span.

II. CLAIMS

Positive:
1) Protective against cancer; 2) protects teeth; 3) prevents sexual impotence; 4) prevents anemia and mobilizes iron.

Negative:
1) Toxic.

III. EVIDENCE

Related to Positive Claims:
1) Protective against cancer—To me, one of the most fascinating programs in the *Nova* television series was "The Cancer Detectives of Lin Xian." Lin Xian is a small region (twenty miles square) in Honan Province in north China, which was documented to have the highest incidence of esophageal cancer in the world. As a result of outstanding scientific investigation, it was determined that the soil in this area was markedly deficient in molybdenum. In order for nitrates in the soil to be reduced to nitrogenous substances (amines) necessary for plant nutrition, a molybdenum-activated enzyme called nitrate reductase (found in nitrogen-fixing bacteria) is required. Molybdenum deficiency decreases the activity of this enzyme, and, instead of being converted to amines, the nitrates get transformed to nitrosamines, known cancer-causing substances. The people of Lin Xian were also deficient in vitamin C, which has been shown to convert nitrosamines to less toxic forms and thus protect us, to some extent, against them. Armed with this knowledge, the Chinese have now enriched the soil with molybdenum, and the inhabitants of Lin Xian are taking supplemental vitamin C. As a result, the incidence of esophageal cancer in the region may be declining for the first time in more than two thousand years. Low levels of molybdenum in the soil and a high incidence of esophageal cancer in the Bantu of the Transkei in South Africa have also been reported.

In experimental work, investigators report that molybdenum supplementation protected rats from chemical carcinogens.

There is no evidence that supplementary molybdenum intake in humans protects against cancer, but molybdenum enrichment of the soil (especially in areas deficient in molybdenum) may very well do so—by decreasing the amount of nitrosamines and their precursors that we consume.

2) Protects teeth—A California study found no difference in the prevalence of cavities among children with high and low intakes of molybdenum. A British study did find a difference—a 20 percent lower incidence of cavities among children with high molybdenum intake. The study was inconclusive, however, particularly in view of the fact that the children with the higher molybdenum intake were also found to have 34 percent more fluoride in their teeth. These skimpy results do not support a role for molybdenum in the prevention of dental cavities.

3) Prevents sexual impotence—This claim has been made, especially with respect to older males. It is purely anecdotal. No studies exist.

4) Prevents anemia and mobilizes iron—There is no evidence that molybdenum deficiency contributes to anemia in humans. Xanthine oxidase, an enzyme dependent upon molybdenum, may participate in the uptake and release of iron from ferritin (storage form of iron), but its role in this regard is not thought to be significant.

Related to Negative Claims:

1) Toxic—Molybdenum toxicity has been noted in some animals that consume feed high in this mineral. This is due to the antagonism of molybdenum to copper. Dietary intake of 10 to 15 milligrams of molybdenum daily has been associated with gout-like symptoms; the molybdenum-activated enzyme xanthine oxidase makes uric acid, high levels of which can produce gout. Daily intake of .54 milligrams has been associated with a significant loss of copper.

IV. RECOMMENDATIONS

A) *Suggested Intake:* The optimal intake of molybdenum is still uncertain. The National Research Council recommends as safe and adequate 0.075 to 0.25 milligrams daily for adults. Dietary intake varies considerably from person to person. This intake, in the American diet, has been estimated at between 0.076 and 0.24 milligrams. The daily adult intake should not exceed 0.5 milligrams, since an intake of 0.54

milligrams daily has been associated with a significant urinary loss of copper.

Since I believe molybdenum is essential for optimal health—and since I do recommend copper supplementation (see copper analysis)—I propose that a daily supplement of from 50 to 100 micrograms (not milligrams) of molybdenum may be useful for "insurance" purposes.

B) *Source/Form:* Molybdenum is found in organ meats (liver, kidney), grains, legumes, leafy vegetables, milk and beans. Sodium molybdate is available as a supplement, usually in combination with other vitamins and minerals. Sodium molybdate gives good bioavailability. Recently a molybdenum-enriched yeast has come on the market. I see no advantage to taking molybdenum in this form, which is considerably more expensive.

C) *Take With:* Best if incorporated into a well-balanced vitamin/ mineral formula. (See Part Three for further recommendations.) Specifically, I suggest taking 1.5 to 3 milligrams of copper daily with molybdenum because of the antagonism of the two.

D) *Cautionary Note:* People with high levels of uric acid and/or gout should consult their physicians before taking molybdenum supplement.

PHOSPHORUS

I. OVERVIEW: Vital for Energy

Phosphorus is a mineral which plays pivotal roles in the structure and function of the body. In the form of phosphate, it is essential for the process of bone mineralization and makes up the structure of bone. Phospholipids, such as phosphatidylcholine or lecithin, are major components of cell membranes. Cell membranes protect cellular integrity, define cellular structure, and mediate all the events that take place from within and without the cell. Integrity of tissue, storage and processing of biologic information, cellular communication, and energy production are the most vital biologic processes, and phosphorus is key to *all* of them.

Phosphorus, mainly in the form of phosphate, is widely distributed in our food supply, and phosphate intake from the normal diet is more than sufficient to meet the body's needs. Consequently, phosphate deficiency states are rare.

The daily intake of phosphorus in the American diet, which ranges between 800 and 1,500 milligrams, has been stable since the beginning of the century. Milk and its products are the richest sources of dietary phosphorus, but phosphorus is widely available in other foods, such as fish, meat, poultry, vegetables, eggs, etc. The major dietary form of phosphorus is inorganic phosphate, but phosphorus is also found in organic (bound to carbon) forms such as lecithin.

Phosphorus deficiency can and does occur. One can predict that the symptoms of such deficiency would affect all of the body's systems, since even mild phosphate deficiency leads to a decrease in the production of energy. Feeling easily fatigued, weak and having a decreased attention span could be symptoms of mild phosphate deficiency. Severe phosphate deficiency could produce seizures, coma, even death. Phosphate deficiency typically requires intensive medical management.

Those at risk for phosphate depletion include patients who are being treated for diabetic ketoacidosis, patients with urinary losses of phosphate due to malfunction of certain kidney structures, those with gastrointestinal malabsorption syndromes (e.g., Crohn's disease, celiac disease, short bowel syndrome and radiation damage of the small intestine) those who are starving and those with acute and chronic alcoholism, as well as alcoholics who are admitted to the hospital for treatment of acute alcoholism or alcohol withdrawal and given intravenous fluids which don't contain phosphate. Many antacids, which are widely used for treatment of peptic ulcer disease, gastritis ("heartburn") and acid reflux, contain magnesium and aluminum, both of which bind to phosphate, preventing its absorption into the body. Several cases have been reported which describe severe phosphate depletion in people who have used these antacids between two and twelve years. An alcoholic who uses such antacids would certainly increase his or her vulnerability to phosphate deficiency.

II. CLAIMS

Positive:
1) Increases endurance in athletes; 2) fights fatigue and is an overall good tonic.

Negative:
1) Toxic.

III. EVIDENCE

Related to Positive Claims:
1) Increases endurance in athletes—The claim is that phosphate supplementation in an athlete with normal phosphate intake can increase athletic endurance and give the athlete a competitive "edge." The argument goes that supplementary phosphate boosts endurance by increasing the synthesis of a substance that enhances production of cellular fuel in muscle. It would be nice if this were so, but it is highly unlikely that anyone with adequate dietary phosphate intake benefits from supplementary phosphate. In those cases where there *are* phosphate deficiencies, as in many alcoholics, supplemental phosphate *will* confer greater energy.

2) Fights fatigue and is an overall good tonic—Homeopathic remedies include many that are phosphate compounds. Kali phosphoricum or potassium phosphate (kali means potassium) is supposed to help with mental fatigue and nervous exhaustion; magnesia phosphorica or magnesium phosphate is reported to help relieve muscle cramps and pain; natrum phosphoricum or sodium phosphate is said to promote a healthier tongue; and a mixture of phosphates (called biochemic phosphates) is thought to be good for nervous conditions and mental fatigue. It is conceivable that some with phosphate deficiencies (alcoholics, long-term users of magnesium-containing and aluminum-containing antacids, etc.) might benefit from these remedies. Adequate research on these homeopathic substances is lacking. Those who wish to try homeopathic remedies are advised to consult a qualified homeopathic physician.

Related to Negative Claims:
1) Toxic—Treatment of phosphate deficiency should be managed by a physician who needs to make the diagnosis and treat accordingly. Severe phosphate deficiency is treated by large doses of phosphate given orally or, if serious symptoms occur, intravenously. Side effects of phosphate treatment include diarrhea (oral phosphate is a mild laxative, especially at doses higher than 1 gram daily). Abnormally elevated serum phosphate can occur in patients with kidney failure. Abnormally

lowered serum calcium and abnormally elevated serum potassium can occur if phosphate is given in the form of potassium phosphate salt to patients with renal failure and some other conditions. Treatment of mild phosphate deficiency, in those who are otherwise healthy, at oral doses of no more than 1 gram daily is much less likely to cause adverse effects.

IV. RECOMMENDATIONS

A) *Suggested Intake:* The intake of phosphorus in the American diet is from 800 to 1,500 milligrams daily. This, typically, provides entirely adequate amounts. *Mild* phosphate deficiency may not be uncommon in chronic users of magnesium-containing or aluminum-containing antacids and in alcoholics. Antacid users who are also alcoholics are in double jeopardy and may, in particular, need to increase their phosphate intake, either through supplementation or through increasing intake of phosphorus-rich foods (after conferring with their physicians). Better yet, of course, they should also consider decreasing or stopping their alcohol use. Also, there are other drugs used in the treatment of gastritis and peptic ulcer disease which are not phosphorus robbers, and those who have been using the kind of antacids discussed above for a year or longer should consult their physicians about alternative drugs.

B) *Source/Form:* Phosphorus is widely present in our food supply. Milk and milk products, preferably no-fat or low-fat, are the richest sources of dietary phosphate. One quart of milk contains about 1,000 milligrams of phosphate. Neutraphos tablets contain 250 milligrams of phosphate per tablet as a sodium or potassium salt. Since potassium deficiency frequently accompanies phosphate deficiency, the potassium salt is usually the desired form. Those with mild phosphate deficiency may profit from taking 1 gram daily of supplementary phosphate. Again, this should be done under a physician's supervision. There are several vitamin-mineral formulations on the market which contain phosphate along with calcium, iron, other trace minerals and all the vitamins. These are *not recommended,* since calcium phosphate may impair the absorption of other minerals (e.g., iron).

C) *Take With:* Those with phosphate deficiency often have deficiencies in other minerals, especially potassium, magnesium and zinc. Alcoholics who are phosphate deficient commonly have deficiencies of *all* vitamins, minerals and trace elements. If you believe that you are at risk for phosphorus deficiency, discuss with your physician a program that will get you back into nutritional balance, using the guidelines discussed throughout this book.

D) *Cautionary Note:* Phosphate supplementation is not a simple matter and requires diagnosis, discussion, and medical supervision.

POTASSIUM
(With Comments on Salt, Sodium, and Chloride)

I. OVERVIEW: Protection Against High Blood Pressure and Strokes

Potassium is a major component of our cells. It plays a major role in many of the most important functions of our bodies, such as muscle contraction, nerve conduction, the beating of the heart, production of energy and the synthesis of nucleic acids and proteins. It is no wonder that potassium deficiency produces global physical problems ranging from easy fatigability, generalized weakness, muscle pains, all the way to death if left untreated. Those mainly at risk for potassium deficiency are diuretic users. It is obligatory that those who use diuretics have their potassium status monitored regularly.

For years, salt (sodium chloride) has been considered a major culprit in causing many of the health problems of modern civilization, such as hypertension (high blood pressure), strokes and other cardiovascular diseases. It is true that, as we have "progressed" from a hunting-gathering existence to our modern industrial society, there has been a large increase in our intake of salt. But, it is also true that our consumption of potassium has gone way down at the same time.

Our liberal use of the salt shaker has caused or aggravated health problems for many. Recent studies indicate, however, that our generally low potassium intake may be an even greater factor in many of these problems. Diets high in potassium appear to be protective against hypertension and stroke-related deaths. Increasing potassium intake, either through diet or supplementation, is also helpful in *treating* hypertension that has already developed.

II. CLAIMS

Positive:
1) Useful in the prevention and treatment of high blood pressure; 2) protective against stroke-related death; 3) improves athletic performance; 4) beneficial in the prevention and treatment of cancer.

Negative:
1) Toxic.

III. EVIDENCE

Related to Positive Claims:
1) Useful in the prevention and treatment of high blood pressure—The most common type of high blood pressure is called essential hypertension. To date, we do not know what causes it. Yet, most hypertension experts advise those with this disorder to restrict salt intake. Salt has become everyone's favorite culprit. In reality, it has yet to be proved that salt really is the bad guy.

Where did the notion that salt has anything to do with hypertension come from in the first place? The strongest evidence for the role of salt in the development of hypertension comes from studies of some primitive cultures, the members of which consume very little salt and rarely have high blood pressure. In industrialized societies, by contrast, salt consumption is very high and so is the incidence of high blood pressure.

When populations *within* industrialized societies are compared, however, the link between salt intake and hypertension is not as strong. Sodium certainly appears to have *something* to do with hypertension and I will discuss this shortly, but there are other factors, as well. The primitive cultures with low-salt intake also have a high intake of potassium. And, when populations within industrialized societies are compared, the link between potassium intake and hypertension is much stronger than the association between sodium and hypertension.

The first important epidemiologic study relating potassium to blood pressure was published in 1959. Researchers reported on two villages in northern Japan where the inhabitants had similar salt intakes but different blood pressures. Interestingly, those living in the village where the blood pressures were lower consumed more potassium in their diets. Studies have shown that vegetarians generally have lower blood pressures than non-vegetarians. Vegetarian diets are richer in potassium than the diets of meat eaters.

This relationship was strengthened in a study reported in 1983. Researchers involved in this work studied ninety-eight adult vegetarians living in Tel Aviv, Israel, and compared them with a matched group of non-vegetarians with regard to blood pressure and potassium intake, as well as other factors that could play a role in hypertension. The average blood pressure was lower in the vegetarian group, and only 2 percent of the vegetarians had hypertension as compared with 26 percent with hypertension in the non-vegetarian group.

Of all the factors that were examined, including family history of hypertension, obesity, coffee drinking, smoking and sodium and potassium intake, *only* potassium consumption was found to be significant. The potassium intake was significantly higher in the vegetarians, while the sodium intake was the same in both groups. The investigators concluded that the protective anti-hypertensive factor in the vegetarian diet was the presence of high amounts of potassium.

There are other epidemiologic studies that also demonstrate the potassium-blood pressure connection. A particularly interesting one examined the fact that the incidence of high blood pressure among blacks in the United States is greater than among whites. No one knows why this is so. The researchers studied blood pressure and dietary habits and performed laboratory studies on a group of blacks and a group of whites living in Evans County, Georgia. The blacks had significantly higher blood pressures than the whites and were also found to be consuming a lot less potassium. Similar studies have yielded the same results. Generally blacks are poorer than whites and so is their health. High-potassium foods, overall, are more expensive than low-potassium foods.

So far so good for the potassium–blood pressure connection. Diets rich in potassium appear to protect against hypertension, at least in certain instances. But, can potassium-rich diets or potassium supplementation lower blood pressure? High potassium intake appears to have no effect on blood pressure in people with normal blood pressure. On the other hand, high-potassium intake does appear to lower blood pressure in many but not all with hypertension.

Many years ago it was reported that adding potassium chloride to the diets of hypertensive patients caused a reduction in blood pressure. More recently, others reported similar results. One group, however, did not find the situation so clear-cut. These researchers reported that sodium restriction led to lower blood pressures in some and higher blood pressures in others. The results with potassium supplementation were similar—lower blood pressures in some, higher blood pressures in others. Apparently there are considerable variations in individual sensitivity and response to salt and potassium, especially with respect to blood pressure. Also, there are indications that the chloride in salt and in some potassium supplements may actually be the factor responsible for some of these confusing results.

So where does this leave us? As I said right at the beginning of this section, we don't understand very much about essential hypertension. We do know that there are many factors associated with it and that people respond differently to these factors. *Overall, diets rich in potassium appear to be protective against essential hypertension.* The frequency of the disorder in those consuming such diets is significantly lower than in those whose diets are poor in potassium.

It is not as clear if restricted salt intake, that is, not adding any salt (sodium chloride) to food, protects against hypertension. However, there are enough other health benefits from restricting salt intake (protection against edema and heart failure in those predisposed, among others) that restricting salt intake is, overall, a good idea.

For those who are hypertensive, increasing potassium intake by diet or through supplementation frequently helps control blood pressure and may lead to less requirement for medication (to be determined *only* by your physician). In most cases, potassium chloride is the form used for potassium supplementation and, as mentioned earlier, some hypertensives may be sensitive to the chloride in the supplement. The chloride may be the reason why these supplements sometimes either have no anti-hypertensive effect or may even raise blood pressure in certain cases. For those, a trial with another type of potassium salt (e.g., potassium citrate or potassium aspartate), under a physician's supervision, might be worth a try. Restricting salt is certainly prudent, since there are many people whose hypertension *is* salt sensitive.

Finally, there are subgroups of hypertensives who do better with increased calcium and/or magnesium intakes in their diets, or with supplements of these nutrients. (See Calcium and Magnesium sections.) Clearly, much more investigation needs to be done to resolve these extremely important and complex issues.

2) Protective against stroke-related deaths—High-potassium intake has been found to protect against death from strokes. This was the conclusion of a recently completed twelve-year study of residents of an affluent community in Southern California. Eight hundred fifty-nine men and women between the ages of fifty and seventy-nine participated in the study. Dietary intake of each participant was carefully determined and the specific nutrients in all food consumed were meticulously analyzed by dieticians. During the twelve years, twenty-four stroke-related deaths occurred in the study group. These twenty-four individuals were found to have significantly lower potassium intake than survivors and individuals who died from causes other than stroke.

Hypertension is considered the most important risk factor for stroke. In the above study, however, the relationship between dietary potassium and stroke mortality was independent of blood pressure, as it also was of obesity, cholesterol level, cigarette smoking, alcohol and blood sugar. It was also independent of the effects of other factors that may confer benefits against stroke such as magnesium, calcium, sodium restriction and fiber. The bottom line of this study is that potassium intake is an independent risk factor for stroke-related death; *increased* intake *lowers* the risk; *decreased* intake *raises* the risk.

Perhaps most significant was the finding that *even one serving of fresh fruit or vegetables daily (high potassium foods) is associated with a 40 percent reduction in risk!* The researchers stress that their findings need confirmation. We certainly hope that they are proven correct.

3) Improves athletic performance—Potassium deficiency does lead to weakness, easy fatigability and most certainly would affect athletic performance. Users of diuretics are particularly at risk for potassium deficiency and must always remain vigilant regarding this.

An athlete who trains for three to four hours daily can lose up to 700 to 800 milligrams of potassium in the sweat. A medium-sized banana and a serving of fresh vegetables are more than enough to make up for this loss.

Extra potassium is not known to improve athletic performance in someone who is *not* deficient in potassium.

4) Beneficial in the prevention and treatment of cancer—These claims originate from the late physician Max Gerson. He postulated that diets low in potassium and high in sodium make sick cells. These sick cells,

according to him, are incapable of producing appropriate quantities of energy for the needs of the body and, he believed, this results in almost all illnesses, including cancer. Gerson thought that the restoration of health in all those suffering from chronic degenerative diseases required the use of, among other things, diets very rich in potassium and supplementation with potassium chloride. The Gerson therapy is most famous as an alternative therapy for the treatment of cancer.

There is no scientific evidence that potassium is protective against cancer or that it is beneficial in the treatment of cancer. The Gerson therapy is not accepted by orthodox medicine. But was Gerson really all wrong? We have already seen that foods rich in potassium are protective against hypertension and probably against stroke-related deaths. Noteworthy, is that foods rich in potassium such as vegetables and fruits also contain other substances (such as beta-carotene, vitamin E, vitamin C, selenium and zinc) that we are discovering might very well protect against cancer. Therefore, Gerson might have been on a right track, after all—though not simply because of potassium.

Related to Negative Claims:

1) Toxic—Diets rich in potassium are unlikely to have adverse effects except for patients with kidney failure. Normally, we can process all the potassium from our diets that our bodies require and excrete the rest. People with kidney failure, however, have problems excreting potassium and, in these individuals, potassium can accumulate to dangerously high levels—levels that can be fatal.

IV. RECOMMENDATIONS

A) *Suggested Intake* (for sodium and potassium): Americans typically consume from 10 to 12 grams of salt daily. Most of this is from salt that has been added to foods either by the manufacturer or from table salt. For many reasons it is desirable to bring our salt intake down to no more than 5 grams daily. Eliminating table salt entirely will knock about 3 grams off the daily intake. Eliminating anything from your diet that contains added salt, such as potato chips, will get you close to the desired goal. Many products are now available that are lightly salted. Many people are now getting used to cooking with herbs and spices, which have no salt but which still add taste and variety to foods.

At the same time that you decrease your salt intake, you should *increase* your potassium intake. This is best done by eating more fresh fruit and vegetables. These foods are richest in potassium. Salt substitutes are available that contain potassium chloride and usually some other ingredients that try to mask the taste of this substance (bitter and metallic). A good half-way substitute is Morton's "Lite Salt," which is essentially one-half potassium chloride and one-half sodium chloride. Many can't distinguish it from regular salt.

Those at particular risk of potassium deficiency are diuretic users and they certainly should subscribe to the above dietary principles. Most diuretic users require an additional 1.5 grams of potassium daily to stay in balance. See sources, below, for how this can be obtained. Further, those with hypertension could do much better on a high-potassium diet.

B) *Source/Form:* The best natural sources of potassium are fresh vegetables and fresh fruits. A medium banana supplies 630 milligrams of potassium or about 75 milligrams per inch; half a cantaloupe, 885 milligrams; a medium orange, 365 milligrams; half an avocado, 385 milligrams; raw spinach, 780 milligrams per three to four ounces; raw cabbage, 230 milligrams a cup; raw celery, 300 milligrams a cup.

There are several potassium supplements available but most of these require a physician's prescription. For those who are interested, most of these are expressed in the chemical unit milliequivalent, or mEq One mEq equals 40 milligrams of potassium. Forms of potassium supplements include potassium chloride, potassium bicarbonate, potassium aspartate and potassium orotate. Those who take diuretics should have their potassium status monitored periodically and use potassium supplements as recommended by their physicians. It is important to note that many on weight-reducing diets may be using diuretics (herbal or otherwise) that they obtain without a physician's prescription. Those individuals should also have their potassium status regularly monitored.

For diuretic users, an extra 1.5 grams or 40 mEq of potassium daily are usually enough to maintain potassium balance. As an alternative to supplementation, this amount may be obtained by eating the foods mentioned above. Incidentally, one level teaspoon of salt substitute is about 1.5 grams of potassium.

Some potassium supplements are available in health food stores at doses of 99 milligrams per tablet. This is equivalent to about one inch of a banana. These do not require prescriptions, but are much lower in strength than those that do.

C) *Take With:* Those taking diuretics are at risk of magnesium and zinc deficiencies as well as potassium deficiency. (See sections on Magnesium and Zinc.) Discuss with your physician the desirability of taking these minerals in supplementary form.

D) *Cautionary Note:* Those who take diuretics should be monitored by a physician and should supplement with potassium according to direction. Those with kidney failure should stay away from potassium-rich foods and potassium supplements, except as advised by their physicians. Those hypertensives who wish to try supplementary potassium to treat their blood pressure should do so under a physician's supervision.

SELENIUM

I. OVERVIEW: The Anti-Aging/Anti-Cancer Element

Selenium is an essential trace mineral required by the body in *minute* quantities. Recognition of its vital importance in human metabolism was long impeded by its very real toxic potential and by fears of carcinogenicity, fears that have now been largely displaced by evidence suggesting just the opposite—that selenium provides *protection* against a large number of cancers and, indeed, against a broad spectrum of diseases.

Once described as "the most maddening, frustrating, nutritional element," selenium was subject to contradictory findings for decades. One group of investigators, for example, casually noted, in one breath, that selenium could dramatically extend the life span of animals (producing the longest-lived laboratory rats in history) but then went on to condemn the element, in the next breath, as the probable carcinogen that ultimately killed the very Methuselahs it had helped create! Eventually, however, it was established that selenium *deficiencies* occur in most warm-blooded animals, giving rise to cataracts, muscular dystrophy, growth depression, liver necrosis, infertility, heart disease, cancer and so on. Veterinarian experience led to officially sanctioned supplementation of animal feeds and helped promote many of the experimental and human epidemiologic selenium studies that are yielding the often promising results summarized below.

That selenium is essential for optimal health is now established. Chronic illnesses, such as arteriosclerosis (coronary artery disease, cerebrovascular disease and peripheral vascular disease), cancer, degenerative joint disease (arthritis), cirrhosis and chronic obstructive pulmonary disease (emphysema), comprise the overwhelming majority of our health problems. The evidence is mounting that selenium is protective against certain of these diseases and should assume a pivotal role in preventive medicine.

A common denominator in the etiology of most of the chronic diseases we associate with the aging process is oxidant damage to cellular membranes, nucleic acids and proteins. A crucial enzyme in the defense against oxidant damage is glutathione peroxidase. This enzyme contains selenium (in the form of selenocysteine) at each of its four catalytic sites. Selenium thus plays a crucial role in this important enzyme's antioxidant function. But, in addition, selenium may also decrease platelet aggregation, making it further protective against coronary artery disease, strokes and heart attacks. Its role in the immune system, especially in enhancing cellular immunity, may explain in part its reported anti-carcinogenicity.

What all the major theories of aging have in common is the "wear and tear" of some vital cellular component or function. Accumulation of mutations contributes to the process of aging in the somatic-mutation hypothesis. The "error-catastrophe" hypothesis states that an accumulation of errors in protein synthesis leads to an ultimately irreversible accumulation of errors and a final, lethal catastrophe—death. Another proposal is that decreased lymphocyte formation accelerates the aging process by predisposing to infection, cancer and degenerative diseases. Lipid peroxidation is thought responsible for some of the changes in hormone production and in the hormone receptors that others believe are central to aging.

Selenium is remarkable in that the best evidence suggests that it can have inhibitory effects on *all* of the major hypothesized aging mechanisms. That it can play a very important role in helping to reduce the incidence of many diseases associated with aging appears certain. Adequate selenium intake is unquestionably necessary if one is to attain optimal health and full life span potential. Man's ability to extend "maximum life span" beyond presently defined limits remains unproved; if there *are* micronutrients that can help break the present "life span barrier," selenium has to be accounted one of the prime contenders.

II. CLAIMS

Positive:

1) Anti-carcinogenic; 2) immunostimulant; 3) protective against heart and circulatory diseases; 4) capable of detoxifying heavy metals, various drugs, alcohol, cigarette smoke, peroxidized fats; 5) cosmetically beneficial to the skin; 6) increases male potency and sex drive; 7) anti-inflammatory and thus useful against arthritis and other autoimmune diseases.

Negative:

1) Highly toxic in even minute doses; 2) mutagenic, i.e., capable of producing potentially harmful mutations in cells; 3) carcinogenic; 4) cannot be effectively utilized by the body in supplement form; 5) rendered useless by concurrent intake of vitamin C.

III. EVIDENCE

Related to Positive Claims:

1) Anti-carcinogenic—A large body of epidemiologic evidence now exists which suggests that cancer mortality goes up when selenium content of soil and thus of crops goes down. Investigators have mapped the selenium content of the various states of the United States and have found its distribution highly uneven, with the highest levels in South Dakota and the lowest in Ohio. These researchers have shown that Rapid City, South Dakota, has the lowest overall cancer mortality rate in the nation, while Ohio has a rate nearly double that of South Dakota.

Others have confirmed these studies and extended them to more than twenty other nations: the lower the selenium intake, they found, the higher the incidence of leukemia and cancers of the colon, rectum, pancreas, breast, ovary, prostate, bladder, skin and (in the male) lungs. Venezuela, with its high selenium soil content, has, to cite one example, a mortality rate from cancer of the large intestine less than one-quarter that of the United States. The low incidence of breast cancer among women in Japan has been attributed to their relatively high selenium intake; Japanese women who emigrate to the United States, however, have a greatly increased incidence of breast cancer. Researchers have found consistently higher levels of selenium in the blood of healthy individuals than in the blood of those suffering from many forms of cancer.

In more recent work, others report a higher incidence of cancer—especially gastrointestinal and prostatic—among those with lower levels of selenium. This was particularly true among those with low blood vitamin E and A levels, as well as low blood levels of selenium. The study is of great importance because this was the first epidemiologic study in which the blood samples were obtained *before* cancer developed. Subsequent similar studies reached similar conclusions. A study out of Finland showed an association between low serum selenium levels and the increased risk of certain cancers, particularly of the gut. A study reported from China at about the same time showed that those living in areas of low selenium were at increased risk for cancer of the stomach, esophagus and liver, while those living in areas of high selenium were at decreased risk for these cancers.

Another Finnish epidemiologic study reported a high risk of fatal cancer in those with low intakes of selenium, especially if they have low intakes of vitamin E. The same study reported that low selenium intake contributes to the increased risk of lung cancer among smoking men with low vitamin A intake.

Selenium also appears to protect against skin cancer. Researchers found that low blood selenium, in the context of low blood vitamin A levels, increases the risk for certain kinds of skin cancer.

The National Research Council of the National Academy of Sciences has asserted that "a large accumulation of evidence indicates that supplementation of the diet or drinking water with selenium protects against tumors induced by a variety of chemical carcinogens and at least one viral agent." This, of course, was done with laboratory animals.

Experimental evidence has shown that selenium added to food or water in doses of 0.5 to 6 ppm (parts per million) has significantly reduced the incidence of liver, skin, mammary and colon cancers in various laboratory animals. In one of these experiments, female mice specially bred to develop spontaneous breast tumors were divided into two groups. The "controls" received normal diet; the "experimentals" were given selenium supplements. Breast cancers occurred, as expected, in 82 percent of the controls but in only 10 percent of the selenium-supplemented experimentals. The evidence is very strong that selenium, in doses that *exceed* the normal nutritional range, inhibits cancer formation in some, perhaps most, animals.

Most of these studies have shown cancer-preventive effects rather than anti-tumor effects. It has been reported, however, that supplemental selenium can retard the recurrence of rat mammary tumors after they have regressed under the influence of other treatment. Others have also reported selenium-induced anti-tumor effects. Selenium has recently been shown to be capable of inhibiting the growth of some human cancer cells in test-tube experiments.

There is some evidence that selenium deficiency is a significantly growing problem. Various explanatory hypotheses have been put forward. One suggests that because sulfur competes with selenium for uptake in plants, increased sulfur-dioxide fallout and "acid rain" may be contributing to selenium loss.

Selenium's anti-cancer mechanisms are not yet well understood. Some research suggests that selenium affects enzymatic processes that may inhibit the activation of some carcinogens. Other research indicates that selenium may increase the efficiency of DNA repair mechanisms in the wake of carcinogenic damage. Whatever the mechanism, there is no longer any doubt that selenium *does* have anti-cancer properties.

2) Immunostimulant—The claim is that selenium given in amounts greater than ordinary nutritional requirements can significantly boost immune responses. Large increases in antibody production following administration of selenium have been demonstrated in animal studies. Up to thirtyfold increases have been related to the administration of combination selenium/vitamin E. Soviet researchers have confirmed some of these findings. Others have reported that selenium added to the drinking water of mice in 2.5 ppm strongly potentiates immune response to malaria vaccine and reduces the fatality rate associated with subsequent re-exposure to malaria. Still others have noted that selenium doubles the immune response to leptospirosis vaccine in calves.

Selenium deficiencies have been associated with marked impairment of the phagocytic cells that normally engulf foreign bodies. The lymphocytes of dogs have similarly shown impaired responses in the presence of selenium deficiency. Increased phagocytic activity is evidenced, on the other hand, in animals given supplemental selenium. Allograft rejection times have been shortened in mice and rabbits following selenium supplementation.

Selenium's immunostimulant mechanisms remain obscure. It has been suggested, however, that these mechanisms may be inferred, in part, from findings related to other antioxidants. High doses of vitamin

E, for example, may have the ability to reduce the synthesis of immunosuppressive prostaglandins. Other research indicates that antioxidant nutrients help protect macrophages against the free radicals they generate to help destroy bacteria. Selenium appears to promote optimal cell membrane function. The responsiveness of immune cells is largely dependent upon the integrity of their membranes. Selenium's immune-stimulating effects and its anti-cancer properties are, no doubt, intimately linked.

There is a report that blood selenium levels were significantly diminished in a group of twelve males with AIDS. This finding is of extreme importance, since AIDS is characterized by an altered state of immunity and selenium appears to be a key element in the immune system. The authors conclude their paper with the statement, "Further data are needed to clarify the contribution of this deficiency as well as the possible interaction with other nutrients related to selenium, such as vitamin E. Until such data is available all AIDS patients should undergo periodic nutritional assessments including attention to selenium status and appropriate therapy to prevent the complications of serious malnutrition."

3) Protective against heart and circulatory diseases—Epidemiologic evidence suggests that many forms of cardiovascular disease increase as selenium intake decreases. The so-called stroke belt of the United States, an area encompassing part of Georgia and the Carolinas, is an area of very low selenium soil content. It has the highest stroke rate in the U.S. as well as a very high incidence of heart disease. In Finland, which also has very low selenium soil content and exceptionally high cardiovascular mortality, a long-term prospective study of 11,000 Finns has revealed that blood levels of selenium of less than 45 micrograms per liter (a condition found in fully 30 percent of those studied) are associated with a death rate from acute coronary disease of nearly three times that of those with higher serum selenium. The rate of non-fatal heart attacks was also increased—to about twice that of those with higher blood levels of selenium.

In patients undergoing cardiac catheterizations to evaluate suspected blockage of the coronary arteries, plasma selenium levels were found to be lowest in those with the greatest degree of blockage. A German study found recent victims of heart attacks to have serum selenium levels significantly lower than controls. Low selenium is associated not only with atherosclerosis. Keshan disease, a cardiomyopathy characterized by enlarged hearts and high death rates, has become endemic in areas of China that have particularly low selenium soil content. This disease has been reported to be responding to oral selenium supplementation.

A number of experimental studies suggest that selenium, especially in combination with vitamin E, may protect against tissue damage related to restricted blood flow or oxygen supply. In a double-blind study, twenty-two of twenty-four patients receiving 1 milligram of selenium and 200 IUs of vitamin E daily obtained significant relief from angina pain while only five of twenty-four patients on placebo were judged to have benefited similarly.

There is some evidence that selenium's potent antioxidant properties may inhibit some of the free-radical mechanisms that have been said to contribute to the sort of tissue damage discussed above. Its anti-clotting effects appear related to its reported ability to inhibit blood platelet aggregation.

4) Capable of detoxifying heavy metals, various drugs, alcohol, cigarette smoke, peroxidized fats—Selenium's ability to detoxify a number of heavy metals, such as mercury and cadmium, has been widely reported. The precise mechanism by which it does this is not known. In combining with the metals it may form inert, harmless selenides.

There is evidence selenium may detoxify peroxidized fats and thus inhibit their carcinogenicity. Several animal studies have shown that selenium can significantly reduce the toxicity of the anti-cancer drug doxorubicin (Adriamycin) without also reducing its anti-tumor activity. Some other studies, however, have failed to confirm this finding. Results are similarly mixed with respect to claims that selenium can protect against alcoholic liver disease. Claims that selenium confers protection against some forms of damage caused by cigarette smoking have not been adequately investigated.

5) Cosmetically beneficial to the skin—Claims that selenium increases the elasticity and "youthfulness" of the skin, removes "age spots" and so on have not been reliably investigated.

Selenium appears, however, to be protective against certain types of skin cancer. Several years ago oral selenium was shown to cause a reduction of chemically induced skin tumors in mice. More recently it was reported that low blood selenium in the context of low blood vitamin A increases the risk for certain types of skin cancer. Another researcher has found that both oral and topical L-selenomethione were effective in retarding some ultraviolet-induced skin cancers in experimental animals. Beneficial effects of selenium-sulfide lotion (Selsun) to counteract dandruff and other exfoliative and seborrheic dermatities have been reported.

6) Increases male potency and sex drive—Selenium is known to contribute significantly to sperm production and sperm motility. Restoration of fertility in some male diabetics has recently been reported following broad-spectrum antioxidant supplementation (including selenium). These reports, and those of increased sexual drive, remain purely anecdotal.

7) Anti-inflammatory and thus useful against arthritis and other autoimmune diseases—Injectable and oral selenium/vitamin E preparations are used, with reported good results, in veterinarian practice to relieve arthritic inflammation in dogs and other animals.

Selenium does have anti-inflammatory properties. Anecdotes abound regarding the use, worldwide, of selenium for aching joints, osteoarthritis, rheumatoid arthritis and other autoimmune diseases. Scientific documentation on the use of selenium in these conditions is, however, lacking at this point.

Kashin-Beck disease afflicts millions in regions of China and Siberia. This disease affects the joints (sometimes called "big joint disease") producing growth retardation, joint enlargement, deformity of the spinal column and muscular atrophy. Selenium deficiency is thought to be a key factor in the causation of the disease, and selenium supplementation can halt the progress of this disease, if given soon enough.

Related to Negative Claims:

1) Highly toxic in even minute doses—The evidence cited above indicates that selenium can be tolerated in doses higher than was previously believed. See Recommendations: Suggested Intake below.

2) Mutagenic, i.e., capable of producing potentially harmful mutations in cells—Selenium in the form of sodium selenite has both mutagenic and anti-mutagenic effects under varying circumstances, but only at doses many times higher than would ordinarily be consumed. Equiv-

alent doses of *organic* forms of selenium are not mutagenic. See Recommendations: Source/Form below.

3) Carcinogenic—See discussion of anti-carcinogenic properties above. Most of the studies showing evidence of carcinogenicity are decades old. One epidemiologic study in 1978, however, reported a higher colorectal-cancer mortality rate related to higher selenium levels in the drinking water. This finding has not been confirmed by other investigators. The National Research Council has concluded that "a critical review of the experimental conditions suggests that the earlier studies demonstrating carcinogenic or (cancer) promoting properties of selenium can be faulted on the basis of experimental design."

4) Cannot be effectively utilized by the body in supplement form—Some forms of selenium now on the market may not, in fact, be effectively absorbed by the body. See Recommendations: Source/Form below.

5) Rendered useless by concurrent intake of vitamin C—See Recommendations: Source/Form below. Vitamin C taken at the same time as sodium selenite may convert the selenium to a non-absorbable form.

IV. RECOMMENDATIONS

A) *Suggested Intake:* The National Research Council recently established the RDA for selenium at 70 micrograms daily for men and 55 micrograms daily for women. That is, roughly, the estimated average for the American diet. Is it adequate? The evidence cited above would suggest that it may not be. According to several researchers, these values are too low. Human doses in the range of 400 to 1,000 micrograms daily and higher correspond to some of those dosages found to be anti-carcinogenic or immunostimulant in animals, though this does not mean that smaller doses cannot also confer some of these same benefits. Some clinicians have reported using up to 1,000 micrograms of organic selenium daily in selected patients for prolonged periods without signs of toxicity.

There is sufficient reason to supplement the diet with 50 to 200 micrograms of selenium daily. (Consult your physician before taking higher doses.) For children below seven years of age, supplemental intake should not exceed 100 micrograms daily. The form of the supplement is important; see Source/Form.

Those who receive food through their veins or by a tube are particularly at risk for selenium deficiency.

B) *Source/Form:* The best natural sources of selenium include broccoli, mushrooms, cabbage, celery, cucumbers, onions, garlic, radishes, brewer's yeast, grains, fish, organ meats. Remember, however, that even these foods may be very low in selenium, depending upon regional conditions. In general, soils in the eastern United States are more lacking in selenium than soils in the western United States.

Selenium supplements can be obtained either in the form of inorganic sodium selenite, sodium selenate or as organic selenium. Organic selenium is actually the major nutritional form of selenium, that is, the form that is present in the foods mentioned above. The organic forms available are usually derived from a special brewer's yeast enriched in selenium. The major food form of selenium is L-selenomethionine. There is evidence that the organic forms of selenium are preferable. According to some, organic selenium yeast has a much lower potential for either toxicity or mutagenicity than the inorganic sodium selenite. Inorganic sodium selenite reacts with vitamin C in a way that may decrease absorption of selenium. This is not true of organic selenium. It has been reported that long-term use of sodium *selenite* at 1 milligram per day or higher for prolonged periods has toxic effects. No toxicity has been reported with organic selenium in similar doses. In any case, it is not recommended that you take more than 200 *micrograms* of selenium daily, in any form.

C) *Take With:* Best if incorporated into a well-balanced vitamin/mineral "insurance" formula. (See Part Three for specific recommendations.) Because of widely reported synergistic effects, a daily 50- to 200-microgram dose of organic selenium may be accompanied by 30 to 400 IUs of vitamin E daily.

D) *Cautionary Note:* Don't take selenium at the same time you take vitamin C if using the *inorganic* form of selenium, as explained above. Discontinue use of selenium if any signs of toxicity occur; these include garlic odor on breath and skin that persists, fragile or black fingernails, metallic taste, dizziness and nausea without other apparent cause. Toxicity is highly unlikely in the recommended dose/form. Be especially careful about high doses of this one.

SILICON

I. OVERVIEW: Element in Search of a Therapeutic Use

Silicon appears to be everywhere. From New Age quartz crystals, which are made up of silicon dioxide, to the semiconductors that created Silicon Valley, to glass, sandy beaches, Silly Putty and breast implants. It is no wonder, because the mineral silicon, next to oxygen, is the second most abundant element in the earth's crust. But only recently has silicon been found to be an essential trace mineral for animals and, although it has not been proven, it undoubtedly is essential for humans, as well.

The highest levels of silicon are found in connective tissue, bone, skin and fingernails. Silicon is thought to play a role in the architecture and metabolism of these structures. It is unfortunate, however, that at the same time so much is being done to exploit silicon commercially so little is being done to try to understand its biologic role.

II. CLAIMS

Positive:
1) Protects against atherosclerosis.

Negative:
1) Toxic.

III. EVIDENCE

Related to Positive Claims:
1) Protects against atherosclerosis—A few researchers have postulated a role for silicon in atherosclerosis. Studies have shown an age-related decline in the silicon content of the aorta and other arteries, as well as the skin, in several different animals and in humans. Some French investigators reported, several years ago, that the level of silicon in the arterial wall decreases with the development of atherosclerosis.

There have not been any confirmatory studies of the above findings nor any recent studies on the role of silicon, if any, in atherosclerosis. This claim needs further research.

Related to Negative Claims:
1) Toxic—Before silicon was known to be an essential trace mineral it was thought of as quite toxic. And toxic it can be, if inhaled. Inhalation

of silica dust can cause silicosis of the lung, a serious disorder. Silicon is widely available in some antacids as magnesium trisilicate. There are a couple of reports of very long-term use of this type of antacid contributing to the formation of kidney stones. This is rare. The silicon in our food is highly unlikely to have adverse effects.

IV. RECOMMENDATIONS

A) *Suggested Intake:* This is not known. The average daily intake of silicon on a mixed diet is about 200 milligrams.

B) *Source/Form:* The best sources of silicon are vegetables, whole grains and seafood. Silicon is available as a nutritional supplement in the forms of magnesium trisilicate and silicon dioxide. Magnesium trisilicate is the form found in widely used antacids. It is unclear at this time what benefit, besides its antacid effect, supplementary silicon can confer. For the time being, get your silicon from food sources. On the other hand, the amounts usually found in supplements are unlikely to cause adverse effects.

Simethicone, a silicon (polymer of silicon and oxygen), is available for the relief of "gas." Activated charcoal usually (see Charcoal) works better in this respect.

Silicea or silicon dioxide is a homeopathic remedy for disorders of bones, joints and skin.

A form of silicon is available called Vegetal Silica. This is an extract of the herb horsetail. It is claimed to be good for the health of bones, the arteries, and the skin and nails. Other horsetail powders are available which are apparently less concentrated in silicon. Although the product is unlikely to be harmful, there is no documentation of its benefits, either.

VANADIUM
(Clues to Manic-Depressive Illness?)

Whether the element vanadium plays any nutritional, biochemical, or biologic role in the human is a question that has been extremely difficult to answer. At present the only thing we can say is, maybe.

At the turn of the century, French physicians used vanadium as a cure-all—but only for a short time, because some thought that it was quite toxic. The question of the role the element plays in humans, if any, has been up in the air ever since.

The vanadium content of most foods is low. Black pepper and dill seed are the richest sources of the element. Fresh fruits, vegetables and beverages contain the least vanadium. In the middle range are whole grains, seafoods, meats and dairy products. The daily intake of vanadium is low in comparison to other essential trace elements and averages about 20 micrograms (1 microgram is 1/1,000th of a milligram).

Although the biologic functions of vanadium are unclear, high doses are known to have pharmacologic action. For example, vanadium has been shown to have an insulin-mimicking effect in rats. Artificially induced diabetes in rats can, in fact, be reversed with a form of vanadium called vanadate.

If and how vanadium affects glucose tolerance and fat and cholesterol levels (as some have suggested) in humans is entirely unclear. Epidemiologic studies have indicated that low vanadium intake may be associated with human cardiovascular disease. Given the fact that vanadium, in pharmacologic doses, does have insulin-like activity in rats, it is conceivable that some form of vanadium could be developed to regulate glucose and lipid metabolism in humans.

Recommendation of vanadium to treat glucose intolerance and elevated cholesterol at this time is inappropriate and unacceptable. Indeed, vanadium may be toxic to some. There is evidence that elevated vanadium levels are associated with manic-depression. Individuals suffering from this disorder improved, in one study, when treated with a low-vanadium diet or when given large doses of vitamin C (which reduces vanadate, an ionic form of vanadium). Drugs used in the treatment of manic-depressive illness are effective in the reduction of vanadate, as well.

We certainly have a lot to learn about vanadium and its intriguing relationship with manic-depressive illness. More study is badly needed.

ZINC

I. OVERVIEW: Immune Stimulator

Zinc, already firmly established as a principal protector of the immune system and a major disease fighter, has recently also demonstrated a dramatic ability to impede a prevalent eye disorder called macular degeneration, which produces irreversible blindness in the elderly. Evidence is mounting that almost all of us become increasingly prone to zinc deficiency as we age.

More than two hundred enzymes (biologic catalysts) require the trace metal zinc for their activity. These include the enzymes involved in the production of the nucleic acids DNA and RNA, the substances that determine our biologic endowment. Zinc lends its hand to form the so-called zinc fingers, which allow proteins to specifically bind to nucleic acids, thereby regulating the expression of our genetic information. Zinc also plays a role in the structure and function of cell membranes.

Signs of moderate to severe zinc deficiency include growth retardation, poor appetite, underfunctioning sex glands, mental lethargy, delayed wound healing, abnormalities of taste, smell and vision, skin changes and increased susceptibility to infection.

Although moderate to severe zinc deficiency is unlikely in developed countries, many groups in the population are at risk for marginal zinc deficiencies. Zinc deficiency is so common among hospital patients who are fed intravenously that hospitals are now adding zinc, along with other minerals, to the intravenous feeding solution.

Intriguing but still contradictory evidence related to zinc's possible role in cancer and cancer protection is slowly emerging. Zinc may be useful in promoting healing of gastric ulcers and can be useful in treating some forms of male infertility and sexual impotence. Reports of zinc's usefulness in some forms of diabetes and in relieving some of the symptoms of rheumatoid arthritis are deserving of further study.

Recently claims have been made that zinc can be helpful in preventing and shortening colds.

Adequate zinc intake is clearly necessary for optimal health and life span.

II. CLAIMS

Positive:

1) Boosts immunity; 2) prevents cancer; 3) prevents blindness as we age; 4) useful in preventing and treating colds; 5) required for maintenance of taste, smell and vision; 6) accelerates wound healing; 7) increases male potency and sex drive; 8) useful in the treatment

and prevention of infertility; 9) prevents prostate problems; 10) useful in the treatment of acne; 11) prevents hair loss; 12) beneficial in diabetics; 13) anti-inflammatory and useful in the treatment of rheumatoid arthritis.

Negative:
1) Toxic.

III. EVIDENCE

Related to Positive Claims:
1) Boosts immunity—There are research indications that adequate supplies of zinc are essential to the development and maintenance of a healthy immune system and that aging is associated with immune impairment that can sometimes be partially repaired with zinc supplementation.

It is clearly established, in fact, that zinc is essential for cell-mediated immunity. The A46 mutant cattle of the Dutch Friesian type have a defect in the absorption of zinc leading to growth arrest, extreme susceptibility to infection and early death. They have impaired cellular immunity, but their humoral immunity is basically intact. The simple, successful treatment is zinc supplementation. Humans with the rare genetic disorder acrodermatitis enteropathica also have a problem with zinc absorption. Their easy susceptibility to infections leads to early death unless they are treated with zinc. The cellular limb of the immune system is mainly affected. They also have reduced antibody response and defects in the immune activity of white blood cells. The thymic wasting associated with protein-calorie malnutrition can be reversed with zinc supplements.

There are many groups in our population at increased risk of at least marginal zinc deficiency. We now know that the elderly, even the middle-to-upper-class elderly, may be getting insufficient zinc in their diets as manifested by decreased zinc levels. The situation is even worse with the low-income elderly, who may be consuming less than 50 percent of the RDA for zinc. As people grow older there are significant alterations in their immune system. These alterations probably account for some aspects of aging. Associated with aging is an increase in the production of antibodies against self, the so-called autoimmune diseases, as well as an increased proneness to infections. Progressive zinc deficiency may play an important part in the gradual breakdown of the aging immune system.

One study showed that zinc supplementation (in the amount of 220 milligrams of zinc sulfate twice a day for one month) increased the number of circulating T-lymphocytes, which fight infection, and improved antibody response in a group of healthy people over seventy years of age. There was no such improvement in a control group that received no supplementation.

It has recently been reported that those with AIDS or LAS (lymphadenopathy syndrome, a pre-AIDS problem) had significantly lower serum zinc levels than a control group. Another report also noted low serum zinc levels in those with AIDS but not other stages of HIV (human immunodeficiency virus) infection. A child with AIDS was found to have all the signs and symptoms of a zinc-deficiency disorder. It is still unclear why these AIDS patients have low serum zinc levels. What is clear is that this aspect of the AIDS problem should be vigorously pursued.

These exciting findings justify further clinical trials to determine the effects of supplementary zinc on the immune system and in the treatment of immune disorders such as AIDS.

2) Prevents cancer—Contradictory findings abound with respect to this claim. Patients with esophageal cancer have been shown to have lower than normal levels of zinc in their blood. Similar findings have been reported for those with bronchogenic cancer. Zinc levels are also significantly lower in men with cancer of the prostate than in men with normal prostates. Zinc deficiency in rats is associated with an increased incidence of chemically induced esophageal cancer. In other reports, adding zinc to hamster and rat diets inhibited chemically induced cancers.

So far, so good. But, unfortunately, there are also reports suggesting that tumor growth is slowed down in animals maintained on diets that are low in zinc. One group found a direct correlation between estimated zinc intake and mortality from several different types of cancer, suggesting that zinc can *increase* some cancer risks.

How do we reconcile these differences? We have seen that zinc plays a pivotal role in immunity. A healthy immune system is undoubtedly important in protection against cancer, as evidenced, for example, by the occurrence of unusual malignancies in patients with AIDS. The reports showing increased susceptibility to chemical carcinogenesis in zinc-deficient animals may relate to a problem of immune deficiency in these animals.

Another partial answer to this puzzle probably relates to zinc's interaction with other metals. When zinc antagonizes cadmium, the result may be *protection* against cancer. On the other hand, when zinc antagonizes selenium, the result may be an *increase* in cancer risk, since selenium is known to be protective against some cancers. Finally, it is not surprising that the rate of tumor growth is slower in zinc-deficient animals. Zinc is essential for nucleic acid synthesis and thus is necessary for *all* growth, including malignant growth.

Since *marginal* zinc deficiency may be widespread, it is very important to clarify the issue of the role of zinc in the prevention of cancer through additional investigation.

3) Prevents blindness as we age—A leading cause of visual loss in the elderly is a condition called macular degeneration. Because this disorder affects parts of the eyes in which zinc is known to have an important impact on the metabolic function of enzymes crucial in vision, investigators hypothesized that zinc deficiencies might play a role in the disease. To test this idea they constructed a double-blind, placebo-controlled trial involving 151 patients afflicted by this condition. In a twelve- to twenty-four-month follow-up they found that the patients given zinc supplements had significantly less visual loss than the group that got placebos. The zinc was given in 100-milligram tablets, twice a day with meals. Side effects were minimal.

These very promising findings deserve immediate follow-up studies to provide confirmation.

4) Useful in preventing and treating colds—This is another new claim for zinc and is based upon still preliminary findings that colds can be aborted or their duration shortened by promptly taking zinc at the first sign of infection. We already know that zinc is capable of boosting immunity. It may also have some direct anti-viral effects. In the small studies that have been conducted to date, cold sufferers took 50 milligrams of zinc gluconate at the first sign of distress and then took 25 milligrams every two hours thereafter until their symptoms abated. The researchers advise that adults should take no more than twelve 25-milligram tablets per day, that teenagers should limit themselves to

nine per day and younger children to no more than six per day. If no benefits are noted after three or four days, I recommend discontinuing this regimen. It is also a good idea to take zinc with food; taken on an empty stomach it can cause nausea. Also be aware that, at these doses, zinc may cause some distortion of taste and smell. These problems go away within a few days of discontinuing zinc. The zinc supplements in this case are not swallowed but are permitted to slowly dissolve, bathing the tissues of the throat for ten to fifteen minutes each time zinc is taken. If the tablets are swallowed, the treatment is said to be largely ineffective. More work is needed before this claim can be substantiated.

5) Required for maintenance of taste, smell and vision—Abnormalities of taste, smell and vision are quite common as we age. Many older people do not have the same good appetite they had when they were young and they often blame this on food not tasting or smelling as good as it once did. The claim has been made that zinc can restore taste for these individuals.

Zinc deficiency can produce impaired taste acuity or unpleasant taste sensations. Altered taste sensitivity has been found to be related to disordered zinc metabolism in Crohn's disease, chronic renal failure, thermal burns, use of the drug penicillamine and in cystic fibrosis.

The clearest evidence that zinc supplementation can correct taste abnormalities is in uremic (kidney) patients on dialysis. But a study on the effect of zinc supplements on taste discrimination among the aged found no significant improvement. It can be concluded that most age-related taste disorders are not due to zinc deficiency *alone,* although such a deficiency may certainly play a role.

Smell may also be impaired by zinc deficiency. Disorders of smell associated with some conditions of acquired zinc deficiency may be responsive to zinc supplementation. However, patients with disorders of smell for which the cause is unknown do not respond to zinc supplementation.

There is no evidence that age-related disturbances in vision can be improved with zinc supplements.

6) Accelerates wound healing—Dramatic acceleration of surgical wound healing has been reported among a group of patients who received zinc supplementation. Complete healing in ten patients receiving 150 milligrams daily of zinc in the form of zinc sulfate required

forty-six days, while in a control group receiving no zinc supplementation, complete healing took eighty days. Another study failed to confirm this effect of zinc supplementation. It would seem that the value of zinc supplementation in wound healing is closely related to the zinc status of the individual. Enhanced wound healing is to be expected in zinc-deficient individuals following zinc therapy, since zinc is necessary for cellular repair. There is still some question, though, if supplemental zinc is useful in this respect in zinc-*sufficient* individuals. In any event, since zinc intake is barely adequate in many groups, it seems reasonable to give zinc supplements for optimal wound healing. To really settle the matter, however, more controlled studies will be required.

Zinc-sufficient patients with gastric-ulcer disease who were given zinc supplements (150 milligrams of zinc per day in the form of zinc sulfate) had an ulcer-healing rate three times that of patients treated with placebos. In addition, complete healing of ulcers occurred more frequently in the patients taking zinc than in the patients given placebos. This work warrants further study.

7) Increase male potency and sex drive—It is claimed that even marginal zinc deficiency can produce impotence. It is certain that moderate to severe deficiency produces regression of the male sex glands, the testes. Mild deficiency leads to low sperm count. Males with moderate to severe zinc deficiency exhibit decreased sexual interest as well as mental lethargy, emotional problems, poor appetite and all the other consequences of zinc deficiency. Researchers, in their studies of sexually impotent males who were suffering from chronic kidney failure and who had low levels of zinc in their blood, reported a marked improvement in sexual potency in those patients who had zinc added to their hemodialysis solutions. This was accompanied by an increase in blood levels of the male sex hormone and in follicle-stimulating hormone. No such changes were observed in patients who got placebos instead of zinc.

Zinc and testosterone, the male sex hormone, are known to be closely interrelated, though the nature of this relationship remains unclear. The prostate gland is one of the organs richest in zinc. Prostatic zinc increases with puberty, and it is thought that testosterone is the main factor governing the zinc level of the prostate. One of the functions of zinc may be to control testosterone metabolism at the cellular level. Zinc is thought to regulate the metabolism of testosterone in the prostate.

It has been found that in males with mild zinc deficiency, zinc supplementation was accompanied by increased sperm count and plasma testosterone. It was not clear if potency was likewise affected. It appears that zinc supplementation is useful in counteracting male impotence only in the context of moderate to severe deficiency of this mineral. Many forms of male impotence have psychologic bases and are otherwise unrelated to zinc. The effect of zinc on female sexual function is purely anecdotal.

8) Useful in the treatment and prevention of infertility—Zinc is known to be essential for sperm formation. Males who are moderately to severely zinc deficient may produce almost no sperm cells, while males who are mildly zinc deficient have reduced sperm counts. Zinc deficiency is also accompanied by a decreased testosterone level. The role of zinc in female fertility is unknown.

Of course, infertility also exists in men who are apparently zinc sufficient. Could zinc supplementation help *them*? Here I will be personal. My wife and I had been married for sixteen years before we had our first child. For at least ten years during that period we tried very hard to make a child. The problem seemed to be me. My sperm count was low, and the motility and morphology (ability to move and overall development) of the sperm cells were abnormal. I had been a cigarette smoker much of that time. I remembered that cadmium was present in cigarette paper. Cadmium is a zinc antagonist and could cause problems with sperm formation. I started taking 50 milligrams of zinc a day in the form of zinc gluconate. Within a few months my sperm count, as well as the morphology and motility of the cells, was normal. In no time our first child was conceived. Admittedly, this is anecdotal. However, cadmium exposure is very common via cigarette smoking and industrial exposure. Heavy exposure to cadmium, research suggests, may lead to softening of the bones, possibly to prostate cancer, renal disease, hypertension, anemia and lung disease. We're all exposed to cadmium. The average American accumulates 30 milligrams, mainly in the kidneys. The effects of mild exposure are unknown. I propose that mild cadmium exposure may lead to problems with sperm production because of its antagonism with zinc. Research of this issue is needed.

9) Prevents prostate problems—As discussed before, there is a great deal of zinc in the prostate. Enlargement of the prostate (benign prostatic hyperplasia) commonly occurs with aging. Supplementary

zinc has been recommended for both the prevention and treatment of this condition. There is no evidence, however, that it does either. More research will have to be done before any definite conclusions can be reached with respect to this claim.

10) Useful in the treatment of acne—Acne vulgaris is a chronic inflammation that primarily affects the adolescent age group. It is argued that adolescents develop an increased need for zinc that is not supplied by the diet and that the marginal zinc deficiency that results contributes to acne. There is no proof this is the case, though zinc therapy has been helpful in the treatment of acne in patients with *severe* zinc deficiency. It has been reported that oral zinc is as good as tetracycline for acne sufferers with severe zinc deficiency. Some others have failed to confirm this, however, so the evidence that oral zinc is helpful in the treatment of acne remains meager. More research is needed.

Topical zinc, on the other hand, does appear to be useful in treating acne, especially when it is combined with the antibiotic erythromycin. Topical zinc may act as an anti-inflammatory agent and help decrease production of the sebum that contributes to clogging the pores and causing acne.

11) Prevents hair loss—A few reports show that supplementary zinc restores hair growth in a few individuals with alopecia areata totalis (complete lack of body hair). There is no evidence that zinc restores hair to those suffering from typical male pattern baldness. And there is no evidence that supplementation with zinc will prevent hair loss.

12) Beneficial in diabetics—Insulin is the major hormone of sugar metabolism. Zinc appears to be involved with insulin at a few stages. Insulin is stored in the beta cells of the pancreas as a zinc crystal; zinc enhances the binding of insulin to liver cells and is involved with insulin in promoting the synthesis of lipids in fat cells. Rats that are deprived of zinc develop glucose intolerance.

It has been reported that 25 percent of a group of diabetics who do not require insulin injections had depressed blood zinc levels as well as excessive zinc excretion in their urine. The authors of this report suggest that these patients have problems absorbing zinc as well as overexcreting it in the urine. Why these patients malabsorb zinc is unclear.

Diabetics suffer from many complications such as poor wound healing and increased susceptibility to infections. Zinc plays an important role in both wound healing and in immune response. If it is true that a large percentage of diabetics are zinc deficient because of zinc malabsorption and hyperexcretion of zinc, then zinc supplementation would certainly be indicated in this group. Zinc supplementation could reduce diabetic complications. High-fiber diets are important in the management of diabetics, and this fact is relevant here because fiber *decreases* the body's ability to absorb zinc. This makes special consideration of zinc supplementation in diabetes an even more urgent matter. More research is needed.

13) Anti-inflammatory and useful in the treatment of rheumatoid arthritis—As indicated above, topical zinc may have anti-inflammatory properties and in that respect may be useful against acne. One researcher has accumulated evidence in animal experiments that zinc supplementation results in the inhibition of several functions of some of the cells involved in immunity and prevents the release of histamine from mast cells. These actions should have anti-inflammatory effects, but more research will have to be done in order to determine the precise role of zinc.

Lower levels of serum zinc have been found in patients with rheumatoid arthritis than in normal individuals. One investigator reported a trial of zinc supplementation in twenty-four patients with chronic rheumatoid arthritis of the sort that had not been helped by other treatments. In a double-blind study comparing zinc sulfate with a placebo, he found that the zinc-treated patients did better than the controls with regard to joint swelling, morning stiffness, walking time and the patients' own impressions of their overall disease activity. It is hypothesized that zinc is essential for the normal function of the joints and that local zinc deficiency is responsible to some extent for rheumatoid condition of joints. Zinc supplementation may lead to increased levels of zinc within the joints where the mineral's possible anti-inflammatory activity can impact directly upon the rheumatoid process. Subsequent studies, however, have failed to confirm these findings. Does this mean that zinc treatment has no role in rheumatoid arthritis or other inflammatory disorders? No, not at all. There probably is a subset of sufferers of rheumatoid arthritis in whom zinc is useful. We are not yet able to identify this subset. Incidentally, oral zinc sulfate was given to a small group of victims of psoriatic arthritis (inflammatory arthritis coupled with the skin disease psoriasis) with benefit.

It is important to note that there exists a bias against the use of nutrients in the treatment of disease by many in the medical profession. This bias, I hope, was diminished to some degree by a report on the effectiveness of oral zinc in the treatment of Wilson's disease. Wilson's disease is an inherited disorder of copper accumulation which is fatal unless treated. Heretofore, penicillamine, which is toxic to many, was the only established treatment. Zinc, it turns out, is as effective and far less toxic.

There has been very little recent investigation of zinc's possible anti-inflammatory capabilities. Perhaps the interest in the non-steroidal anti-inflammatory drugs has crowded out any follow-up work on zinc in this area. This is too bad; zinc deserves further study to define the possible role it may play in rheumatoid arthritis, its treatment and prevention, as well as in other rheumatologic disorders.

Related to Negative Claims:

1) Toxic—Zinc is thought to be relatively non-toxic. Some people have been taking up to 150 milligrams of zinc each day for a few months (e.g., for rheumatoid arthritis, wound healing) with only occasional complaints of gastrointestinal problems, such as nausea, vomiting, diarrhea, epigastric distress and colic. However, recently some side effects have been observed in patients taking large doses of zinc over extended periods of time. One group reported that in young men large doses of zinc (150 milligrams of zinc daily) depress high-density lipoprotein (HDL) cholesterol levels. This is undesirable, because high-density lipoprotein cholesterol is thought to protect against coronary heart disease.

Subsequent reports showed that 100 milligrams a day of elemental zinc caused a reversible lowering of HDL in healthy women after several weeks, while about 30 milligrams a day of zinc given over a period of several weeks had no adverse effect on the lipid profiles of either sedentary or active men.

Zinc competes with copper for intestinal absorption; thus high doses of zinc may create a copper deficiency. Copper deficiency in rats causes an increase in low-density lipoprotein cholesterol, also bad because this form of cholesterol *increases* the risks of coronary heart disease, and a relative decrease in high-density lipoprotein cholesterol. Some believe that an elevated zinc/copper ratio, which could occur in the context of a patient taking large amounts of zinc, is an important risk factor for coronary heart disease. It has been reported that a woman treated with zinc (150 milligrams of zinc daily) for fourteen months developed a profound anemia due to copper deficiency. Thus, patients who need to take large doses of zinc, for medical reasons, should be given copper supplementation (unless zinc is being used to block copper, as in Wilson's disease).

Megadose zinc supplementation may also have adverse effects on the immune system. It has been reported that 300 milligrams of zinc given daily to healthy men for six weeks resulted in several reversible findings, including reduction in lymphocyte responsiveness. The subjects involved in this study, however, never noted any symptoms. The adverse effects were strictly laboratory findings. Follow-up work is needed.

There are no reports of long-term adverse effects of low-dose supplementation with zinc. Many people take 30 to 50 milligrams of zinc daily. Even in this dose range, however, it is advisable to include supplemental copper whenever zinc is taken.

IV. RECOMMENDATIONS

A) *Suggested Intake:* The National Research Council's Recommended Daily Allowances (RDAs) for zinc are: 15 milligrams for men, 12 milligrams for women, 3 milligrams for infants, 10 milligrams for children from one year to ten years of age, 15 milligrams for pregnant women and 16 to 19 milligrams for those lactating (nursing infants). The optimal zinc intake for maximal longevity with minimal disease has not been defined.

There are many factors that make it difficult for us to be sure that we are getting enough zinc in our diets. Zinc content varies a great deal among different foods. And the amount of zinc that we absorb from these foods is influenced by many different things. The aged appear to be at particular risk of marginal zinc deficiency. They—and particularly those who eat mainly vegetarian diets—may be getting less than two-thirds, and in some cases less than one-half, the RDA. Our ability to absorb zinc decreases with age. Fiber, phytates (found in plants), iron and calcium also diminish the amount of zinc we are able to absorb and utilize in our bodies. Athletes and dieters are at higher risk of zinc deficiency than most others, except for the aged and the vegetarians. Certain drugs (such as diuretics) and various disease states (such as diabetes and chronic alcoholism) lead to increased zinc excretion and thus to a need for increased zinc intake. Excessive sweating (as in the case of runners, athletes, etc.) can also cause significant zinc loss. There are compensatory mechanisms in the body that try to make up for these losses, but it is unclear if they are always adequate.

We can reasonably conclude that zinc intake may be barely adequate in many people, even in "healthy" and "well-fed" people. This inadequate or borderline-adequate intake may prove particularly troublesome in situations where increased zinc is required, e.g., the growing child, pregnancy, infection or convalescence.

I believe that a zinc supplement is a prudent form of health "insurance." I recommend between 15 to 30 milligrams daily for adults and 10 milligrams daily for children. Consult your physician before taking higher doses. It is noteworthy that many of the currently available children's and pregnant women's vitamin/mineral formulas do not contain zinc. Only recently has zinc been added to some children's cereals; this is fortunate in view of the fact that some children seem to eat almost nothing but cereals.

B) *Source/Form:* Dietary sources of zinc include whole-grain products, brewer's yeast, wheat bran and germ; seafoods and animal meats are, in general, much better sources of bioavailable (easily absorbed) zinc than are vegetables. There are several zinc supplements on the market: zinc sulfate, zinc acetate, zinc gluconate, zinc citrate, amino acid chelates of zinc, zinc dipicolinate, zinc aspartate and zinc orotate. There is some evidence that the protein breakdown products (amino acids and their derivatives) naturally facilitate the absorption of zinc. Zinc sulfate often causes gastric irritation. The amount of zinc is commonly listed on the product label as the "zinc equivalent."

C) *Take With:* Best if incorporated into a well-balanced vitamin/mineral formula. Specifically, I suggest that a daily 15- to 30-milligram dose of zinc be accompanied by 1.5–3 milligrams of copper and 50–200 micrograms of selenium for the reasons already discussed. The ratio of zinc to copper should be about 10:1 (milligram to milligram). Therefore, if a physician recommends higher intakes of zinc, the copper dose can be adjusted using this ratio.

D) *Cautionary Note:* Toxicity at the recommended dose is highly unlikely. See discussion under Related to Negative Claims with respect to higher doses.

SIX

Amino Acids

Amino acids are being marketed widely as individual food supplements. In order to make sense of these substances it is important to define some terms. In principle, an amino acid is any compound that contains an amino group and an acidic function. This definition includes a wide variety of substances, many of which have no known biologic function. When biologists talk about amino acids, they usually mean the twenty amino acids that are necessary for the synthesis of proteins. Proteins are large molecules that are crucial to life; they are involved in the formation of living structure and they catalyze the chemical reactions necessary for the maintenance of life.

The twenty amino acids that form the building blocks of all proteins are alanine, arginine, asparagine, aspartic acid, cysteine, glutamic acid, glutamine, glycine, histidine, isoleucine, leucine, lysine, methionine, phenylalanine, proline, serine, threonine, tryptophan, tyrosine, and valine. There are other amino acids found in our bodies such as taurine and ornithine, but these amino acids are not involved in the synthesis of proteins.

In addition to participating in the synthesis of proteins, amino acids are involved in other important biologic processes such as the formation of the brain neurotransmitters. There are some recent studies which suggest that certain amino acids may play important roles in enhancing the immune system and protecting against cancer.

The twenty amino acids involved in protein biosynthesis are divided into two broad groups—essential and non-essential. Healthy human adults required dietary intake of eight of these amino acids to maintain good health; phenylalanine, valine, threonine, tryptophan, isoleucine, methionine, lysine and leucine. The remaining twelve—the non-essential amino acids—can be made by the body from other substances. Healthy children require, in addition to the eight amino acids listed above, histidine and arginine. Situations exist in which non-essential amino acids become essential. For example, a physically traumatized adult requires arginine for optimal repair processes to occur.

Some promising pharmacologic applications are emerging for amino-acid supplements, especially in the realms of psychiatry and neurology.

L-ARGININE
(With a Note on Ornithine)

I. OVERVIEW: Growth vs. Anti-Growth

Despite all the hype and anti-hype surrounding L-arginine, this substance remains one of the most intriguing of the amino acids and, potentially, one of the most useful. It has marked effects on several major endocrine hormones, plays very significant roles in muscle, growth and healing, helps regulate and support key components of the immune system and has exhibited important liver-protective and anti-cancer properties. It is also of critical importance in male fertility.

Both too much and too little have been claimed for L-arginine (and its cousin, ornithine). The hype surrounding its reputed fat-burning/muscle-building properties has no doubt been excessive, although there is *some* foundation for these claims. Meanwhile, some potentially much greater benefits—in the realm of cancer and immunity—have been largely overlooked.

L-arginine and ornithine are classified as "non-essential" amino acids. This means that the body is capable of synthesizing these particular amino acids, with the result that it is not essential that we get additional amounts in our daily diet. L-arginine, incidentally, *is* an essential amino acid for children.

That, at least, has been the "common wisdom." There is a growing body of evidence, however, that L-arginine and ornithine are actually conditionally-essential, that is, we may need to get them via diet under some circumstances. There are, for example, rare genetic disorders in which synthesis of these amino acids is impaired. More important, though, are findings of relative deficiency states related to injury, surgical trauma and some other forms of stress. Reproductive health can also be adversely affected by inadequate dietary intake of these so-called non-essential amino acids.

These are exciting substances that warrant far more serious investigation. Touted for their growth-promoting capabilities (in the realm of body building), these nutrients may turn out to be more important for their *anti*-growth properties (in the realm of cancer treatment).

II. CLAIMS

Positive:

1) Boosts immunity; 2) fights cancer; 3) builds muscle and burns fat; 4) promotes healing of burns and other wounds; 5) protects the liver and detoxifies harmful substances; 6) enhances male fertility.

Negative:

1) Causes bone and skin disorders in large doses; 2) produces nausea and diarrhea; 3) causes mental and metabolic disturbances; 4) promotes herpes.

II. EVIDENCE

1) Boosts immunity—Research to date indicates very clearly that supplemental arginine stimulates the thymus gland and promotes production of lymphocytes in that gland. Lymphocytes are crucial for immunity. Arginine (and ornithine, discussed below) produce not only more lymphocytes but also more active and effective lymphocytes. This has been demonstrated both in a number of different animals and in humans, both in injured/sick subjects and in healthy subjects. What is especially worth noting is that beneficial effects have been observed

even in subjects *not* deficient in arginine by conventional standards. This suggests that supplemental arginine in excess of nutritional needs (the exact or even approximate amounts of which have yet to be established) may be helpful in some cases.

The precise amounts needed to stimulate heightened immunity, under varying circumstances, has not been determined either. Most of the studies suggest that once a desired effect is observed at a particular dose level, giving more will *not* produce an even greater or more sustained effect. Oral administration requires higher doses (to achieve a given effect) than does delivery by injection. In one human study, healthy volunteers received 30 grams of arginine daily for a week. That oral dose (considered very high) was sufficient to produce dramatically enhanced lymphocyte activity within three days.

The immune-stimulating effects of arginine appear almost certain to be related to its effects on the secretion of various endocrine hormones. And its ability to fight infection and boost immunity is also, undoubtedly, related to its anti-tumor and enhanced wound-healing properties.

I have previously called attention to the urgent need for further investigation of arginine's immune-stimulating capabilities. I am gratified that more research is being done. A group of Japanese investigators recently reported, for example, that immune cells from healthy humans, incubated with excess arginine in the test-tube, demonstrated a *threefold* increase in natural killer cell activity and equally significant increases in other desirable immune activities. These experiments showed not only increased immune response but direct anti-tumor cell activity.

Much more work still remains to be done.

2) Fights cancer—There's increasing credence, accumulating in animal work, that arginine can inhibit the growth of a number of tumors (see also discussion of immunity above). More than two dozen different tumors have been inhibited (in terms of regression, slower growth and/or decreased incidence) by the use of arginine, in animal work. Some of these results have been extremely dramatic, and there are now *fifty years* of accumulated evidence attesting to arginine's anti-tumor potential. It is high time (and past time) that some serious human investigations begin. Unfortunately, researchers who have wanted to pursue this human work have not been able to obtain ade-

quate funding. This is, unquestionably, due in large part to the fact that arginine is a freely available nutritional substance and not a patentable drug.

3) Builds muscle and burns fat—This is the claim that is most often made these days for arginine and ornithine. A still-increasing number of athletes, body builders and dieters are using these amino acids. It is true that arginine stimulates the pituitary gland in ways that increases secretion of growth hormone (GH). This hormone, once in the bloodstream, is said to help burn fat and build muscle. GH release has been verified in humans after administration of both oral and injected arginine. There is no real evidence, however, that arginine (or ornithine) supplements can either "burn fat" or "build muscle" in humans. This lack of evidence, however, may simply be due to the fact that, as of yet, no one has done sound, controlled studies to test these claims. In one human study, 1,200 milligrams of arginine combined with 1,200 milligrams of lysine, an amino acid similar to ornithine, *did* cause the release of biologically active quantities of GH, but no follow-up was done to see if this had any effect on fat or muscle. Without the lysine combination, incidentally, little GH was released. Given what we know about arginine, it is not unreasonable to expect that it might have some of these capabilities—though to what extent and at what possible risk remain unknown.

One thing appears reasonably certain: The small amounts of arginine available in most oral supplements are highly unlikely to have any effect. This is not to suggest that you start megadosing on arginine; though arginine has low toxicity high doses can definitely be risky in some cases. (See Negative Claims.) Here, again, we need more work to find out what the precise risks and benefits with respect to these claims are.

4) Promotes healing of burns and other wounds—Arginine's ability to stimulate secretion of human growth hormone undoubtedly accounts for its capacity to accelerate wound healing and inhibit loss of muscle mass after surgery or injury. Numerous animal studies have documented these beneficial effects. Preliminary work in humans suggests that high-dose supplemental arginine (via intravenous feeding) can probably inhibit postinjury wasting or weight loss and speed wound healing in many cases.

Some of arginine's positive effects in this regard may be due to immune-stimulating effects, increasing resistance to infections that could slow the healing of burns and other wounds. In a study of children with severe burns, researchers found that higher concentrations of arginine in the blood of these children correlated with greater resistance to infection.

We already know enough to begin using supplemental arginine in many postinjury and postsurgical cases, particularly since high doses can be conveniently administered in a hospital setting where continual monitoring is also more easily achieved.

5) Protects the liver and detoxifies harmful substances—It was shown many years ago that supplemental arginine could prevent the toxic and usually deadly effects of giving ammonia to rats. Ornithine was also shown to have this detoxifying effect. In the wake of these findings humans suffering from some serious forms of liver disease were also given arginine, sometimes with excellent results. Other treatments (not necessarily superior) ultimately supplanted arginine in this context, at least in the United States. The early data were strong, certainly sufficient to warrant renewed interest in arginine as a liver-detoxifying agent. It is possible that it has some additional, hitherto unsuspected, detoxifying properties.

6) Enhances male fertility—Arginine's importance in normal sperm production in the human male is well established. A number of studies have shown a relationship between low sperm count and diets deficient in arginine, studies that occurred owing to the discovery that human semen is particularly rich in arginine under normal circumstances. Studies in which men with low sperm counts were given arginine supplements have met with mixed results, although more have shown benefit than have not. In one study, for example, men who had been given a wide range of other treatments in unsuccessful efforts to overcome their low sperm counts responded favorably to arginine supplementation. More than 80 percent of them showed significant improvement when given 4 grams of oral arginine daily. Improvement was great enough in many of these to result in pregnancies.

Related to Negative Claims:

1) Causes bone and skin disorders in large doses—There is no proof that this is so, but I do not recommend that young people, in whom long-bone growth is still incomplete, take supplementary arginine or

ornithine under any circumstances. The risks in adults, in this context, appears negligible.

2) Produces nausea and diarrhea—Some report this with very high doses. These effects quickly recede when arginine is discontinued or the dose lowered.

3) Causes mental and metabolic disturbances—It has been suggested but never demonstrated that very high doses of arginine might aggravate mental disturbances in schizophrenics. Prolonged high doses might pose some peril to those with some forms of kidney and liver failure. Such individuals should use arginine only while under medical supervision.

4) Promotes herpes—The relative intake of lysine and arginine have been reported, anecdotally, to have some effect on the incidence of herpes outbreaks. There is no scientific proof of this. (See discussion on lysine in this section for more details.) Those worried about this might want to take equal amounts of lysine and arginine.

IV. RECOMMENDATIONS

A) *Suggested Intake:* Optimal intake is unknown. Doses of arginine up to 1.5 grams per day appear to be safe (unless you have kidney or liver failure or are a non-adult). Those with infections, injuries, burns, male fertility problems or those scheduled for surgery may want to consider taking supplementary arginine. Discuss the use of this amino acid for these problems with your physician.

B) *Source/Form:* Natural sources of arginine include raw cereals, chocolate, various nuts. There are many arginine supplements available, including some in which arginine is combined with lysine.

C) *Take With:* There *may* be valid reasons to take arginine with lysine. If arginine promotes herpes growth (something that has never been demonstrated) and lysine inhibits herpes (as some believe) then taking the two amino acids together in roughly equal doses may inhibit any adverse effect arginine might have in this context. In addition, as was noted earlier, in one study arginine was more effective in releasing GH when teamed with lysine. Take on an empty stomach and do not combine with other amino acids.

D) *Cautionary Note:* Do not take arginine if you have kidney or liver disorders—unless you first receive the permission of your physician. Non-adults should not take arginine, as explained above under Negative Claims. Note that *some* liver disorders may actually benefit from arginine supplementation—but only your physician can determine this.

NOTE ON ORNITHINE—Ornithine shares many of arginine's properties. It is also capable of stimulating GH release and, like arginine, can increase the weight and activity of the thymus gland, possibly enhancing immune response in the process. In addition, it has shown liver-regenerating effects in animals. Doses of up to 1.5 grams per day appear to be safe in adults without liver or kidney problems.

L-ASPARTIC ACID
(Fatigue Fighter?)

L-Aspartic acid is a non-essential amino acid that was used some years ago in the treatment of chronic fatigue. Eighty-five percent of the 145 patients who were given the potassium and magnesium salts of aspartic acid in one study felt significantly more energetic with this treatment. This was a double-blind, placebo-controlled study conducted over an eighteen-month period. Unfortunately, there has been no recent work to further elucidate this possible benefit of aspartic acid, although there are now products being sold as "workout formulas" and "aerobic enhancers" that include aspartic acid.

More recent work with aspartic acid suggests, in a very preliminary way, that this substance might be helpful in overcoming the rigors of opiate withdrawal. It was found to be more useful, in this context, than some major tranquilizing drugs.

I don't recommend using this amino acid in doses greater than 1.5 grams daily except under a doctor's supervision.

BRANCHED-CHAIN AMINO ACIDS
L-LEUCINE/L-ISOLEUCINE/L-VALINE
(New Treatment for Neurologic Disorders?)

Leucine, isoleucine and valine are three essential amino acids of the so-called branched-chain category that are, increasingly, in evidence in the supplement supermarket. Some body-building enthusiasts have been promoting these amino acids as potent anabolics (muscle builders) and energizers. Unfortunately, there is little scientific evidence to support those claims. There *is* some evidence suggesting that these substances might be able to help restore muscle mass in those who have liver disease, those who have undergone surgery and those who have suffered injury or other trauma, but no one has shown that they are effective in this regard in healthy individuals.

On the other hand, the branched-chain amino acids appear to be quite useful in treating and, in some cases, even reversing hepatic encephalopathy, a form of liver damage that is a frequent feature of alcoholism. The branched-chain amino acids help curb muscle wasting in individuals with this disease and, through their actions on brain neurotransmitters, help prevent a number of the adverse neurologic effects of chronic liver disease.

Other recent reports suggest possible additional roles for the branched-chain amino acids in the treatment of some neurologic disorders. One researcher has reported that a subset of sufferers of Parkinson's disease can be helped by doses of 10 grams of leucine daily. This very preliminary report needs follow-up.

A much better and more recent study suggests that leucine, isoleucine and valine may be helpful in amyotrophic lateral sclerosis (ALS), better known as Lou Gehrig disease. Since this is a potentially fatal disease for which no effective treatment has hitherto been found, this report must be considered potentially very significant.

This pilot study involved nine ALS patients, eight of whom reportedly benefited from supplementation with these branched-chain amino acids, to the extent that, over the one-year period of the study, they maintained muscle strength and the ability to walk. By contrast, five of nine control subjects with ALS, all of whom received placebos instead of the amino acids, lost their ability to walk within the one-year period.

Those receiving the amino acids got (daily) 12 grams of leucine, 8 grams of isoleucine and 6.4 grams of valine. These were divided into four doses taken between meals.

The researchers in this study, funded by the National Institutes of Health, decided to try the branched-chain amino acids in part because of leucine's and isoleucine's ability to promote the enzymatic breakdown of glutamate, another amino acid, which appears to be overactive and possibly toxic in the brains of ALS victims. Valine was added to the regimen, as well, because levels of this amino acid are severely reduced in the blood and cerebrospinal fluid of ALS patients. No significant side effects were noted.

Owing to the importance of these findings, a much more ambitious three-year follow-up study is now underway involving one hundred ALS patients.

L-CYSTEINE
(and Glutathione)

I. OVERVIEW: Anti-Toxin

Cysteine is one of the amino acids that contain sulfur in a form that is said to inactivate free radicals and thus protect and preserve cells. Claims are made that various sulfur-containing antioxidants can extend life span and protect against various toxic substances. (Methionine and taurine, discussed later in this chapter, are other sulfur-containing amino acids.) Cysteine is a precursor of glutathione, a tripeptide, that can, it is claimed, protect the body against various pollutants. Glutathione is a major antioxidant in the body but is unlikely to be useful in supplement form.

II. CLAIMS

Positive:
1) Extends life span; 2) protects against toxins and pollutants, including some found in cigarette smoke and alcohol; 3) combats arthritis.

Negative:
1) Contributes to kidney stones; 2) dangerous for diabetics; 3) toxic.

III. EVIDENCE

Related to Positive Claims:
1) Extends life span—Several years ago, researchers injected guinea pigs and mice with cysteine every other day for more than a month. They reported significantly increased survival times in these animals. Another investigator similarly noted marked increases in survival time among cysteine-supplemented mice. Others have noted an age-related decrease in those sulfur-containing substances that are hypothesized to protect against degenerative diseases linked to aging through antioxi-

dant and other influences. It has been suggested that cysteine may participate in some forms of DNA repair, another mechanism that, theoretically, could help inhibit these degenerative changes. Cysteine is an established antioxidant, but its anti-aging effects remain to be demonstrated in humans. Even the animal work, though intriguing, is far from conclusive. More work needs to be done.

2) Protects against toxins and pollutants, including some found in cigarette smoke and alcohol—Aldehydes, toxic products of some fats, alcohol, smoke, smog, etc., are said to be partially neutralized by cysteine. One group reported that large doses of alcohol-derived acetaldehyde killed 90 percent of the rats to which it was given. Another group of rats were first given quantities of vitamins C and B_1, along with cysteine, then were exposed to the same doses of acetaldehyde that had proved fatal in most of the other group of rats. *None* of the vitamin/cysteine-augmented rats died. There have been other reports that cysteine can protect against other potentially toxic substances. Cysteine is a precursor of glutathione, a tripeptide (made from three amino acids) that has been reported to eliminate certain toxic chemicals by binding to them and thus rendering them harmless. There is a report that rats fed methionine-deficient and cysteine-deficient diets have lower levels of enzymes that are protective against carcinogens. Further research is indicated.

3) Combats arthritis—British research indicated that cysteine given in conjunction with pantothenic acid (see discussion of pantothenic acid and royal jelly elsewhere in this book) had positive effects on patients suffering from osteoarthritis and rheumatoid arthritis. At this point, however, there is insufficient evidence to support the claim that cysteine can alleviate the symptoms of any form of arthritis, though the preliminary British study deserves follow-up.

Related to Negative Claims:
1) Contributes to kidney stones—There have been no studies showing that cysteine supplementation will result in kidney stones, though the fear that it might is not entirely without foundation. Even most of the cysteine enthusiasts caution people on this score, urging that vitamin C be taken along with cysteine to help prevent it from converting to cystine, a close relative, which could, in fact, cause bladder and kidney

stones. The recommended combination is two to three times as much vitamin C as cysteine.

2) Dangerous for diabetics—There is some evidence that cysteine may interfere with insulin; diabetics are therefore advised not to use cysteine supplements without consulting their physicians.

3) Toxic—There are anecdotal reports that cysteine can increase the toxicity of monosodium glutamate in individuals who suffer from the so-called Chinese restaurant syndrome, a set of symptoms, including headache, burning sensations, and sometimes dizziness and disorientation, that follows the ingestion of monosodium-glutamate-laced foods.

IV. RECOMMENDATIONS

A) *Suggested Intake:* Optimal intake is unknown. I do not recommend taking cysteine supplements in amounts greater than 1.5 grams per day. If you have problems that you believe might be helped by cysteine supplementation in doses higher than 1.5 grams daily, consult your physician, calling attention to data cited above.

B) *Source/Form:* Good dietary sources of cysteine include eggs, meat, dairy products and some cereals.

C) *Take With:* If you do take cysteine supplements, take with vitamin C (two to three times as much vitamin C as cysteine, milligram to milligram) as a precaution against kidney-stone and bladder-stone formation.

D) *Cautionary Note:* Diabetics should not take cysteine supplements unless directed to do so by a physician who is aware of the diabetes. (Also see information related to kidney stones and "Chinese restaurant syndrome" under Evidence: Related to Negative Claims above.)

L-GLUTAMINE/L-GLUTAMIC ACID
(Alcohol Curb?)

L-glutamic acid and L-glutamine are closely related amino acids. Glutamine is a derivative of glutamic acid. Research some years ago suggested that glutamine, but not glutamic acid, might help curb alcohol craving. Other equally inconclusive studies have suggested glutamine can speed the healing of peptic ulcers, energize the mind, inhibit senility and counter depression. Glutamic acid was once reported to be capable of boosting the IQs of mentally retarded individuals. Numerous studies related to these and other claims have consistently contradicted one another.

Glutamine's possible favorable effects in alcoholics, however, seem particularly worthy of further investigation. Recent animal work showing that glutamine-supplemented diet can significantly improve survival from a deadly form of colitis also deserves follow-up.

I do not recommend use of glutamine or glutamic acid in doses greater then 1.5 grams per day except under a physician's supervision.

GLYCINE
(Spastic Control?)

There are preliminary indications that supplementation with this amino acid may help dampen the sort of overactive brain processes that produce certain forms of spastic movement. In a pilot study investigating this possibility, ten patients with severe chronic spasticity of both legs were given 1 gram of glycine daily for six months to one year. Seven of these patients were suffering from chronic multiple sclerosis. Overall improvement was rated at 25 percent. All patients benefited to some degree, and no toxicity or other adverse side effects were noted. More work is warranted. At this time we still have too little useful information about L-glycine to justify using it without medical indications and supervision.

L-HISTIDINE
(Arthritis Treatment)

L-Histidine is one of the lesser known amino acids in the supplement marketplace, and few claims have been made for it. One researcher who was studying rheumatoid arthritis found abnormally low levels of this amino acid in the blood of those suffering from that disease. He gave some of his arthritic patients up to 6 grams of histidine daily.

Benefits were observed in many; some were said to be helped with as little as 1 gram daily.

A subsequent study found lesser benefits—but enough to justify further investigation, according to the researchers involved.

More recent reports suggest that supplementary histidine may boost the activity of suppressor T cells. This is intriguing, particularly in view of those earlier reports on histidine's possible usefulness in rheumatoid arthritis—which is one of many autoimmune diseases in which suppressor T-cell activity is subnormal. These recent studies lend further support to the idea that histidine may be helpful in rheumatoid arthritis and suggest the pathway by which it may work in that disease. Again, more work is needed and warranted.

Histidine should not be used in doses greater than 1.5 grams daily except under a doctor's supervision.

L-LYSINE

I. OVERVIEW: Herpes Control?

Lysine is an essential amino acid humans must obtain from diet. Interest in lysine focuses on its reputed usefulness in the prevention and treatment of herpes. There is also interest in it now as a possible muscle-building adjunct.

II. CLAIMS

Positive:
1) Inhibits herpes; 2) builds muscle.

Negative:
1) Suppresses growth in infants.

III. EVIDENCE

Related to Positive Claims:
1) Inhibits herpes—In view of the fact that 50 to 70 percent of the world's population is afflicted with recurrent attacks by the herpes simplex virus (which causes painful lesions, especially in the oral and genital areas), any claim that a largely non-toxic, relatively inexpensive

substance such as lysine is an effective preventive must be taken seriously and be carefully investigated.

Unfortunately, this is a difficult subject to research, because herpes can be easily activated by emotional factors and, by the same token, may be particularly vulnerable to placebo effects. Despite this, a succession of researchers have investigated a possible role for lysine in the prevention and treatment of herpes and have produced very mixed results, with good studies reporting both positive and negative findings.

Researchers have hypothesized for some time that the amino acid arginine promotes herpes, while lysine inhibits it. Herpes sufferers, therefore, have often been advised to cut back on such arginine-rich foods as chocolate, beer, cola drinks, peanuts, cashews, barley and peas and to consume, instead, a lot of lysine-rich foods such as milk and other dairy products, potatoes and brewer's yeast, in addition to taking lysine supplements (up to 1 gram a day during active viral outbreak).

Early studies were small and poorly controlled. They were not conducted double-blind; nor did they use placebos. Their positive results were, therefore, given little weight.

The first good study came out of Denmark. It was a placebo-controlled, double-blind study that utilized 1 gram of lysine daily in the experimental subjects. It failed to find any evidence that lysine can reduce the recurrence rate of herpes outbreaks. The investigators acknowledged, however, that larger doses might still prove to be useful. A more recent double-blind, placebo-controlled study utilizing 1,200 milligrams of lysine also failed to find any benefit. This study, however, involved only twenty-one patients.

A still more recent, larger, better designed study of greater duration *did* find significant benefit from lysine supplementation. This Mayo Clinic study utilized 1,248 milligrams of lysine daily and was also conducted double-blind and placebo-controlled. Various groups of herpes sufferers alternated between high- and low-dose (624 milligrams daily) lysine and placebo. Low-dose lysine and placebo were found to be completely ineffective. The higher dose lysine regimen was consistently and significantly effective in reducing the recurrence rate of herpes outbreaks. Lysine did not, however, reduce the duration or severity of attacks once underway.

Both of these more recent studies, incidentally, found that avoidance of arginine-rich foods did nothing to alter recurrence rates or severity of attacks.

It appears possible that lysine may be able to reduce the recurrence rate of herpes in some individuals, far less likely that it can appreciably reduce the severity of an established attack.

There may be virtue in conducting further tests with still higher doses. Given lysine's low toxicity there is little to lose and potentially much to gain in doing so.

2) Builds muscle—The claim is that lysine, combined with the amino acid arginine, can help build muscle mass. This claim is based upon a study that demonstrated a significant human-growth-hormone (GH) releasing effect with an oral daily dose of 1,200 milligrams of lysine combined with 1,200 milligrams of arginine, both taken on an empty stomach. This study, however, was designed only to see if such a combination could induce secretion of biologically active amounts of GH and there was no follow-up to see if such doses would result in muscle building. There is only anecdotal evidence that arginine and lysine, when used as adjuncts in a program of body-building exercises, can have this effect. More research is needed.

Related to Negative Claims:
1) Suppresses growth in infants—This fear is based upon observations that lysine supplementation can result in growth suppression in immature rats and chicks. There is no evidence that this is true in humans, as well, but, to be entirely on the safe side, lysine supplementation is not recommended for children.

IV. RECOMMENDATIONS

A) *Suggested Intake:* Intake for optimal health is unknown. Adults in good health may take up to 1.5 grams daily in an effort to prevent herpes. Higher doses should be taken only with medical consent and monitoring.

B) *Source/Form:* There are many lysine supplements now on the market.

C) *Take With:* Those who wish to use lysine as an adjunct in a body-building exercise program may want to take lysine with an equal amount of arginine. There are supplements available that combine these two amino acids, or they may be purchased separately and taken at the same time. Best if taken on an empty stomach and not in combination with other amino acids.

D) *Cautionary Note:* Not recommended for children.

L-METHIONINE AND TAURINE
(Nervous System Regulators)

These are both sulfur-containing amino acids (see discussion of same under the analysis of cysteine, earlier in this chapter). There are unproved claims that methionine, which can be found in eggs, milk, liver, fish and many other foods, has therapeutic lipotropic activities similar to those of choline (see discussion of choline later in this book), which help eliminate fatty substances that might otherwise clog the arteries. Little useful research has been done on the possible therapeutic effects of methionine supplementation in humans. There is one study that indirectly suggests that methionine is destroyed by excessive use of alcohol. But, in any event, there is no doubt that methionine is very important in numerous processes in humans. Both cysteine (see discussion earlier) and taurine, two other important amino acids, depend upon adequate levels of methionine for their biosynthesis in the body.

There is increasing evidence that taurine is an important regulator of various nerve and muscle systems and that it may be essential for proper growth. Mammalian species apparently differ to some extent in their relative abilities to biosynthesize (produce in their own bodies) taurine; most seem to require at least some in their diets. Human work is largely lacking, but cats have been shown to suffer a tenfold reduction in tissue taurine levels a few months after having been placed on taurine-deficient diets. Some taurine is synthesized from methionine and cysteine, but eventually these sources prove inadequate and retinal degeneration is one of the consequences. (Very large quantities of taurine are found in the retina of the eye of many mammals.) Retarded growth has been noted in young monkeys fed taurine-free diets. More study will be required before any conclusions can be drawn about possible taurine deficiencies in humans and the consequences thereof.

Those who are considering taurine supplements—and some are on the market—are advised that numerous studies have shown that taurine has a *depressant* effect on the central nervous system and may adversely affect short-term memory. It is the nerve-depressant aspect of taurine that has attracted the interest of those concerned with epilepsy, which involves a state of neural *over*excitation. Taurine seems to inhibit and modulate various of the neurotransmitters, the chemical messengers of the brain. There have been reports on the benefits of oral taurine in the treatment of human epilepsy. Studies are ongoing to see whether taurine may be more useful in some instances than the standard anti-convulsants. Preliminary work also suggests taurine may eventually have some role in the treatment of cystic fibrosis and congestive heart failure.

For now, supplementation with either taurine or methionine appears ill-advised, though these substances may be useful in certain individuals, when prescribed by physicians. Taurine is present in meats and animal products but not in plant products.

L-PHENYLALANINE, D-PHENYLALANINE, DL-PHENYLALANINE

I. OVERVIEW: Pain Reliever?

The essential amino acid, L-Phenylalanine, is involved in a number of biochemical processes related to the brain synthesis of various neurotransmitters, principally dopamine, norepinephrine and epinephrine. It is claimed that L-phenylalanine can increase mental alertness, help control addictive-substance abuse, promote sexual arousal and release hormones that help control appetite. D-phenylalanine is a non-nutrient amino acid that has been shown to inhibit the breakdown of opiatelike substances called enkephalins in the brain. It is claimed that D-phenylalanine can help alleviate chronic pain.

II. CLAIMS

Positive:

1) Provides pain relief; 2) increases mental alertness and dispels depression; 3) suppresses appetite; 4) controls addictive behavior/cravings; 5) sexually stimulating.

Negative:

1) Can dangerously elevate blood pressure; 2) dangerous in combination with some anti-depressant drugs; 3) may promote growth of pigmented malignant melanoma; 4) contraindicated in persons with PKU.

III. EVIDENCE

Related to Positive Claims:

1) Provides pain relief—The non-nutrient D-phenylalanine has been shown to have analgesic as well as antiinflammatory effects in both animals and in humans. Studies have shown that D-phenylalanine helps alleviate back pain and dental pain. It is thought to work by inhibiting the breakdown of opiatelike substances called enkephalins in the brain. The nutrient L-phenylalanine does not have these properties. DL-phenylalanine which is available in health food stores consists of an equal mixture of D-phenylalanine and L-phenylalanine. There are many anecdotal claims that DL-phenylalanine is effective in the treatment of chronic pain in such conditions as arthritis and fibrositis. It is likely that the D-phenylalanine part of the mixture has something to do with these effects. However, DL-phenylalanine has not been scientifically tested in this regard. Since chronic pain is such a widespread problem and since D-phenylalanine and DL-phenylalanine are unlikely to have significant adverse effects for most people, further investigation of these substances is urgently needed.

2) Increases mental alertness and dispels depression—There have been anecdotal claims to this effect of L-phenylalanine for some time. With respect to depression, at least, there is now some supporting experimental evidence. In one study, forty depressed patients were given L-phenylalanine daily for up to six months in doses that began at 500 milligrams and gradually built up to, typically, 3 to 4 grams daily. They were also given 100 to 200 milligrams of vitamin B_6 daily to enhance the activity of the amino acid.

Thirty-one of these patients were said to have benefited to some extent from this treatment, and ten were reported to be completely relieved of depression. The principal investigator reported that those who responded positively did so "almost immediately."

This very promising study needs a placebo-controlled, double-blind follow-up.

3) Suppresses appetite—There is no sound evidence to support this claim.

4) Controls addictive behavior/cravings—There is some preliminary evidence that L-phenylalanine, in combination with other substances,

may help curb some addictive cravings (for alcohol and possibly some other drugs). Far more research will have to be done, however, before this claim can be taken seriously.

5) Sexually stimulating—Support for this claim is entirely lacking.

Related to Negative Claims:

1) Can dangerously elevate blood pressure—This has been reported in a few individuals taking L-phenylalanine. If you have high blood pressure consult your physician before using phenylalanine.

2) Dangerous in combination with some anti-depressant drugs—Persons taking anti-depressants containing monoamine oxidase inhibitors should definitely avoid L-phenylalanine supplements. The combination could cause dangerously high blood pressure.

3) May promote growth of pigmented melanoma—If you have a melanoma (form of skin cancer), consult your physician before using L-phenylalanine. L-phenylalanine does not produce melanomas but may help nourish them once they develop.

4) Contraindicated in persons with PKU—People suffering from PKU (phenylketonuria) have an inherited inability to metabolize L-phenylalanine and should, of course, avoid phenylalanine supplements.

IV. RECOMMENDATIONS

A) *Suggested Intake:* Intake for optimal health is unknown. Those who wish to try DL-phenylalanine for chronic pain may take up to 1.5 grams per day. At higher doses consult a physician. The same applies to L-phenylalanine for depression.

B) *Source/Form:* DL-phenylalanine typically comes in 375-milligram doses, L-phenylalanine usually in 500-milligram doses. There are many different brands available.

C) *Take With:* If you use L-phenylalanine for depression you may want to take 20–30 milligrams of vitamin B_6 with the L-phenylalanine. Do not take more than 50 milligrams of B_6 daily. Otherwise take alone and on an empty stomach for maximum effect.

D) *Cautionary Note:* Persons with high blood pressure should use phenylalanine only with a doctor's permission. Persons with PKU, malignant melanoma and those using anti-depressants containing monoamine oxidase inhibitors should not use phenylalanine.

L-TRYPTOPHAN

I. OVERVIEW: Mind/Mood Regulator

L-tryptophan is one of the essential amino acids. (You must get it in your diet.) It was one of the first amino acids to be marketed as an individual supplement—in this case as a "natural sleeping aid." Tryptophan is particularly important in the biosynthesis of a brain neurotransmitter called serotonin, thought to be an inducer and regulator of certain stages of sleep, among other things. Some preliminary research suggests that serotonin may also reduce sensitivity to pain and have tranquilizing effects. There are also claims that tryptophan is an appetite suppressor and that it can reduce cravings for alcohol and some other drugs. It may even help prevent panic attacks. The bad news is that in November, 1989 the FDA recalled supplementary tryptophan because of several reports associating the amino acid with some severe side effects.

II. CLAIMS

Positive:
1) Natural sleeping aid and jet lag treatment; 2) mood/behavior regulator; 3) pain reliever; 4) suppresses appetite; 5) suppresses alcohol and amphetamine cravings; 6) inhibits hyperventilation and panic attacks.

Negative:
1) May contribute to bladder cancer; 2) may, in high doses, lead to liver abnormalities; 3) toxic.

III. EVIDENCE

Related to Positive Claims:
1) Natural sleeping aid and jet lag treatment—This is the most persistent claim made for tryptophan, and what few studies have been done related to this issue seem to substantiate it, at least to some degree. In

general, tryptophan seems to have gentle sedative effects and, in some, induces drowsiness and sleep. It does this without the adverse effects typical "sleeping pill" medications often produce. Tryptophan is particularly useful as a sleeping aid if taken just before bedtime with carbohydrates. Even some who suffer from chronic insomnia may benefit from tryptophan, according to Swiss researchers who gave such patients 2 grams of the amino acid thirty minutes before bedtime for three days followed by four days without supplementation, then by three days with supplementation and so on until benefits were experienced. After three months of this "interval" treatment, a significant number of these victims of severe insomnia were said to have recovered completely. Most of the others were also helped substantially with continued tryptophan treatment. The benefits have persisted in many two years after they were first treated, according to the report.

Tryptophan's ability to induce natural-seeming sleep also led to a recent investigation of its possible use in reducing the harmful effects of jet lag. In this University of California (San Diego) School of Medicine study, fifty-one U.S. marines flown across eight time zones were divided into two groups. Half got tryptophan and the other half got placebos. Those who got the amino acid were able to sleep more, not only during their long flight but also during the first night upon arrival at their destination. (They continued to get tryptophan for three days after arrival.) And on several tests involving performance, such as reaction times, the tryptophan-treated marines did better.

Tryptophan appears to work well as an alternative to the standard hypnotic sleeping drugs.

2) Mood/behavior regulator—There is evidence that tryptophan, through its effects on serotonin, has an impact on human behavior in a number of ways. Preliminary studies suggest that supplemental tryptophan may have anti-anxiety and other calming effects that could, among other things, help control aggressive behavior in *some* individuals without resort to the sort of major tranquilizing drugs that have so many serious side effects. There is anecdotal evidence that the manic phase of the manic-depressive disorder can be partially or wholly controlled in some cases. There are, in addition, preliminary indications that some types of depression may be helped by supplementation with this amino acid.

3) Pain reliever—Some recent studies lend support to earlier findings of pain relief via tryptophan supplementation. Some sufferers of chronic pain have been found to have decreased levels of serotonin in their cerebrospinal fluid. The combination of tryptophan and a high-carbohydrate diet reportedly boosts serotonin and diminishes pain in some of these chronic cases.

4) Suppresses appetite—Because tryptophan can alleviate some forms of anxiety and depression, some assumed it could be useful in favorably altering behavior that may contribute to overeating. Studies involving tryptophan have shown appetite suppression in animals. Results in humans have been mixed. One of the positive studies utilized doses of tryptophan in the 2–3-gram range. This resulted in a subjective decrease in hunger and a short-term reduction in food intake. The subjects in this study, however, were men who were lean to begin with. In a better designed and more relevant study, markedly obese individuals were given 3 grams of tryptophan daily supplemented by psychologic therapy and behavior modification designed to reinforce caloric restriction. Despite all this, these subjects did *not* lose more weight than other obese patients treated in the same way but with placebo instead of tryptophan. The researchers in this study conceded, however, that these extremely obese individuals may require doses higher than 3 grams per day, since doses in that range did, in fact, seem to have appetite-suppressing effects in lean individuals, as noted above, and, to some extent, in more mildly obese people.

5) Suppresses alcohol and amphetamine cravings—Tryptophan itself has not been shown to have any measurable effect on alcohol craving but this has not been directly investigated. The idea that tryptophan might thus be effective apparently springs from recent research indicating that some newly emerging drugs that affect brain serotonin activity can inhibit alcohol craving. Tryptophan is the precursor of brain serotonin. Some work suggests that these drugs may be able to reverse Korsakoff's psychosis, memory loss due to alcohol and the cause of one of the most prevalent forms of dementia in the United States. One of the drugs that is being developed for use in alcoholism, the antidepressant Prozac, which maintains brain levels of serotonin, also, incidentally, inhibits binge eating in bulimics. More studies are needed and are currently underway in this exciting area of research.

Amphetamine craving has been markedly diminished, in rats, with the use of tryptophan. The rats, in this experiment, were surgically implanted with jugular catheters through which, by pressing levers with their paws, they could self-administer injections of d-amphetamine, a powerfully stimulating drug. When pretreated with tryptophan, rats injected themselves with far less amphetamine. The researchers tested the idea that the tryptophan might simply be sedating the rats and found that this could be largely ruled out. The animals exhibited no signs of decreased motor ability. It is hypothesized that tryptophan, through its effects on brain neurotransmitters, alters perception of drug effects in ways that make the drug no longer or less rewarding. Possibly the tryptophan itself provides a substitute reward.

6) Inhibits hyperventilation and panic attacks—Hyperventilation (overbreathing) has long been thought to be the result of anxiety or panic. It is now known that it also may be the other way around, that improper breathing (usually of long standing and originating early in life) can lead to dramatic intermittent episodes of hyperventilation, feelings of anxiety and even full-fledged panic attacks. Some very preliminary research suggests that vitamin B_6 and tryptophan may help reduce the severity of hyperventilation and the anxiety and panic it can produce.

Related to Negative Claims:
1) May contribute to bladder cancer—A study done many years ago gave rise to this claim. More recent studies, however, show no relationship between tryptophan and bladder cancer.

2) May, in high doses, lead to liver abnormalities—An animal study, using doses of tryptophan equivalent to 4 to 5 grams daily in humans, found evidence of fatty deposits in the livers of these animals. There have been no reports of liver damage in humans taking tryptophan at high doses for prolonged periods, but this possibility should be further investigated.

3) Toxic—In December, 1989 the FDA and CDC reported over 600 cases of a flu-like syndrome associated with a blood abnormality (eosinophilia) in those taking tryptophan. It is unclear as of this writing whether this was a rare reaction from the tryptophan, or, *more likely,* from a contaminant in the preparation. However, because of these adverse effects, the FDA recalled supplementary tryptophan in November, 1989.

IV. RECOMMENDATIONS

To be completely on the safe side, do not use supplementary L-tryptophan until it has been determined that the available products are completely safe to take (see Toxic—above). *And when this occurs, use only under a physician's guidance.*

L-TYROSINE

I. OVERVIEW: Anti-Depressant

L-tyrosine is not an essential amino acid since it is synthesized (from phenylalanine) in the body. Like phenylalanine, tyrosine is intimately involved with the important brain neurotransmitters epinephrine, norepinephrine and dopamine. Claims for tyrosine are similar to those being made for L-phenylalanine, although, in some respects, tyrosine appears to be more useful.

II. CLAIMS

Positive:
1) Psychic energizer and stress reliever; 2) anti-depressant; 3) effective in the treatment of PMS; 4) addictive-drug detoxifier.

Negative:
1) May elevate blood pressure; 2) dangerous if combined with anti-depressants containing monoamine oxidase inhibitors; 3) might trigger migraine headaches; 4) might promote growth of malignant melanoma.

III. EVIDENCE

Related to Positive Claims:
1) Psychic energizer and stress reliever—Animals subjected to stress in the laboratory have been found to have reduced levels of the brain neurotransmitter norepinephrine. Treating with tyrosine prior to stressing the animals prevents reduction of norepinephrine.

Findings such as these led to human tyrosine experiments in which soldiers undergoing various forms of stress were given tyrosine to see what effect it might have on their performance. In one of these experiments conditions were created that simulate rapid ascent to 15,500 feet in light clothing. This dramatically stresses the mind and body and significantly diminishes the oxygen supply to the brain.

Some of the soldiers thus stressed were given tyrosine supplements prior to this challenge and some were not. Those who got the tyrosine performed much better on a variety of tests than those who did not get the supplements. The tyrosine-dosed soldiers were more alert, efficient, less anxious and had fewer complaints about the physical discomforts of their sudden "ascent." They complained less of such things as muscle soreness and headaches and were more resistant to cold.

These intriguing studies need follow-up and suggest that tyrosine may provide an attractive alternative to some of the psychiatric drugs now commonly used—since tyrosine, by comparison, is much safer.

2) Anti-depressant—Studies such as those cited above, as well as growing anecdotal evidence and clinical observation, suggest that tyrosine may be an effective anti-depressant in some major forms of depression. Well-controlled studies remain to be done.

3) Effective in the treatment of PMS (premenstrual syndrome)—Again, there is a growing body of anecdotal evidence and accumulating clinical observation that tyrosine supplements can be quite helpful in reducing the irritation, depression and tiredness of PMS. This claim needs to be evaluated in a well-designed study.

4) Addictive-drug detoxifier—Tyrosine is now being used, reportedly with some success, to aid in the treatment of and withdrawal from cocaine abuse. In one study, tryptophan and tyrosine were used in conjunction with the anti-depressant imipramine to treat chronic cocaine abuse with a reported 75–80 percent success rate. Success was judged to be a reduction of at least 50 percent in cocaine use up to complete discontinuance. Most of those participating in the study said this combination not only blocked the cocaine high but also warded off the severe depression that typically accompanies discontinuance or marked reduction in cocaine intake. A placebo-controlled, double-blind follow-up of this study is planned.

Other researchers at UCLA and elsewhere, have also reported favorably on regimens containing tryptophan and tyrosine for the treatment of cocaine abuse.

Related to Negative Claims:

1) May elevate blood pressure—This has been reported in a few cases.

2) Dangerous if combined with anti-depressants containing monoamine oxidase inhibitors—This combination can produce dangerously elevated blood pressure.

3) Might trigger migraine headaches—There is only scant anecdotal evidence that this might be the case in some migraine sufferers.

4) Might promote growth of malignant melanoma—There is no proof of this but it remains a possibility. This does not mean that tyrosine produces melanoma, a skin cancer, but only that if a melanoma develops due to other reasons, a lot of tyrosine might help nourish the growth.

IV. RECOMMENDATIONS

A) *Suggested Intake:* Optimal intake is unknown. For PMS (with depression and fatigue as the major symptoms), I recommend 500-milligram doses before each of three meals. If that is ineffective, try 1,000-milligram (1 gram) doses before each meal. For depression I recommend the same regimen. If results are inadequate you may, with the consent of your physician, gradually work up to as much as 12 grams of tyrosine (in divided, premeal doses) daily. To counteract stress, see what results you can get with 1,500 milligrams daily. If more is required, again first consult your physician.

B) *Source/Form:* There are now many tyrosine supplements on the market.

C) *Take With:* Take on an empty stomach. Do not combine with other amino acids. Taking with up to 25 milligrams (no more than 50 milligrams *total* daily) vitamin B_6 may be helpful.

D) *Cautionary Note:* Do not take tyrosine if you suffer from migraine headaches and find that this amino acid triggers migraine attacks. Do not take tyrosine with anti-depressants containing monoamine oxidase inhibitors. If you develop a malignant melanoma, do not take tyrosine without your physician's approval. If you suffer from high blood pressure, don't take tyrosine without your doctor's approval.

SEVEN

Nucleic Acids and

Derivatives

Some of the most important biomedical discoveries of all time were made during this century. They concern substances we call the nucleic acids. These are large biologic molecules within which are encoded the genetic instructions that determine biologic specificity, that is, whether we will be a bacterium, a cat, a human being or any number of other life forms. Nucleic acid genetic material also helps determine what color and size we will be and even, to a certain extent, whether we will have a sweet or a sour disposition, an analytical or a creative frame of mind.

There are essentially two major categories of nucleic acids: deoxyribonucleic acid, or DNA, and ribonucleic acid, or RNA. The information that these acids impart depends upon the arrangement—the sequence— of molecules called the purine and pyrimidine bases. The bases that combine in various sequences to make up the "messages" of DNA are called adenine, guanine, thymine and cytosine. Adenine, guanine and cytosine are also found in RNA, but thymine is replaced by uracil. These individual bases are strung together along a backbone comprised of phosphate and a sugar called deoxyribose in the case of DNA and ribose in the case of RNA.

The genetic instructions contained within DNA are transferred to RNA by a process known as "transcription." Once information is transferred or transcribed from DNA to RNA it is utilized to build biologic matter by causing the twenty amino acids to line up in the proper sequences required to make protein. This process is called translation. The formation of life thus depends upon the proper translation of the original genetic code contained in the DNA. The continuity of the DNA code is ensured by repair processes and by DNA replication. Cellular aging has been attributed to errors that occur during DNA repair, DNA replication, the synthesis of RNA (transcription) and the synthesis of proteins (translation).

It is not difficult to understand, then, why nucleic acids and various nucleic derivatives have become staples in the food-supplement supermarket. The makers of cosmetics, too, have been quick to incorporate RNA, DNA and derivatives into hair and skin products. The idea is that as we age, our DNA/RNA become depleted or, in any event, are prone to increasing "error." Thus, it is argued, we must "replace" our lost or ineffective nucleic acids with supplemental forms. This is, in a sense, an offshoot of "cellular therapy," where oral and injected preparations of young cells—from various tissues and organs—were given to replace "worn-out" tissues and organs in aging bodies.

The physician who is mainly responsible for the popularity of dietary and cosmetic nucleic acids is the late Dr. Benjamin S. Frank, who believed that *dietary* nucleic acids were essential for optimal health. His ideas were not widely accepted, however, because his results were largely anecdotal. We probably do experience breakdowns and shortages in nucleic acids and their machinery as we age, but oral supplements are not likely to do us much good. There is some evidence that synthetic preparations may have some pharmacologic effects (discussed below), but these are not really related to the claims made in the popular literature. Perhaps one day we *will* be able to dramatically retard aging via nucleic acid manipulation, but that will require sophisticated gene surgery.

DNA AND RNA

I. OVERVIEW: Life and Longer Life

Given the fact that the nucleic acids DNA and RNA are equated with life itself, it is hardly surprising that these substances and their various derivatives are well represented in the supplement supermarket. DNA and RNA are widely incorporated into shampoos and cosmetics, as well, attended by claims, implied or explicit, that these substances will add "life" to skin and hair.

The idea is promoted that as we age our DNA/RNA become depleted or defective. It is argued, then, that we must replace our lost or ineffective nucleic acids with supplemental forms. This is, in a sense, an extension of "cell therapy" in which preparations of cells from various tissues and organs of young animals are given, by injections or orally, in an effort to replace "worn-out" tissues and organs in our aging bodies.

Cell therapy has been widely rejected by the scientific community and, for the most part, rightly so. Some of the cellular substances that have been injected are hazardous and, in any case, show no sign of working.

There have been widespread, almost universal, doubts that taking oral RNA/DNA supplements could benefit us, either, since it has always been assumed that these substances would be destroyed in the gut before they could get to target organs and tissues. It has only been very recently that the first scientific evidence has emerged that nucleic acid supplementation might be beneficial, after all. This work opens up several exciting possibilities.

II. CLAIMS

Positive:

1) Retard aging; 2) improve memory and mental functioning; 3) stimulate immunity; 4) fight cancer.

Negative:

1) Produce excessive uric acid and may promote or aggravate gout.

III. EVIDENCE

Related to Positive Claims:

1) Retard aging—It was first reported some years ago that nucleic acid supplements can retard aging, in general, and most of the degenerative

diseases that go along with aging. These claims were based on a few animal experiments and upon largely undocumented studies, short on controls and high in subjectivity.

There were, however, a very few studies, even some years ago, suggestive of possibly genuine efforts using RNA/DNA *injections*. In one of these studies, rats injected once a week with DNA and RNA reportedly lived twice as long as control rats that did not get these nucleic acid injections. This was a very small study, however, and apparently was never followed up. In another, somewhat more recent study, mice with induced tumors lived significantly longer when given RNA. The possible life-prolonging effects of supplemental RNA and DNA should be further investigated, scant though the evidence in support of this claim is.

2) Improve memory and mental functioning—There is a report that *injections* of RNA can be of some benefit in senility. Follow-up on this work has been inconclusive and not very promising.

3) Stimulate immunity—If DNA and RNA supplements really are anti-aging substances they would almost certainly have to exhibit some immune-stimulating properties. Until very recently there was little evidence that they possess these properties (except in derivative and synthetic forms—see below).

Now papers, based upon well-designed research, have been appearing in the medical literature reporting, for the first time, that nucleic acid supplementation can boost resistance to both fungal and bacterial infections. In these experiments animals were fed diets devoid of the nucleotides that are the building blocks of nucleic acids and were compared with other groups of animals fed diets enriched with varying amounts of these RNA/DNA nucleotides. The nucleotide-free diets were found to suppress immunity and shorten survival times significantly. The nucleotide-enriched diets, on the other hand, decreased susceptibility to infection.

These promising studies need to be confirmed and expanded. They provide us with the first real evidence that RNA/DNA supplements might actually be of benefit.

There are, in addition, a number of studies attesting to the validity of some synthetic forms of nucleic acids (currently being used as experimental drugs) to favorably affect immunity.

One of these is a synthetic polyribonucleotide called Poly(A)/Poly(U). Another is called Poly(I,C). These potentiate various components of the immune system and are being investigated as anti-cancer agents, as well (see below). Early research indicates that these unique and quite potent substances may be useful against a broad spectrum of bacterial, viral and fungal diseases. There is even very preliminary evidence that they may be helpful in such autoimmune disorders as multiple sclerosis and have been suggested for experimental use against AIDS.

Meanwhile, another synthetic polynucleotide, called Ampligen, is already being investigated as an experimental AIDS treatment. A chemically modified form of DNA, called apurinic acid, has also been shown to inhibit the virus believed to be a major component in AIDS.

Clearly, the immune-stimulating properties of both natural and synthetic nucleic acids deserve further research.

4) Fight cancer—There has been only very little investigation of RNA and DNA, in their natural forms, as possible anti-cancer agents. In one study, cited earlier, mice with induced cancers did live significantly longer than controls when given RNA.

Most work, however, has involved synthetic forms of the nucleic acids. Poly(A)/Poly(U), for example, has been used, with considerable promise, in the treatment of breast cancer. More work is proceeding in this area.

Related to Negative Claims:
1) Produce excessive uric acid and may promote or aggravate gout—The danger here appears to be slight, but anyone with gout or a tendency to develop gout should use nucleic acid supplements only with a physician's approval.

IV. RECOMMENDATIONS

A) *Suggested Intake:* If you want to try nucleic acids to see if they have any effect on your immunity or energy, I suggest taking up to 1.5 grams daily.

B) *Source/Form:* There are several RNA supplements on the market. You can also get RNA in nutritional yeasts (which are about 10 percent RNA). You'll get about 1.5 grams in a tablespoon of brewer's yeast.

C) *Cautionary Note:* Don't use nucleic acid supplements without your physician's approval if you have a tendency to develop gout.

ADENOSINE
(From Heart to Herpes)

There has been quite a flurry of interest lately in adenosine and its derivatives. Adenosine has been used with some apparent success in helping control irregular heart rhythms, in strengthening cardiac muscle and in relieving the pain of angina pectoris. There's some evidence to suggest it may be of benefit in congestive heart failure and in reducing the death rate from recurrent heart attack.

There are also preliminary reports that adenosine may lower cholesterol, reduce the stiffness of arthritis, protect against radiation and some neurologic disorders.

That an adenosine drug is useful in the treatment of herpes zoster has been reported based upon a double-blind, placebo-controlled study. Herpes zoster, popularly known as shingles, is characterized by painful blisters and most frequently afflicts those over age fifty and those who are immunocompromised.

In this study, seventeen herpes zoster patients got adenosine monophosphate (AMP) injections three times a week for four weeks; fifteen control subjects got placebo injections. At the end of the four weeks, 88 percent of the AMP-treated patients were reportedly free of their symptoms, while only 43 percent of the controls were. The investigators reported, moreover, that two years after the conclusion of the study there had been no recurrences of herpes zoster among those successfully treated in the study.

Adenosine's role in immunity is just beginning to be investigated. In the meantime, until more is known, I don't recommend supplementation.

INOSINE AND ISOPRINOSINE
(Immune Stimulator)

Inosine has been used overseas for a variety of things, but most of the interest is directed at a derivative of this substance: isoprinosine. Marketed as a drug in many nations (but not yet in the United States), isoprinosine has established an impressive record for itself as an immune stimulator in a variety of circumstances. It is possible that it also has direct anti-viral properties.

Isoprinosine has been used for many years, with reported good results, in some cases of subacute sclerosing panencephalitis, believed to be caused by measles or a related virus. In test-tube studies, many of them quite recent, isoprinosine has demonstrated positive effects on several of the most important components of the immune system. This substance has also been shown to increase the anti-tumor effects of interferon, to inactivate some of the herpes viruses and to significantly help sufferers of aphthous stomatitis resistant to all other treatments.

Lately, isoprinosine has been exciting attention in some AIDS research circles. In a double-blind, placebo-controlled study of male homosexuals with prolonged generalized lymph-gland swelling and various depressed immune parameters, twenty-eight days of isoprinosine treatment resulted in clinical improvement in 29 percent of the treated patients as opposed to only 5 percent of the placebo patients, an improvement that persisted at least six months, when the patients were examined again.

Further research on the possible role of isoprinosine in HIV (human immunodeficiency virus) disease is underway.

Isoprinosine can be used in the United States under some circumstances. Consult your physician and use it only under medical supervision. Those with gout or a predisposition to develop gout should not use inosine or isoprinosine.

OROTIC ACID

Russian researchers reported that orotic acid is helpful in post-heart-attack treatment. Others have found that it increases the strength of contraction of damaged cardiac muscle in experimental animals and have speculated it might have some future use in the management of congestive heart failure, particularly since it is relatively non-toxic compared to the currently used drugs, such as digitalis. A study conducted many years ago that attributed a cholesterol-lowering effect to orotic acid was not confirmed in a more recent investigation of this issue.

I do not recommend supplementation with orotic acid.

EIGHT

Lipids and Derivatives

The 1980s can be called the decade of fat (lipid) consciousness. Several prestigious medical and scientific organizations decided that there is ample evidence that a high-fat and high-cholesterol diet is not healthy and that it is time that people lowered fat and cholesterol intakes. In 1988 the Surgeon General joined this battle, making it a top health priority.

Actually, not all lipids are our enemies; as you'll soon learn, some are looking downright friendly.

Lipids are a heterogeneous group of biologic compounds that in contrast to carbohydrates and proteins are defined according to their solubility rather than their chemical structure. Of all the biologic substances, the lipids are those that are least soluble in water. Lipids are commonly called fats, although in stricter usage fat comprises the most abundant kinds of lipids called triglycerides or neutral fats. In addition to triglycerides, substances classified as lipids include phospholipids, (phosphatidylcholine, phosphatidylethanolamine, phosphatidylserine and phosphatidylinositol), cholesterol, steroids (cortisone, testosterone, estrogen, progesterone), sphingolipids (glycosphingolipids, sphingomyelin and cerebrosides), fatty acids (saturated, monounsaturated, polyunsaturated, prostaglandins and leukotrienes) and vitamins A, D, E and K.

High cholesterol levels are associated with an increased incidence of coronary heart disease and heart attacks. Diets of Western societies have had a tendency to be high in triglyceride (common fats), cholesterol and fatty acids, especially of the saturated types. We now know that increased intake of fatty acids of the *mono*unsaturated types (e.g., oleic acid—found in olive oil) and of the *poly*unsaturated types (linoleic acid, linolenic acid) can lower serum cholesterol levels and protect against coronary heart disease.

Recently some evidence has emerged that even one of the saturated fatty acids, stearic acid, can lower serum cholesterol levels. Long-chain fatty acids, found in cold-water oily fish, can decrease platelet stickiness, which is also considered beneficial in the prevention of coronary heart disease. The so-called fish oils can lower cholesterol levels in those who also have elevated triglyceride levels and they also have anti-inflammatory properties.

Linoleic acid, which is an omega-6 polyunsaturated fatty acid, was considered, until recently, the only essential fatty acid for humans. That is, humans cannot make linoleic acid and are thus absolutely dependent on dietary sources for it. The omega-3 fatty acid, alpha-linolenic acid, which is found in certain plants, is now also considered essential.

An important concept that has now become popular is that of "membrane fluidity." This refers to the responsiveness and resiliency of cells. As cells age, their membranes become less fluid and more rigid. The ratio of cholesterol to phospholipids (mainly phosphatidylcholine) in the cell membrane is associated with its fluidity. The higher the ratio the lower the fluidity and vice versa. Also, the greater the degree of saturation of fatty acids in the membrane structure, the less its fluidity. By the same token, the greater the degree of unsaturation of fatty acid, the greater its fluidity.

Cellular membrane fluidity can be influenced by diet. Nutrients that increase membrane fluidity include fish oils and phosphatidylcholine (of the type that contain polyunsaturated fatty acids). Diets low in saturated fats and cholesterol maintain membrane fluidity; diets high in these substances produce rigid membranes. Thus, we see that cholesterol not only plugs up our arteries but also our very cells. A new field is emerging called membrane engineering. Substances are now available, made from lipids, which can fluidize cell membranes and potentially rejuvenate cells. "Fats" may, ironically, turn out to be some of the most exciting "anti-aging," disease-fighting nutritional and pharmacologic substances of the next decade.

AL 721
(Useful in AIDS?)

In late 1986 reports began circulating in the popular press and, then, in some medical magazines about a substance that was being used in Israel for the treatment of ARC (AIDS-related complex) and AIDS. The substance is called AL 721. In most cases, letters and/or numbers are code terms for experimental medicines to hide their true identities. This was not the case for AL 721. AL 721 stands for *a*ctive *l*ipid made up of 70 percent or *7* parts of neutral lipids, 20 percent or *2* parts of phosphatidylcholine and 10 percent or *1* part of phosphatidylethanolamine. The lipids are derived from egg yolk, which means that their fatty acids are mainly of the saturated variety.

AL 721 exists as an aggregate of the above lipids, a kind of soap bubble, if you will. It is thought to work by modifying the structure and fluidity of cell membranes by removing cholesterol and possibly adding phosphatidylcholine and phosphatidylethanolamine to the membranes. Membrane fluidity, which is crucial to the cell's responsiveness and processing of nutrients and information, is determined by the ratio of *c*holesterol and *p*hospholipid (mainly phosphatidylcholine), or the C/PL ratio of the membrane. The greater the C/PL ratio, the more rigid or less fluid the membrane, and vice versa. Typically the C/PL ratio increases with aging and this is associated with certain cells, such as immune cells, losing their special functions. AL 721 was developed by the Israeli scientist Meier Schinitzky and colleagues at the Weizmann Institute in 1981, and was shown to lower the C/PL ratios of several different types of cells, even though its phosphatidylcholine utilizes saturated fatty acids. Its reported benefits, if confirmed, seem to hinge on its unusual geometry.

Many pathogenic human viruses contain lipid membranes as part of their structure. Such viruses include herpes simplex I and II, herpes zoster, cytomegalovirus (CMV), Epstein-Barr virus (EBV), the influenza viruses and HIV (human immunodeficiency virus), which is the prime player in AIDS. In November, 1985, a letter appeared in the *New England Journal of Medicine* demonstrating that AL 721 clearly interfered with the infection of cells by HIV *in vitro* (in the test tube). Presumably, it did this by altering the lipid membrane of the virus. Others have reported that AL 721 interferes with the infectivity of herpes virus in animals, as well.

In 1986 it was reported that several AIDS patients who were being treated with AL 721 in Israel appeared to do better clinically. Since the method of making AL 721 was published and the patent readily obtainable, it wasn't too long before copycat or "work-alike" versions of AL 721 became available in the United States. In fact, the company that holds the patent on AL 721 decided against pursuing FDA approval of the substance as a drug and instead, at this writing, plans to sell it as a food supplement.

AL 721 or, more commonly, one of the AL 721 "work-alikes" have been, or are being, used by many who are infected with the HIV virus including those with lymphadenopathy syndrome (LAS), ARC and AIDS. Those who use these substances usually start with 10 grams twice a day for a month and then 10 grams daily. Some report feeling better when taking this substance, some report improvement in their T-helper lymphocyte counts (these cells decrease as the disease progresses), some report no difference and some say they do worse. But, overall, those taking these substances appear to be doing better clinically than before they started taking them. No one, however, believes AL 721 is a cure for AIDS.

There are a few studies going on looking at the effects of AL 721, in LAS, ARC and AIDS patients, either alone or in combination with the anti-viral agent AZT. A 1988 study looked at the effects of AL 721 in eight patients with LAS. AL 721 given at 10 grams twice daily was found to reduce the extent of HIV proliferation in five of the patients and to improve immune-cell responsiveness in four of the patients. No change was noted in the number of T-helper lymphocytes. AL 721 was stopped after eight weeks and then restarted after a four-month period at 15 grams twice daily. The results were not nearly as positive in the follow-up study. A "rebound effect" had earlier been reported, suggesting that those starting the substance should continue it without interruption.

It is possible that AL 721 will play a useful role, even if a small one, in the fight against AIDS.

In addition, AL 721 may have immune-enhancing effects. The Israeli scientists withdrew lymphocytes from men between seventy and seventy-five years old and found that treatment of these cells *in vitro* (in the test tube) with AL 721 produced a marked increase in immune responsiveness. In another experiment, blood taken from elderly subjects was found to have significantly greater anti-bacterial activity if the subjects were first treated with AL 721. AL 721 did not stimulate lymphocyte activity of young subjects, nor did it increase anti-bacterial activity of blood from young donors. Immune responsiveness is known to decrease with age, and the Israeli researchers believe that AL 721 has a rejuvenating effect on the immune system of the elderly. Much more research is needed to verify this. It is possible that whatever benefits this substance may have in HIV-infected individuals are due to immune enhancement, though AL 721 may also have direct anti-viral activity.

The Israeli researchers found that AL 721, given orally or by injection, reduced, or almost completely eliminated, withdrawal symptoms in morphine-addicted mice. (See discussion of this in analysis of lecithin in this section.) More research on the possible role of AL 721 and phosphatidylcholine in the treatment of drug addiction is urgently needed. AL 721 has also been suggested for the treatment of Chronic Fatigue Syndrome, which appears to be increasingly prevalent these days. In some cases of chronic fatigue, viruses as well as immune dysfunctions are involved. Some with these disorders are trying AL 721 at doses of 10 grams daily or 10 grams twice a day, and in a few cases those who are taking it claim that it makes them feel less tired. These are all anecdotal reports. There have not been any controlled studies on the effects of AL 721 in this illness.

Reversal of aging of cells, rejuvenating the immune system, anti-viral activity, abolishing the withdrawal symptoms of drug and alcohol dependence, and more—such are the claims for AL 721. Will it turn out to be a miracle substance or will it fizzle out as many have before? Only time and continued research will tell the story. It is apparent, however, that various lipids look very promising as potential therapies in a wide range of ailments. Perhaps AL 721, even if it doesn't live up to its promises, will help point the way to new lipid preparations that will.

FISH OILS/EPA AND DHA

I. OVERVIEW: Wonders from the Sea

If the fish oils were causing excitement a few years ago, they're inciting something akin to a revolution today. Originally touted, with justification, for their cardiovascular protective effects, the fish oils are now the subjects of feverish research, some of which suggests that these remarkable oils may also be helpful in arthritis and other inflammatory disorders, in hypertension, psoriasis, possibly even in some forms of cancer and kidney disease.

These oils contain two long-chain fatty acids called eicosopentaenoic acid (EPA) and docosahexaenoic acid (DHA) that affect the synthesis of prostaglandins, a complex family of hormone-like substances that have far-reaching regulatory effects in the body. Most of the interest has thus far focused on EPA. The two fatty acids have similar and distinct functions. EPA is the precursor of DHA, and some believe the latter can "convert back" to EPA when body needs so require.

People began getting excited about fish oils when epidemiologic studies of Eskimos and Japanese, who consume large quantities of fish and other marine life rich in these oils, were completed and the results analyzed. Researchers found that both groups studied are at far lower risk than most other populations of suffering from various heart and circulatory disorders, which are among the major killers of our time.

II. CLAIMS

Positive:
1) Protects against cardiovascular disease; 2) protects against hypertension; 3) useful in the treatment of arthritis and other inflammatory disorders; 4) helpful in the treatment of psoriasis and other skin problems; 5) helps prevent/treat cancer; 6) therapeutic in kidney disease.

Negative:
1) Toxic; 2) harmful in diabetics; 3) can cause vitamin deficiencies.

III. EVIDENCE

Related to Positive Claims:
1) Protects against cardiovascular disease—It is a striking fact that despite a diet high in protein, fat and cholesterol and very low in carbo-

hydrate, fiber and vitamin C, many Eskimos have a remarkably low incidence of blood clots, narrowing of the arteries, heart attacks and other manifestations of cardiovascular disease. Greenland Eskimos, whose diet consists primarily of fish, seal and whale meat, have low blood levels of triglycerides and total cholesterol, high levels of high-density lipoprotein (HDL) cholesterol, which is known to have a cardiovascular protective effect, and decreased platelet aggregation, which makes them resistant to clotting disorders. In coastal villages of Japan where fish is the main dietary staple, similar epidemiologic findings have been noted.

The primary protective component of this diet has been identified as EPA, which is believed to exert its favorable effects through prostaglandin activity. Among other things, EPA inhibits prostaglandin effects that promote blood-clotting mechanisms. DHA apparently has similar effects through a separate pathway.

There have now been numerous clinical studies to assess the cardioprotective effects of fish diets, fish oils and supplements. Nearly all of these human studies have revealed benefits. The fish oils have been demonstrated to reduce blood levels of low-density lipoproteins (LDL) and very-low-density lipoproteins (VLDL). LDL and VLDL are harmful forms of cholesterol. These effects have not always been consistent, however, a fact some attribute to doses of fish oils they say have been inadequate in some studies.

A triglyceride-lowering effect is seen more consistently. Reduction in elevated blood levels of this fat are beneficial to cardiac health.

There is more agreement over the anti-clotting effects of fish oils. The oils inhibit blood platelet "stickiness" of the sort that contributes to clots. It takes fairly large doses of fish oils to get this effect, however—3.6 grams per day for two weeks in one study.

In one long-term (two-year) trial, fish oil supplements reduced angina pain and diminished the need, among these patients, for nitroglycerin. This effect was not confirmed in two small, short-term (twelve-week) studies, which have, however, been faulted for their design. More long-term work will have to be done.

Overall, the fish oils appear to have a promising future in the cardiovascular realm.

2) Protects against hypertension—This claim relates to the foregoing claim. Hypertension—high blood pressure—is the leading cause of stroke. Again, through effects in prostaglandins, this time leading to

events that promote vasodilation, the opening up of vessels so that blood can flow through with less constriction, the fish oils can lower blood pressure in some patients. In one study, hypertensive patients were fed mackerel (supplying 2.2 grams of EPA daily) for two weeks. This resulted in significant reductions in blood pressure. Several studies have now documented this effect, but the definitive long-term investigation still remains to be done.

For now it must be said that the fish oils appear to be useful in lowering blood pressure.

3) Useful in the treatment of arthritis—Recent investigation of this claim are yielding promising results. Fish oils have an anti-inflammatory effect, as demonstrated in both animal and human experiments. In one study, rheumatoid arthritis patients were given fish oil supplements containing 1.8 grams of EPA daily. This seemed to stop further progression of the disease in those getting the EPA, while progression continued in controls who received only placebos. Subsequent studies have also shown benefits. In one of these the daily dosage was 2.7 grams of EPA and 0.125 grams of DHA, continued for fourteen weeks. Side effects were minimal (stomach upsets, in some cases) and usually disappeared within two weeks.

It should be stressed that while the fish oils are showing promise as agents that can reduce the symptoms of rheumatoid arthritis and perhaps even slow its progression in some cases, it is not a cure for the disease.

There are suggestions that fish oils may be useful in treating some other inflammatory processes, as well. A study is in progress, for example, to see what effect fish oil can have on bronchial asthma. Other studies have already been conducted, with reported good results, on the use of fish oils in inflammatory processes involving the skin. (See below.)

4) Helpful in the treatment of psoriasis and other skin problems—In a recent double-blind, placebo-controlled study, 1.8 grams daily of EPA were shown to confer significant improvement in patients with psoriasis. Patients also continued to use the topical medications they had been using; at both eight-week and twelve-week evaluation periods, the fish oil-treated patients were found to be significantly improving compared with the controls, in whom there was no change.

There has also been one report, involving a single patient, that the fish oils can help control the rarer, even more severe pustular form of psoriasis, and there has been a well-controlled study reporting benefit from fish oils in the treatment of atopic dermatitis. All of this work, while very promising, needs confirmation.

5) Helps prevent/treat cancer—There have been several animal studies suggesting that very large doses of fish oils can inhibit some cancers. Breast cancers have thus been slowed and survival time significantly extended in rats. More work is urgently needed to further explore a possible anti-cancer role for fish oils.

6) Therapeutic in kidney disease—A number of animal experiments have suggested that the fish oils may eventually prove useful in some forms of kidney disease. There is enough evidence to warrant human clinical trials in patients with chronic renal disease. Meanwhile, a study has already begun to see whether fish oil can help prevent some of the damage to the kidneys that frequently results from the use of immunosuppressive drugs in connection with organ transplants. The preliminary studies, showing that the fish oils can counteract some of the blood vessel constriction caused by the immunosuppressive drugs (used to keep the body from rejecting the transplanted organ), have yielded promising results.

Related to Negative Claims:

1) Toxic—Natural fish oils contain almost no vitamin E and, therefore, peroxidize (become rancid) easily and quickly. So make sure your fish oil preparation contains vitamin E. Most do. Fears that the cetoleic acid component of fish oil might be toxic to heart muscle have been found to have no basis. Very high doses of fish oil may reduce blood-clotting capabilities to the point that hemorrhage becomes a possibility. This is rarely seen, however, even in those who do consume lots of fish oils. *Those with a tendency to hemorrhage or bleed very easily should, nonetheless, use fish oil supplements only under a doctor's supervision.*

2) Harmful in diabetics—Several research groups have now reported that fish oil supplements produce notable increases in blood sugar and sharp declines in insulin secretion in diabetic patients of both the type I and type II categories. These adverse metabolic effects are reversible when supplements are discontinued. *No diabetic should take fish oil*

supplements except with the knowledge, consent and monitoring of his/her physician.

3) Can cause vitamin deficiencies—Mice, fed on fish oil-enriched diets, have been found to have dramatically reduced levels of vitamin E in their blood and tissues. Studies are underway to see if this occurs in humans, as well. Vitamin E acts as an antioxidant in these oils. So, the more of these substances you consume, the more vitamin E you need. (See Recommendations below.)

IV. RECOMMENDATIONS

A) *Suggested Intake:* I do not recommend fish oil supplements for everyone. I do recommend that most people increase their consumption of fish since considerable benefit can be derived in that fashion, as suggested by a number of epidemiologic studies. Any increase in fish consumption will be useful; having fish two or three times a week (or even more often if you really love fish/seafood) is ideal.

For those with hypertension, ischemic heart disease or any condition (e.g., by-pass or other vessel surgery) that predisposes to potentially dangerous clotting, psoriasis, rheumatoid arthritis or other inflammatory process, I suggest fish oil supplementation in the range of 2 to 4 grams daily. Consult your doctor, however, before beginning this supplementation. There are some conditions that can benefit from higher daily doses but those definitely need a doctor's supervision.

B) *Source/Form:* The best way to get your fish oils are the way nature packaged them in fish. Here's how much of these fish oils (total of EPA and DHA) you can get in each seven ounce serving of the following fish:

Herring	3,200 milligrams (3.2 grams)
Salmon	2,400 milligrams (2.4 grams)
Bluefish	2,400 milligrams (2.4 grams)
Tuna	1,000 milligrams (1 gram)
Cod	600 milligrams (.6 gram)
Shrimp	800 milligrams (.8 gram)
Flounder	600 milligrams (.6 gram)
Swordfish	400 milligrams (.4 gram)

Adapted from *Journal of the American Dietetic Association* 86:788, 1986.

Almost *all* fish and seafood have some EPA and DHA. The table gives just some of the examples. Herring, salmon and bluefish are particularly rich. As you can see, it *is* possible to get quite a lot of these oils in fish itself.

If you don't like fish, however, and want to use supplements instead, these usually come in capsule form and are easily swallowed. There are many fish oil products on the market now. The capsule size is often 1,000 milligrams or 1,200 milligrams. You must look carefully at the labels, however, to see how much of that oil is actually EPA and/or DHA. The doses recommended in Suggested Intake are the combined EPA and DHA.

Thus, in a typical product that offers 1,000-milligram capsules, you'll find when you look at the label that each capsule contains 180 milligrams of EPA and 120 milligrams of DHA. This varies, of course; some 1,000-milligram capsules contain up to 350 milligrams or even more of EPA and 150 milligrams or more of DHA.

If the product you're buying contains 180 milligrams of EPA and 120 milligrams of DHA, then you are getting 300 milligrams of the fatty acids. If you are aiming for a 3-gram daily dose, then you would have to take ten of these particular capsules a day to achieve that dose. Take them in divided doses with each meal.

C) *Take With:* It is best to take your fish oil supplements with a vitamin/mineral preparation that provides 30 to 200 IUs of vitamin E and 50 to 200 micrograms of selenium daily. Also, check to make sure the fish oil supplements you are using also contain vitamin E. It is *not* necessary to take your additional vitamin E and selenium supplementation at the same time you take your fish oil supplements.

D) *Cautionary Note:* Diabetics should not use fish oil supplements under any circumstances unless advised to do so by their physicians. Those predisposed to easy bleeding or hemorrhage should use fish oil supplements only with their physician's approval. Supplement fish oils with 30 to 200 IUs of vitamin E and 50 to 200 micrograms of selenium daily. Make sure that the fish oil supplement that you use does not contain vitamin A and D as these vitamins are toxic in large doses (see sections on vitamin A and D).

GAMMA-LINOLENIC ACID AND OIL OF EVENING PRIMROSE

I. OVERVIEW: Will a Fading Rose Bloom Again?

A few years ago the claims for oil of evening primrose (a particularly rich source of gamma-linolenic acid, better known as GLA) seemed boundless. The promises made for GLA/oil of evening primrose just haven't panned out, with one possible exception, a potentially very important one.

The body makes GLA from essential fatty acids. Linoleic acid is the primary dietary source of the essential fatty acids, which have numerous functions in the body; among other things, they are precursors of an important family of substances, collectively known as the prostaglandins, which have complex and profound effects throughout the body, such as regulation of platelet aggregation, blood vessel tone, salt and water balance, gastrointestinal function, neurotransmitter function and secretion of insulin.

Linoleic acid is converted in the body to GLA, via enzymatic action, and thereafter can contribute to prostaglandin synthesis and regulation. Thus the claim has been that the more GLA you get, the more beneficial prostaglandins you'll have and the healthier you will be in every respect. This claim overlooks the fact that we have a great deal to learn about the prostaglandins; it also overlooks the fact that different varieties of these substances can have markedly contrary effects.

More is not always better. Given our present level of knowledge, trying to "fine tune" our prostaglandin biochemistry with high doses of oil of evening primrose is a little like trying to modify a microchip with a mallet. We *may,* however, have discovered *one* manifestation that might work. Read on.

II. CLAIMS

Positive:

1) Combats arthritis; 2) protects against cardiovascular disease; 3) fights cancer; 4) helpful in skin disorders; 5) useful in PMS; 6) immune modulator; 7) helpful in psychiatric and neurologic disorders.

Negative:
1) Toxic; 2) carcinogenic; 3) immune depressant; 4) dangerous in epilepsy and manic disorders.

III. EVIDENCE

Related to Positive Claims:
1) Combats arthritis—Research related to this claim has been underway for some time. GLA is known to increase production of a series of prostaglandins that have inflammatory lowering effects, so it is not unreasonable to expect that it might be helpful in the treatment of arthritis. And, in fact, one group has reported that evening primrose oil supplements resulted in significant improvement in several rheumatoid arthritis patients.

The same researchers followed their pilot work with a more ambitious double-blind, placebo-controlled study and reported in 1988 more evidence of evening primrose oil's effectiveness in the treatment of rheumatoid arthritis. Those who got 540 milligrams of GLA per day, in the form of evening primrose oil, showed significant improvement at the end of the year-long treatment period. Those who received placebo did not show improvement. When those who had been receiving GLA were switched to placebo for three months they relapsed.

Improvement was measured subjectively and in terms of nonsteroidal anti-inflammatory drug use. Those who got GLA needed significantly less of these drugs. This promising work needs follow-up and confirmation from others. GLA may yet claim an important therapeutic role.

2) Protects against cardiovascular disease—GLA affects prostaglandins that are active in the regulation of the cardiovascular system. It has been claimed that GLA can help prevent heart attacks by inhibiting blood clots and arterial spasms. Research related to this claim has failed to produce any compelling supportive evidence, but more work is probably warranted.

3) Fights cancer—There is no evidence that GLA/evening primrose oil has any usefulness in the treatment of cancer. Findings that GLA can kill some cancer cells in tissue culture seem to be the basis for this claim. Far from sufficient.

4) Helpful in skin disorders—Most of the studies related to this claim have failed to confirm that GLA is useful in skin disorders. When used in a cream, as opposed to oral supplements, however, it makes a good moisturizer.

5) Useful in PMS—There have been studies showing that GLA may be useful in the treatment of premenstrual syndrome. I must report, however, that this has not been my experience, nor that of any of my colleagues who have tried GLA/evening primrose oil in this context.

6) Immune modulator—GLA may actually have immune-suppressive, not immune-stimulating effects. If this is the case it might conceivably find use in some autoimmune disorders to help dampen overactive immune components. We are a long way, however, from knowing precisely what role, if any, GLA plays in immunity.

7) Helpful in psychiatric and neurologic disorders—Here again we find inconclusive evidence, at best.

Related to Negative Claims:
1) Toxic—There is no evidence of toxicity.

2) Carcinogenic—There is no evidence GLA is carcinogenic.

3) Immune depressant—There is only scant and inconclusive evidence of this. The claim is unproved.

4) Dangerous in epilepsy and manic disorders—GLA/evening primrose oil has been reported to aggravate temporal lobe epilepsy and should definitely be avoided by those with this disorder. It has been suggested, but not proved, that GLA/evening primrose oil may also have adverse effects in those suffering from manic-depressive disorder.

IV. RECOMMENDATIONS

If you want to try GLA/evening primrose oil for symptomatic relief from rheumatoid arthritis, do so only with a doctor's supervision. Those with temporal-lobe epilepsy should avoid GLA/evening primrose oil altogether. Manic-depressives should also avoid these substances. As noted above, evening primrose oil cream is a good moisturizer.

GLYCOSPHINGOLIPIDS
(Skin Rejuvenator?)

Glycosphingolipids, sometimes abbreviated GSL, are found in cell membranes, especially those of nerve cells. They are also found in the epidermis (outer layer) of the skin and, along with some other lipids found in this layer, are thought to be important to the integrity of the skin.

Claims are made that a skin cream containing GSL can rejuvenate the skin. Advertisements for this product said that GSL production in the skin decreases with age, starting at puberty, and that GSL could restore skin to youthfulness, rid it of wrinkles and increase its elasticity.

As with most cosmetics, all this would be wonderful, if it were true. Alas, GSL molecules are too large to penetrate into the regenerating lower layers of skin tissue. This is the only area where GSL would work for skin regeneration, if it worked at all. At best, GSL works as a moisturizer, temporarily trapping water in the top layers of skin, which does briefly smooth out some lines and wrinkles, as do dozens of other skin creams, devoid of "miracle" ingredients.

INOSITOL (MYO-INOSITOL) AND PHOSPHATIDYLINOSITOL
(For the Nervous System)

Myo-inositol, the nutritionally active form of inositol, is a constituent of the phospholipid phosphatidylinositol. Phosphatidylinositol is a minor phospholipid constituent of cell membranes. However, phosphatidylinositol molecules are storage forms for several derivatives of myo-inositol which serve as messenger molecules within the nervous system, transmitting signals that control functions of a number of cells within the system.

Although clear-cut deficiency states of myo-inositol have not been identified in humans, they have been described in other animals. In the early 1940s, it was recognized as an anti-hair loss factor in certain rodents. Additionally, it was found to have lipotropic activity (that is, prevent fatty liver formation) in various animals.

Several health claims have been made for myo-inositol. It has long been claimed to lower blood concentrations of triglycerides and cholesterol and to generally protect against cardiovascular disease. There is, however, no evidence that supplementary myo-inositol lowers serum lipid levels or protects against cardiovascular disease in humans.

Some people take from 1 to 2 grams of myo-inositol either to help them sleep or to relieve anxiety. There are many anecdotes that myo-inositol helps with insomnia or serves as a tranquilizer, but there are no studies that document this. Myo-inositol intake can influence the phosphatidylinositol levels in the membranes of brain cells. The myo-inositol compounds derived from this phospholipid could conceivably have some beneficial effects on insomnia and anxiety. Since myo-inositol is so much safer than most of the drugs used to treat these problems, controlled studies of myo-inositol are very much needed.

Diabetic peripheral neuropathy is one of the most crippling complications of diabetes. It has been thought for several years that decreased levels of myo-inositol in the nerves of diabetics suffering from this complication are associated with the damage to nerve fibers. One report suggests that the adverse effects of chronic high blood sugar on these fibers may be heightened by reduced myo-inositol concentrations in the nerves. One investigation found that myo-inositol given in doses of 500 milligrams twice a day for two weeks increased the amplitude of the evoked action potential of certain nerves, suggesting that a greater number of nerves were firing after stimulating. No such apparent improvement was noted when placebo was given.

Researchers also reported improved sensory nerve function in twenty diabetics with peripheral neuropathy in whom dietary intake of myo-inositol was increased from 770 to 1,650 milligrams daily. However, a recent study showed *normal* levels of myo-inositol in nerves from diabetics with neuropathy. Further research is definitely indicated to determine if myo-inositol does play a role in this disorder and its treatment.

Adult Americans consume about 1 gram daily of myo-inositol mainly in the phospholipid form and as phytic acid present in plant sources. Foods richest in myo-inositol are fruits, nuts, beans and grains. Fresh vegetables and fruits generally contain more myo-inositol than do frozen, canned, or salt-free products. A quarter of a fresh cantaloupe of average size contains 335 milligrams; one orange contains 307 milligrams; one-half of a grapefruit has 200 milligrams; one-half cup of frozen concentrate of grapefruit juice contains 456 milligrams; one-half cup of frozen concentrate of orange juice has 245 milligrams; one slice of whole-wheat bread contains 288 milligrams.

Myo-inositol is available in health food stores. For those who want to use this substance, *insist* on *myo*-inositol, which is the only nutritionally active form. This is the form usually sold in health food stores. Commercial lecithin contains, in addition to phosphatidylcholine, *a small amount* of phosphatidylinositol. No adverse effects have been noted in humans taking 3 grams of oral myo-inositol daily for short periods of time. Diabetics who wish to take supplementary myo-inositol for possible benefit in diabetic neuropathy should do so only under a physician's supervision.

LECITHIN/PHOSPHATIDYLCHOLINE/CHOLINE

I. OVERVIEW: New Life for Lecithin

Lecithin has been one of the most popular dietary supplements for a long time. Claims and anecdotes abound regarding its ability to lower blood cholesterol levels, to protect against heart disease, to enhance memory and to increase energy levels, among other things. Many in the medical community have completely rejected any beneficial effects of lecithin as old wives' tales. Some actually become incensed at the mere suggestion that lecithin can lower blood cholesterol levels.

Lecithin is enjoying a rebirth, however, with an accumulation of evidence in the last few years that lecithin and choline may be very important in the treatment of some major neurologic, psychiatric and infectious disease problems. And, yes, these substances may yet prove to be helpful in cardiovascular disease.

One of the most confusing issues surrounding lecithin is the term itself. Lecithin means different things to different people. To chemists and biochemists, lecithin refers to phosphatidylcholine. Phosphatidylcholine is a molecule composed of saturated, unsaturated and/or polyunsaturated acids. It also contains glycerin, phosphorus and the nitrogen-containing base choline.

The lecithin sold in health food stores and as a food additive is not pure phosphatidylcholine. This type of lecithin is a mixture of phospholipids containing only 10 to 20 percent pure lecithin, by which I mean phosphatidylcholine. The other substances in food-form lecithin include phospholipids containing myo-inositol, ethanolamine and serine. Recently some health food stores began selling a phosphatidylcholine of higher purity. For example, a substance called PC-55 contains 55 percent phosphatidylcholine.

To avoid further confusion (I hope), I will use the term *phosphatidylcholine* when I mean pure lecithin, and lecithin when I refer to the typical product sold in health food stores and used as a food additive. This lecithin, as mentioned above, usually contains 10 to 20 percent of the real thing: phosphatidylcholine.

Lecithin is a widely used food additive found in ice cream, margarine and mayonnaise, among others. It is the bridge that joins water to the fats in these products and thus helps maintain their consistency. This is because phospholipids have the ability to associate with both water and lipids which are not soluble in water. Lecithin is one of the few truly nutritious agents used as a food additive. It is also a protector against oxidant damage.

Phosphatidylcholine in food is our major source for the nutrient choline. Choline is extremely important for human health. Its role in phosphatidylcholine is crucial in the maintenance of cellular membrane fluidity, key to the normal and healthy working of our cells. In addition to contributing to the structure of phosphatidylcholine, choline is involved in the synthesis of acetylcholine, a molecule fundamental to the proper functioning of the nervous system. Acetylcholine is one of the neurotransmitters that mediate our emotions and behavior.

Alzheimer's disease, the most common cause of dementia characterized by deterioration of memory, judgment, orientation and personality, appears due in part to a relative deficiency of acetylcholine in the brain. Attempts to treat Alzheimer's disease with supplemental phosphatidylcholine or choline have met with disappointing or inconclusive results to date, though this substance may still turn out to be helpful in *preventing* the disease.

Supplemental choline and phosphatidylcholine have been found to be very beneficial in the treatment of tardive dyskinesia (which may result as a side effect of anti-psychotic medications) and affective disorders, such as manic-depressive illness.

There is a lot of excitement building around these substances, as you are about to discover. Some of the therapeutic effects of these substances verge on the "miraculous."

II. CLAIMS

Positive:

1) Protects against cardiovascular disease; 2) prevents/treats memory loss and diseases of the nervous system; 3) helpful in the treatment of

affective disorders, such as manic-depressive illness; 4) helpful in the treatment of hepatitis; 5) has anti-viral activity and is useful in the treatment of AIDS; 6) can prevent morphine dependence and facilitate morphine recovery; 7) has anti-aging properties; 8) helpful in the prevention and treatment of gallstones.

Negative:
1) Produces a fish odor in the body; 2) causes depression.

III. EVIDENCE

Related to Positive Claims:
1) Protects against cardiovascular disease—This is a relatively old claim, though one that has persisted. Both choline and lecithin have been said to affect lipid metabolism. This claim dates back many years, to when it was discovered that both lecithin and dietary choline can alleviate fatty livers in animals. In humans, however, no one was able to demonstrate similar effects. Neither choline nor lecithin has been found to alleviate fatty liver disease (mostly caused by alcoholism) in humans. Choline has never been shown to lower cholesterol or triglyceride levels in humans and the evidence that lecithin can favorably modify blood lipid levels is inconsistent. But hold on. This doesn't necessarily mean these substances are of no value in human cardiovascular disease.

The problem has been a total lack of consistency in the type of lecithin used in these studies. Each molecule of phosphatidylcholine has two molecules of fatty acid. It is known that certain fatty acids, e.g., polyunsaturated fatty acids, some monounsaturated fatty acids and even a saturated fatty acid, stearic acid, can lower cholesterol levels. Phosphatidylcholine containing cholesterol-lowering fatty acids can be expected to lower cholesterol levels, at least in some cases. To establish whether phosphatidylcholine can affect lipid metabolism, it is mandatory that the fatty acid makeup of this substance be known. Recently there have been reports that supplemental phosphatidylcholine rich in polyunsaturated fatty acids can elevate the *HDL-cholesterol* ratio. HDL-cholesterol represents "good" or desirable blood cholesterol.

Although oral choline does not affect blood pressure, intravenous choline *can* lower blood pressure in humans and a variety of experimental animals. There is at present no convincing evidence that lecithin, phosphatidylcholine or choline protect against cardiovascular disease. But in truth, the proper studies have not yet been done to resolve this issue. It would be particularly interesting to study phosphatidylcholine of known fatty acid makeup in this context, as suggested above.

2) Prevents/treats memory loss and diseases of the nervous system— Choline and phosphatidylcholine have been used in the experimental treatment of a number of neurologic disorders. Both supplements can increase choline levels as well as brain acetylcholine levels. Acetylcholine is a major neurotransmitter, and nutritional maneuvers to increase the amount of acetylcholine or other neurotransmitters are called precursor therapies.

There is evidence that cholinergic neurons, that is, nerve cells that use acetylcholine as their neurotransmitters, are involved in memory processing and storage in certain regions of the brain. A study reported in *Science* in 1980 demonstrated evidence of choline-induced memory enhancement in mice. Choline-enriched diets improved memory in the animals, while choline-deficient diets seemed to contribute to memory loss. Healthy humans given drugs which are antagonistic to acetylcholine, such as certain tricyclic anti-depressants, antihistamines, and anti-spasmodics, have been shown to develop impaired short-term memory. This is particularly true of the elderly who may develop reversible dementia following use of these drugs.

A few reports show that humans given supplemental choline exhibit increased short-term memory skills. Some clinical anecdotes suggest that supplementary phosphatidylcholine enhances short-term memory skills, as well. In my own practice, I have noticed that a few patients taking phosphatidylcholine at 9 grams daily (which raises serum choline levels twofold) showed improved short-term memory. Interestingly, these patients complained of short-term memory problems when they ran out of phosphatidylcholine and noted improvement again when they restarted it.

Since there is some evidence that choline and phosphatidylcholine supplements help memory, it is important to continue this line of research to determine which groups would be helped by these substances and at what optimal doses.

Sufferers of Alzheimer's disease have exhibited reduced ability to synthesize the neurotransmitter acetylcholine and/or the ability to utilize this substance especially, it appears, in those areas of the cerebral cortex associated with memory. This being the case, researchers hoped that supplemental choline or phosphatidylcholine might boost acetylcholine activity in victims of this disease and thus improve their memories. Although there have been a few reports that such supplementation improves memory in some cases, most of the studies have, unfortunately, been negative. The overall consensus by investigators in this area is that neither supplemental phosphatidylcholine nor choline can by themselves alter the course of Alzheimer's disease.

More recently phosphatidylcholine in combination with other drugs such as physostigmine, an anti-cholinesterase (prevents the breakdown of acetylcholine), and piracetam and hydergine (two drugs which are reputed to improve memory in some, see analyses elsewhere), have been studied. One report demonstrated a significant improvement in memory in Alzheimer's patients taking 10.5 grams daily of phosphatidylcholine as well as the drug physostigmine. Another study, however, found no improvement in patients taking 18 grams of phosphatidylcholine and physostigmine.

Choline and piracetam were reported to improve mood in Alzheimer's patients in one study, and phosphatidylcholine and piracetam improved cognitive functions in another. In the largest study to date, no improvement was detected in eighteen patients treated with 14.5 grams daily of phosphatidylcholine plus piracetam. That was a double-blind study. Phosphatidylcholine plus hydergine has not been found effective.

The lack of effectiveness of phosphatidylcholine and choline in the treatment of Alzheimer's disease is disappointing, since these substances are so appealing at least from a theoretical view. It is still likely, however, that phosphatidylcholine, plus some other substance which we have not yet tried, *will* be helpful—and for this reason alone the research should continue. Perhaps if we could identify those who are likely to develop Alzheimer's disease, then *pretreatment* with phosphatidylcholine might protect against it.

It is also possible that the composition of the phosphatidylcholine in these studies varied and thus gave varying results. If the amelioration of Alzheimer's depends upon membrane fluidization in addition to neurotransmitter boosting, then it is vital that unsaturated fatty acids be used in the phosphatidylcholine. (See below for more discussion of this crucial issue.)

There are a number of neurologic disorders that are characterized by abnormal muscular movements (so-called movement disorders) and which are thought to be due to, at least in part, abnormalities of the acetylcholine neurotransmitter system. These disorders include tardive dyskinesia, Parkinson's disease, Huntington's disease, Tourette syndrome and familial spinocerebellar degeneration (also known as Friedreich's ataxia). Supplemental choline and phosphatidylcholine have proved effective in the treatment of tardive dyskinesia. Equivocal or negative results have been reported for the others, but more research is warranted, particularly using combinations of these substances with drugs.

Tardive dyskinesia is a neurologic disorder which is a side effect found in 10–15 percent of those taking antipsychotic medications. The disorder is characterized by twitching and jerking movements of the facial muscles and tongue and sometimes of the muscles in the trunk and extremities. Most studies have demonstrated that supplementary choline, as well as phosphatidylcholine, reduces the abnormal movements by about 50 percent. Consequently, phosphatidylcholine is now the first drug of choice for treatment of this disorder.

3) Helpful in the treatment of affective disorders such as manic-depressive disease—There is evidence that acetylcholine can influence mood. Those who already have a tendency to depression may become depressed if given high-dose choline supplements. On the other hand, choline and phosphatidylcholine supplementation appears to improve manic symptoms. One group of researchers gave 13.5 to 27 grams of phosphatidylcholine daily (actually 15 to 30 grams of 90 percent phosphatidylcholine) to four patients with manic symptoms. In addition to phosphatidylcholine, two of the four patients received lithium (standard therapy for manic-depressive illness) and the other two, in addition to the phosphatidylcholine, received lithium and another psychiatric drug. All four patients improved. But when the phosphatidylcholine was withdrawn, manic symptoms reappeared in three of the four, even though they continued on the other medications.

In a later study, these researchers found that manic symptoms improved significantly more with phosphatidylcholine than with placebo in five of six patients treated. Another study demonstrated that phosphatidylcholine by itself relieved the symptoms of a thirteen-year-old girl with mania who improved with 13.5 grams daily, whereas other psychiatric medicines, including lithium, did *not* help.

I have a few patients in my practice whose manic symptoms are controlled very nicely with 1 to 1.5 grams of choline or 10 to 15 grams of phosphatidylcholine daily. These are also patients, I must add, who did not respond well to lithium or other psychiatric medicines. They continue to do well after four years of treatment. Considering the toxic side effects of lithium and most psychiatric medications, it is urgent that research on the effects of phosphatidylcholine and choline in manic-depressive illness be energetically pursued.

4) Helpful in the treatment of hepatitis—This will probably come as a surprise to most, including physicians, but there are at least four reports in the medical literature on the treatment of viral hepatitis with polyunsaturated phosphatidylcholine. One of the first publications was in the *Journal of Czech Medicine* in 1981. In this paper, the authors examined the effects of polyunsaturated phosphatidylcholine given at 1.8 grams daily to patients with viral hepatitis type A and type B. Those given phosphatidylcholine were compared with control groups who were not given the substance. The phospholipid helped achieve a faster resolution of symptoms, a shorter time for the normalization of abnormal laboratory results (mainly liver tests) and a reduction in the number of relapses, as compared with the control groups. The authors believe that the phosphatidylcholine works by repairing the membranes of the liver cells.

Chronic active hepatitis is a serious disease and can be life-threatening. The most common causes of the disorder are hepatitis B and hepatitis non-A non-B (aka hepatitis C) viruses. Researchers at the King's College Hospital and Medical School in Great Britain reported on the use of 3 grams daily of phosphatidylcholine in the treatment of chronic active hepatitis caused by hepatitis non-A non-B virus. The study was a prospective double-blind trial (meaning a good one), and the authors found that patients treated with the phospholipid had significantly reduced and, in some cases, totally absent histologic evidence of disease activity. They, too, believe that the phosphatidylcholine works by repairing the membranes of the liver cells.

A report has also appeared in an Italian medical journal which demonstrated that patients with acute viral hepatitis B cleared the hepatitis B surface antigen much more quickly when given 1.8 grams of phosphatidylcholine daily. The trial was a double-blind and randomized one. Another report from the College of Medicine in Ibadan, Nigeria, similarly showed that treatment of patients with acute hepatitis B with 1.8 grams of phosphatidylcholine hastened recovery from this some-times fatal disease when compared to those patients not treated with the phospholipid.

These exciting and important findings urgently warrant trials of phos-phatidylcholine on not only viral hepatitis but non-viral forms as well, such as alcohol-induced hepatitis. It is likely that only phosphatidyl-choline utilizing *unsaturated* fatty acids will be useful in this context.

5) Has anti-viral activity and is useful in the treatment of AIDS—A phosphatidylcholine-containing lipid aggregate known as AL 721 does inhibit the replication of the AIDS virus, HIV, in the test tube and is being used clinically in the treatment of AIDS. (See section in this chapter on AL 721 for further discussion.) Phosphatidylcholine itself has not been demonstrated to have direct anti-viral activity.

6) Can prevent morphine dependence and facilitate morphine recovery—This claim goes back to a publication more than a half century old. In 1931 a Chinese scientist reported in the *Chinese Jour-nal of Physiology* that lecithin could prevent morphine dependence and facilitate morphine recovery in mice. Years later, in 1982, a few Israeli scientists repeated this work and reported their results. They found that phosphatidylcholine did *not* alleviate withdrawal symptoms in morphine-addicted mice and actually made them worse. They did find, however, that a phosphatidylcholine-containing substance called AL 721 was highly beneficial in alleviating withdrawal symptoms of morphine-addicted mice. (For further discussion, see section on AL 721.) The Israeli authors believe that although phosphatidylcholine may be the active substance producing this effect, it must be presented in the right delivery form such as AL 721.

The fact that the Israelis could not get the same results with phos-phatidylcholine the Chinese researcher did may be accounted for in this way: The Chinese investigator was using a lecithin that utilized polyunsaturated fatty acids, which are membrane fluidizers. The Is-raelis used a phosphatidylcholine that uses highly saturated fats, which are membrane rigidifiers. This could account for the opposite results.

Harder to account for are the Israeli claims for AL 721, which also contains saturated fats. If this substance really does have any efficacy (see analysis of AL 721 in this section), then perhaps its unique structure is the key.

7) Has anti-aging properties—In 1975 German scientists reported on the administration of oral polyunsaturated phosphatidylcholine to young and old rats. They found that the older rats incorporated more of the lipid into their cell membranes than did the younger rats. When they looked at the cell membranes of liver cells, they found that the older rats that were fed phosphatidylcholine had membrane structures and functions more like younger rats than older rats.

As cellular membranes age, they become less fluid and more rigid. This is associated chemically with a decrease in phosphatidylcholine and an increase in cholesterol in the membrane. The rejuvenating effect of phosphatidylcholine appears to be in the reversal of this condition of aging. Whatever beneficial effects phosphatidylcholine has in the treatment of viral hepatitis, as discussed above, are probably related to this phenomenon. That is, repair and fluidization of the membranes of the liver cells.

The Israeli scientists mentioned earlier in this section found that phosphatidylcholine by itself *decreased* the fluidity of mouse brain membranes, but, again, this appears to be because they were using phosphatidylcholine with saturated fatty acid content, which is, as explained earlier, membrane rigidifying.

8) Helpful in the prevention and treatment of gallstones—Two scientists recently reported on the effects of dietary phosphatidylcholine upon the bile composition in the gerbil. It is well known that the ratio of phosphatidylcholine to cholesterol in the bile is crucial to the maintenance of soluble bile. When the ratio gets too low, that is, when the amount of cholesterol increases or the amount of phosphatidylcholine decreases, cholesterol can precipitate and form gallstones. Other substances that keep cholesterol from precipitating are the bile salts.

The two scientists found that feeding phosphatidylcholine to gerbils produced a much more soluble bile, that is, a bile much less likely to form gallstones. This was mainly due to the production of more solubilizing bile salts, as well as to increased bile phosphatidylcholine.

A large number of adults are at risk for forming gallstones, many of them requiring surgery to remove the gallbladder. Human trials with supplementary phosphatidylcholine may lead to ways of preventing and even treating gallstones.

Related to Negative Claims:

1) Produces a fish odor in the body—The very rare fish odor syndrome (fishy odor is especially bad in the summer) is due to an enzyme deficiency that impairs choline metabolism. Those few who have this problem should not take choline supplements and should restrict choline intake in their diets. Phosphatidylcholine should not cause the problem. Those who develop a fishy body odor after they consume small amounts of choline supplements should stop taking these supplements and determine if they have the enzyme deficiency. Those with liver failure may develop the fish odor syndrome, as may those who have normal livers but consume 20 grams or more of choline daily, an amount which exceeds the capacity of even the normal liver enzyme to metabolize it.

2) Causes depression—There are a few, with *preexisting* tendency to depression, who may become depressed if given high doses of choline. They may also become depressed if given high doses of phosphatidylcholine. Depressed individuals who want to use choline or phosphatidylcholine supplements should be monitored by a physician.

IV. RECOMMENDATIONS

A) *Suggested Intake:* For years it was thought that the dietary intake of phosphatidylcholine from the American diet ranged between 4 to 9 grams daily. This corresponds to 400 to 900 milligrams daily of choline (choline makes up about 10 percent of phosphatidylcholine). A more rigorous calculation performed in 1979 by Richard Wurtman demonstrated that the average intake of phosphatidylcholine by Americans is 3.1 grams, corresponding to 300 milligrams of choline. In Europe, the numbers are even lower. For example, in Sweden daily intake of phosphatidylcholine is 1.8 grams. The optimal intakes of phosphatidylcholine and choline are unknown. However, some believe that daily intake of these nutrients, at least for certain groups, should be higher. Research is urgently needed to determine the amount of these nutrients we really need for optimum health. Refer to the appropriate sections in this article for suggested intakes for certain conditions.

Generally, supplementary phosphatidylcholine can be taken in doses up to 10 grams daily without adverse effects and choline in doses up to 1,000 milligrams or 1 gram daily without adverse effects.

B) *Source/Form:* Phosphatidylcholine, and hence choline, is found in all animal and plant products. The foods richest in phosphatidylcholine include egg yolks, soybeans, cauliflower and cabbage. The plant phosphatidylcholines, such as those found in soybean products, are rich in polyunsaturated fatty acids, while those found in egg yolks and other animal products are rich in the saturated fatty acid. Try to get your phosphatidylcholine from soybean products (e.g., tofu, tempeh, and miso), and cauliflower and cabbage.

Lecithin, phosphatidylcholine and choline are available in health food stores and certain drug stores and supermarkets. Lecithin is available in granular form and typically contains 20 percent phosphatidylcholine plus other phospholipids. Therefore, every 5 grams of lecithin contains about 1 gram of phosphatidylcholine, and every 50 grams contains 10 grams of the nutrient. It is important to note that 1 gram of lecithin is equivalent to 9 calories and the ingestion of 50 grams would yield 450 calories.

Recently phosphatidylcholine of higher purity has become available. One product contains 55 percent phosphatidylcholine. Another is 90 percent phosphatidylcholine, available in 0.9-gram capsules. Choline itself is available in tablet and liquid form.

Phosphatidylcholine-rich supplements are the preferred supplementary forms, since they are longer acting and less likely to produce adverse effects than choline. You can use either "regular" lecithin or one of the purer forms that deliver more phosphatidylcholine per given dose.

C) *Cautionary Note:* Those who develop a fishy odor from choline should stop taking it and see their physicians. Those who become depressed following ingestion of large amounts of phosphatidylcholine or choline should likewise stop taking these supplements and see their physicians. Those who wish to take higher daily doses of phosphatidylcholine or choline than 10 grams or 1,000 milligrams respectively should do so under a physician's supervision. *Very* high doses of choline have produced nausea, vomiting, dizziness and a fishy odor in some people (taking up to 20 grams daily for several weeks). There is no evidence that these high doses are any more beneficial than lower doses (1 to 2 grams daily).

LIPOSOMES
(Miracle Membranes)

Liposomes are artificial vesicles or sacs made up of the same phospholipids that constitute cell membranes. Liposomes were inadvertently discovered by an English scientist in 1961, but it wasn't until the 1980s that interest developed in the use of liposomes in the field of medical therapeutics. The inner space of liposomes (sort of like the inside of a soap bubble) can be loaded with drugs and used as delivery systems to get the drugs to where they will do the most good in the body. Drugs such as anti-microbials, anti-parasitics, anti-fungals, anti-cancers and superoxide dismutase are all being studied in this context. Liposomes hold great promise for improving the effectiveness and safety of a large number of drugs, and it is likely that these substances will be highly popular in the 1990s.

Recently a researcher at Columbia University found that even "empty" liposomes, phospholipid sacs *not* loaded with any drug, are capable of shrinking atherosclerotic plaques in the blood vessels of animals. The liposomes appear to work by mopping up cholesterol from cells in the plaques. Remarkably, the liposomes, combined with this cholesterol from the plaque, behave like HDL particles ("good" serum cholesterol) and get processed in the liver. Human experiments are planned and the results eagerly awaited.

The ability of liposomes to remove cholesterol from cell membranes makes them potentially very important tools for the fluidization of cell membranes. Such fluidization can have rejuvenating effects on cells, enhance immune responsiveness, be useful for the treatment of drug addiction, have anti-viral effects (on membrane viruses), and so on. I would imagine that whatever AL 721 (see discussion this section) is reported to do, liposomes would do better. Incidentally, liposomes do not appear to be absorbed very well if given orally and need to be given by injection.

Never believe that the cosmetic industry doesn't know a good thing when it sees it. A few cosmetics already contain liposomes. One of these products was actually developed in consultation with scientists at the Pasteur Institute. The claim is that the liposomes have "anti-aging" properties, fusing with membranes of the skin, restoring fluidity and promoting the reactivation of skin cells. It is not inconceivable that removing cholesterol from the skin cells *would* rejuvenate them. However, it is highly unlikely that the liposomes in these cosmetics could penetrate deep enough in the skin for this to happen. The theory is interesting, but lacking in proof. For now, as noted above, it appears that liposomes must be injected to have any appreciable effect.

LIPOTROPES/ACTIVATED LIPOTROPES
(Toward New Drugs)

Lipotropes, substances which have an affinity for fat, are important in lipid metabolism. The four lipotropes most significant for humans are choline, methionine, folic acid and vitamin B_{12}. All of these participate in the synthesis of phosphatidylcholine, a major player in cell membrane fluidity. It was recognized many years ago that these substances are effective in helping prevent fat accumulation in the liver.

We now know that these substances play major roles in other biologic activities besides lipid metabolism. They play central roles in many metabolic processes at the cellular and subcellular levels, including DNA synthesis, maintenance of immune competence and protection against transformation of normal cells to cancer cells. Involvement with phosphatidylcholine and cell membrane fluidity probably account for their activity in these functions. (See sections on choline, methionine, folic acid and vitamin B_{12} for more information.)

Active forms of the lipotropes choline and methionine are cytidine diphosphate choline, or CDP-choline, and S-adenosylmethionine, or SAM. CDP-choline is available as an injectable drug in Japan and Italy. It is used as a brain-circulation stimulator to treat disturbances of consciousness that may follow a brain injury or brain surgery. The drug has also been used in Alzheimer's disease, severe depression, Parkinson's disease and other degenerative brain disorders. It is thought that the drug works by increasing blood flow and oxygen use in brain tissue. The drug has several adverse effects including dizziness, agitation, headaches, nausea and blood-pressure lowering if given too quickly. There is some ongoing research with this drug overseas but none that I know of in the United States.

SAM is now being researched in several centers, and early work suggests that it may be helpful in the treatment of osteoarthritis, fibromyalgia and depression. It looks like a very promising new drug.

MONOLAURIN AND CAPRYLIC ACID
(Antimicrobials?)

There have been reports that some fatty acids have anti-bacterial, anti-fungal and anti-viral activities. Monolaurin is one of these and is now being used by some of those infected with the HIV virus, including some AIDS patients. Monolaurin comprises glycerin and the 12-carbon saturated fatty acid lauric acid. It has been shown to have anti-viral activity against a number of membraned viruses, including influenza viruses and herpes viruses *in vitro,* i.e., in the test tube. Apparently it works by affecting the lipid membrane of these viruses. The HIV virus is also a membraned virus. No adverse effects have been reported in those taking 600 milligrams of monolaurin for fourteen days. Whether it works *in vivo* (in the body) as it works *in vitro* remains to be seen.

Caprylic acid is an 8-carbon fatty acid which appears to have activity *in vitro* against the yeast *Candida albicans*. Many who believe that they have candidiasis use caprylic acid along with other substances. I would caution against its use as the sole agent for the treatment of documented candidiasis because of its relatively low potency. You'll probably need something stronger.

PHOSPHATIDYLSERINE AND PHOSPHATIDYLETHANOLAMINE
(Promising Preliminary Results)

Phosphatidylserine and phosphatidylethanolamine are phospholipids present in the structure of cell membranes. (Phosphatidylcholine, as discussed earlier, is the major phospholipid found in human cell membranes). A 1987 report by an Italian scientist showed that when phosphatidylserine was given orally to rats with known age-dependent declines in cerebral function it improved memory deficits, prevented the decline in learning capacity observed in aged rats, restored age-dependent electroencephalogram (EEG) abnormalities and prevented some degenerative nerve cell changes in certain parts of the brain.

Other reports show similar behavioral benefits in animals, and there are reports that phosphatidylserine can activate cells of the immune system. Phosphatidylserine is thought to work by stimulating repair of cell membranes.

Preliminary results of a multicenter trial in Italy on phosphatidylserine in Alzheimer's disease patients have now been reported. It appears that after the first six months of the study, improvements in memory and overall decrease in dementia were observed, but only in the most severely demented patients. Phosphatidylserine does not appear to have any adverse side effects. Future results of this study are eagerly awaited and will, perhaps, be confirmed by others.

Capsules containing phosphatidylcholine, phosphatidylethanolamine and phosphatidylserine are available in Europe and are used for the enhancement of memory. There are only anecdotes regarding their benefits.

Finally, it should be noted, phosphatidylethanolamine is part of the structure of AL 721 (discussed in this section).

NINE

Herbs

(Yielding Some

Startling Therapeutic

Secrets)

There has been a resurgence of interest recently in herbs here in the United States. Most health food stores now carry a multitude of herbal products, and herbal remedies are increasingly being used by alternate health practitioners, including acupuncturists, naturopaths and chiropractors. Colleges teaching herbal medicine are more prominent and magazines discussing herbs, as well as advertising them, are being seen more frequently on the newsstands. In fact, there have been some very positive articles on herbs in conservative newspapers and medical journals. And it is no longer just a handful of familiar herbs that is being discussed. Chinese traditional herbs, as well as herbs used in Ayurvedic (traditional Indian) medicine, have now also entered the U.S. marketplace.

There are many reasons for the increased interest in herbs. Some of these have to do with the increasing incidence of immune-deficiency disorders (such as ARC, AIDS, and the Chronic Fatigue Syndrome) and the search by those with these afflictions for anything that may help them. There are reports, including some good ones, that certain substances contained in herbs are immune enhancing and anti-viral.

That herbs may contain powerful pharmacologic agents should not come as a surprise. Many of the most important drugs in use today are derived from herbs. The white willow bark led to aspirin; the birth-control pill had its origins in the Mexican wild yam; the opium poppy is the basis of all the opiate narcotic drugs; from foxglove came the digitalis drugs; the ephedra plant was the original source for ephedrine and pseudoephedrine; bark from the cinchona tree gave us quinine and quinidine; from the periwinkle comes vinblastine and vincristine, two very important anti-cancer drugs; atropine was derived from the deadly nightshade; podophyllin (used to treat venereal warts) and podophyllotoxin (cancer drug) comes from the mandrake root or May apple; colchicine comes from the meadow saffron; physostigmine is derived from a cousin of the pea, the calabar bean; chymopapain, used for the treatment of herniated spinal disks, comes from the papaya. These are just a few examples.

What is an herb? It is a plant or plant part valued for its medicinal, savory and aromatic qualities. Those prized for their savory and aromatic qualities are the culinary herbs and spices. The medicinal herbs are valued not only for their ability to treat illness but also for their capacity to *prevent* illness. There is increasing evidence that certain plant foods, such as the cruciferous vegetables (cabbage, broccoli, brussels sprouts and cauliflower), high dietary fiber foods, carrots, green leafy vegetables, garlic and onions, among others, can protect us against certain forms of cancer and heart disease.

The medical and scientific communities have, until recently, generally been negative about medicinal herbs and, in most cases, with good reason. Folk medicines which use herbs are based almost exclusively on anecdotal observations. The effectiveness of herbal remedies has seldom been proven via adequately controlled scientific trials. And in many cases, we have better medications today to treat conditions previously treated only by herbs. In addition, there is tremendous variability in the potency and quantity of the active ingredients found in different samples of herbs. This is true even when they are not adulterated or diluted. A recent study at the Philadelphia College of Pharmacy and Science revealed that most of the ginseng samples tested were adulterated or diluted.

In spite of all of the negatives, though, there are many productive things happening in the world of medicinal herbs. Good studies are finally taking place. I already spoke about the disease preventive qualities of many of our food plants. Feverfew appears beneficial in the treatment of migraine headaches and arthritis, according to recent research. Extracts of some herbs, such as licorice and Saint John's wort, have definite anti-viral activity, including activity against the AIDS virus, HIV (human immunodeficiency virus). Substances found in such herbs as echinacea are potent immunostimulants. The ginkgo tree has yielded at least one substance which is a circulation enhancer and may be helpful in the treatment of Alzheimer's disease. Anti-allergic bioflavonoids are being discovered in many herbs. Orange berries of the African medicinal shrub *Maesa lanceolata* are yielding antibiotic agents. Substances from herbs show promise for the treatment of cancer, rheumatoid arthritis, angina, high blood pressure and diabetes. The future of medicinal herbs is looking brighter all the time.

ACONITE
(Warning: Highly Toxic)

Aconite, also known as monkshood and botanically as *Aconitum napellus,* has been a long time favorite in Chinese traditional medicine, Mexican folk medicine and homeopathic medicine. It is claimed to be effective in treating cancer, heart disease, kidney disease and diseases of the liver and spleen, among other ailments. Homeopathic physicians use it in low doses to treat flu, congestive disorders, colds and rheumatism.

Aconite is a very toxic herb. One of its principal ingredients, aconitine, is an extremely potent, fast-acting poison. Aconite affects both the heart and central nervous system, and toxic doses can cause the heart to stop beating and respiration to cease. Topical application of aconite liniments were once used in medicine to treat rheumatism and sciatica. Even in liniment form the poison can be absorbed and lead to serious consequences. This herb should never be used without medical advice, supervision and careful monitoring. Frankly, I would avoid aconite altogether.

ALFALFA
(Good Source of Chlorophyll and Vitamins)

Alfalfa (*Medicago sativa*) belongs to the legume family, which includes beans, peas and clover. It is not a grass as some believe. Claims abound regarding its health benefits with very little or no documentation to support them. It has been called the "great healer" by some. Health benefits attributed to alfalfa include: good for the treatment of allergic disorders, helpful in the treatment of arthritis, protects against hemorrhages, useful in the treatment of stomach disorders, peptic ulcer disease and gas pains. It is said to work as an appetite stimulant, a laxative and a diuretic.

Alfalfa leaves are used as a vegetable in parts of China and Russia, and alfalfa sprouts are widely consumed in many countries including the United States. Alfalfa is a good source of chlorophyll and vitamins especially beta-carotene and vitamin E. Extracts of alfalfa have been shown to have anti-bacterial activity against some gram-positive bacteria. Alfalfa seeds are used in India to make a cooling poultice for the treatment of boils. In Colombia, the mucilaginous fruits of the alfalfa plant are used to treat coughs.

Alfalfa seeds and sprouts contain the amino acid L-canaverine, which is structurally related to the amino acid L-arginine. L-canaverine has been shown to have anti-tumor activity against certain types of leukemia cells in mice and selective toxicity in dog cancer cells grown *in vitro*. L-canaverine inhibits the growth of certain bacteria and this could be the basis for the anti-bacterial action of alfalfa extracts. The amino acid has also been found to inhibit the growth of some viruses, including herpes simplex. On the downside, L-canaverine is thought to cause a lupus-like disease in monkeys, and there have been two reports of patients who experienced aggravation of their systemic lupus erythematosus (SLE) symptoms associated with chronic consumption of alfalfa tablets. The L-canaverine in the tablets was thought to be responsible. Since alfalfa is widely consumed, further research on the beneficial and toxic effects of L-canaverine is urgently needed.

Alfalfa leaves and extracts of alfalfa are readily available in health food stores. These are sold as supplementary sources of beta-carotene and chlorophyll. For the reasons previously stated, those with SLE should not take either supplementary alfalfa or consume alfalfa sprouts on a regular basis. Those who are allergic to grass pollens are unlikely to be sensitive to alfalfa (unless they are specifically allergic to it) since alfalfa is not a member of the grass family. There is no evidence that alfalfa can help with allergy problems.

ALOE VERA AND DERIVATIVES
(More Points for "The Miracle Plant")

Aloe plants have been used for centuries for a variety of claimed curative powers. There are more than 300 species of this yucca-like plant, but the ones most frequently used are *Aloe vera, Aloe barbandensis, Aloe perryi* and *Aloe ferrox.* Extracts of these plants are also widely used today in cosmetics, soaps, skin lotions, shampoos and suntan preparations. Current claims for aloe vera and derivatives range from skin moisturizer to a possible treatment for AIDS. Aloe vera is not a panacea but it does have some very useful therapeutic properties.

There are many anecdotes and some clinical evidence that aloe vera gel can alleviate certain skin conditions, such as radiation dermatitis. There are also clinical reports that these gels can promote healing of chronic leg ulcers. Controlled studies are generally lacking in humans, but in some well-designed animal experiments, aloe gels sped up healing of surgical wounds, burns, pressure sores and frostbite.

Aloe juices and gels have also been shown to have anti-bacterial and anti-fungal properties. They appear to be active against a broad spectrum of microbes. Recently an extract of aloe called Carrisyn, has exhibited anti-viral activity, inhibiting reproduction of herpes, measles and the HIV virus *in vitro.* Further studies are underway to determine whether Carrisyn, which is being developed as a drug, may be helpful in the treatment of AIDS. The same company that makes Carrisyn has marketed several other aloe products, including a "wound gel" that combines aloe with some other substances. Good clinical results are reported.

There are a number of ways in which aloe vera may produce therapeutic effects. Salicylates, which have both anti-inflammatory and pain-killing characteristics, are found in aloe. So is magnesium lactate, a substance which can inhibit histamine reactions of the sort that can cause, among many other things, itching and irritation of the skin. In addition, an enzyme in aloe has been found to be a bradykinin inhibitor in test-tube experiments. Bradykinin produces pain in inflamed tissue.

The antimicrobial and perhaps immune-stimulating effects of aloe are less well understood. Carrisyn (mentioned above) appears to stimulate the body to produce more immune-protective substances and more T-lymphocyte helper cells.

Most people use the aloe products that are currently being sold without side effects, but a few people have hypersensitivity reactions in the form of skin rashes. They should avoid aloe products. Long-term studies have not been performed to determine whether it is safe to drink aloe juices and gels, as many people are now doing. Some HIV-infected and AIDS patients are now regularly drinking an aloe beverage that has a high Carrisyn content. I suggest that this be done only with a doctor's supervision.

The aloe plants have looked interesting for some time and look more promising than ever today. They deserve a lot more scientific and medical attention in the form of further research and clinical trials.

ANGELICA/DONG QUAI
("Blood Tonic")

Angelica has recently become very popular in the American health food marketplace. There are several different species of angelica, but the one most sought after these days comes from China and is commonly known as Dong quai and botanically as *Angelica sinensis*. This species is used in China as a spice in Oriental dishes, such as Dong quai chicken. It is also widely used in China as an herbal medicine. Other species of angelica which come from Europe are used for flavoring wines, perfumes and liqueurs. These are also used in folk medicine.

Dong quai has been used in traditional Chinese medicine for thousands of years, mainly for female disorders. It is used to treat menstrual disturbances, such as infrequent menstruation and abnormal menstrual bleeding. It is thought to work as a blood tonic, that is, to "build up" the blood and "invigorate" the circulation. Other benefits attributed to Dong quai are a laxative action for chronic constipation of the aged and debilitated and usefulness in the treatment of headaches, abdominal pain and arthritis.

Many pharmacologically active substances have been isolated from Dong quai. These include some that are anti-inflammatory, analgesic, antiseptic, bactericidal, fungicidal, anti-allergic, anti-spasmodic, vasodilative and immune enhancing. This herb *is,* in fact a great treasure trove of pharmacologic chemicals. But there is a great variability in the quantity and potency of these substances among different samples of the herb. Thus it is unpredictable as to what benefits, if any, can be derived from taking Dong quai. Some claim that it helps bring up mucus from the respiratory tract, others that it causes them to sweat. It is a relatively safe herb.

ASTRAGALUS
("Body Energizer" and Immune Stimulant)

Astragalus, derived from the root of *Astragalus membranaceus,* a perennial of northern China, is a mainstay of traditional Chinese medicine. It is used in nearly half of all Chinese prescriptions. It has a reputation for being a potent energizer and immune stimulant. Chinese researchers report success in using it in cancer patients—to offset some of the immune-suppressing effect of many Western cancer drugs and radiation.

In two studies, survival times reportedly doubled among those patients receiving herbal therapy that included astragalus, as compared with those who got only standard chemotherapies and radiation. Test-tube studies with astragalus show that the herb can have positive immune modulating effects. Researchers in the U.S. have confirmed some of these findings. Investigators at the University of Texas have reported strong immune-restorative effects in test-tube studies of cancer cells treated with astragalus extracts. And certain cells treated with astragalus extracts in culture survive 50 percent longer, according to some U.S. researchers.

Chinese studies suggest that astragalus, in addition to boosting immunity and detoxifying a number of drugs and some metals, is also an anti-viral, a diuretic and a coronary artery dilator. They believe it is particularly effective in warding off flu and some other respiratory infections.

Well-controlled studies on astragalus are largely lacking, but it does contain a number of potentially therapeutic substances, including a polysaccharide called astragalan B, a bioflavonoid and choline. Astragalan B, tested in animals, protects against some toxins, stimulates components of the immune system and protects against a number of bacterial infections. The structure of astragalan B suggests that it might bind to cholesterol and thus *could* destabilize the membranes of certain viruses, including HIV. How potent it might be in this respect has not been determined.

How well astragalus is absorbed in the body when taken orally also remains an issue of conjecture. Even if its activity is limited to the gut, though, it might still exert therapeutic effects by detoxifying substances such as heavy metals or by inhibiting intestinal reservoirs of viruses. Astragalus is usually prepared by boiling the roots of the herb to produce a decoction; in China, the usual dosage is 9–16 grams of this decoction daily. Up to 30 grams are used in cancer patients in China. Astragalus powders are also available. The typical Chinese dosage of the powders is 9 grams per day. The powder is about 15–20 percent astragalus.

BAYBERRY ROOT BARK
(Favorite of Native Americans)

Bayberry is an evergreen shrub or tree which is also known as wax myrtle and candleberry. The botanical name is *Myrica cerifera*. The berries have a waxy coating and the American settlers used them to make wax and candles.

Bayberry is a folk remedy for the treatment of a wide array of ailments, including boils, cankers, carbuncles, colds, cholera, diarrhea, dysentery, fever, goiter, headaches, coughing up blood, blood in the stool, jaundice, abnormal menstrual bleeding, sore throat, typhoid and ulcers. The herb has been one of the favorites of Native Americans. There have never been controlled trials of the medical effects of bayberry. Bayberry may give symptomatic relief in some ailments, such as sore throats and colds, but it is highly unlikely that it does anything more than that.

Bayberry does have astringent properties. Astringents precipitate proteins and when applied to mucous membranes or to damaged skin they form a superficial protective layer and are not usually absorbed. This dries the mucous membranes or hardens the skin and keeps exudative secretions and minor hemorrhages in check. Bayberry root bark contains a few astringent substances such as tannic acid, gallic acid and a resin. It can be used to prepare a gargle that may be helpful for relief of a sore throat. It may also help in the symptomatic treatment of colds and diarrhea. Bayberry root bark is a relatively safe substance.

Black Cohosh
(Lydia Pinkham Revisited)

Black cohosh, black snakeroot, bugbane and squawroot are the common names for the plant *Cimicifuga racemosa*. The plant is native to North America and was a favorite herbal remedy of the Native Americans. Those of you who remember Lydia Pinkham's Vegetable Compound may be interested to know that black cohosh was one of its main components.

Native Americans have used the herb for the treatment of chronic fatigue, malaria, rheumatism, kidney problems, female disorders and sore throat. It has also been used as a folk remedy for bronchitis, fever, itching, high blood pressure, anxiety, menstrual cramps and the symptoms of menopause. Substances extracted from black cohosh have been found to have anti-inflammatory, sedative and blood-pressure-lowering activity in animals. Human data are lacking.

A few claim that consumption of black cohosh root produces a mild relaxant effect. Ingestion of large amounts could produce nausea, vomiting, perspiration and dizziness. Large doses during pregnancy have been suspected of causing premature birth.

Blessed Thistle
(The Monks' Tonic)

Blessed thistle (*Cnicus benedictus*) is also known commonly as St. Benedict thistle, holy thistle and spotted thistle. The plant is native to southern Europe and western Asia. The common names of the herb are derived from its popular use during the Middle Ages as a tonic by monks in the monasteries.

Blessed thistle is mainly used as a folk remedy to stimulate the appetite and as a tonic. It is also claimed to act as a mild diuretic and to be helpful in the treatment of constipation, flatulence, liver disorders, headaches and fever.

The dried flowering tops of blessed thistle are most commonly used as bitters. Usually of vegetable origin, bitters have been traditional remedies for loss of appetite and are still used in many tonics. They are usually taken before meals and are thought to work (if they work at all) by stimulating stomach and small-intestine activity. The herb can cause nausea and vomiting in some.

BUCHU
(Used in Wine and Brandy)

Buchu, bucco and boochoo are the common names for the plant *Agathosma betulina,* also known as *Bartosma betulina.* Buchu is native to South Africa where it is used in brandies and wines, imparting to these alcoholic beverages their characteristic peppermint-like flavor.

Buchu has been widely used as a folk remedy, particularly in Europe and Africa. It is said to be helpful in the treatment of kidney stones, cholera, blood in the urine and rheumatism, among other disorders. These claims have not been substantiated.

Buchu is a weak diuretic and urinary antiseptic and was used in the past by physicians to treat urinary tract infections. There are now much better agents for the treatment of these infections.

BURDOCK
(Mild Diuretic)

Burdock (*Arctium lappa*) is also known in Europe as lappa. It has been used as a vegetable as well as a folk remedy for the treatment of a large number of disorders. In Japan the root is eaten as a vegetable called gobo.

Burdock has been used as a folk remedy for the treatment of various cancers in China, India, Russia and Chile. Homeopathic medicine uses tinctures of the burdock root to treat acne and other skin disorders, gonorrhea, gout, impotence, rheumatism, sterility, peptic ulcer disease and more. It is said to neutralize and eliminate poisons from the body and to be helpful in the treatment of liver problems, arthritis, syphilis, kidney stones, gallstones, flu and vertigo. An essential oil derived from burdock is said to promote hair growth. Lots of claims, but no evidence that it does any of the above.

As is the case for many of the herbs being sold today, burdock may have mild diuretic properties. There is a report of poisoning in a woman who used burdock root tea. However, it was determined that the burdock was contaminated with atropine and that the atropine, not the burdock, was the culprit.

BUTCHER'S BROOM
("Circulatory Tonic")

"Butcher's Broom Sweeps Away Circulation Problems." So reads the headline of a recent flyer on this product. The use of butcher's broom as an herbal remedy dates back to the early Greeks who used it as a tonic and diuretic. However, butcher's broom was essentially an un-known during most of our century until the 1980s when it re-emerged on the health food scene accompanied by some sweeping claims, as evidenced by the above headline.

Butcher's broom (*Ruscus aculaetus*) is a short evergreen shrub be-longing to the lily family. It grows in southern Europe and is a close relative of asparagus. The herb is also known as sweet broom, knee holly and box holly. Butcher's broom was thus named because butch-ers often used the leaf-like twigs of the plant to scrub their chopping blocks.

Butcher's broom is said to be highly effective in the treatment of a wide range of problems related to the circulatory system including varicose veins, postoperative thrombosis, phlebitis (inflammation of the veins) and hemorrhoids. It is often referred to as a circulatory tonic. In addition, it is said to have anti-inflammatory and diuretic properties.

The formation of blood clots following surgery is not uncommon and can lead to serious complications. A French report indicated that surgical patients receiving butcher's broom, which was administered several days prior to surgery and was continued until discharge from the hospital, had a significantly lower incidence of thrombosis (blood clots) than those who did not get the herb. A more rigorous trial is needed to determine if the herb really has any beneficial effect in this condition. Other reports from Europe, which also require verification, suggest that butcher's broom is helpful in the treatment of hemor-rhoids and varicose veins.

Butcher's broom does appear to have a mild diuretic action. Swelling of the lower extremities is frequently associated with varicose veins. The symptoms that go along with varicose veins are often due to the swelling. Any substance which has a diuretic action could reduce the swelling. It is likely that the reports of butcher's broom helping with varicose veins, phlebitis and hemorrhoids can be explained by the mild diuretic action of the herb.

Butcher's broom, now available in the U.S. health food marketplace, is reported to occasionally cause an increase in blood pressure. Thus those with hypertension should use it only under a physician's supervision. Those who require anticoagulation medicine for the treatment or prevention of blood clots should not substitute the herb for these medicines. There are many who prefer taking "natural" remedies to drugs. However, it has not been established that butcher's broom is an anticoagulant.

CAPSICUM/HOT PEPPERS
(The Heat That Cools)

Hot red chili peppers (*Capsicum frutescens*) are hot subjects in the medical literature these days. The big news a few years ago was research showing that capsicum can help prevent dangerous blood clots. Now there's evidence that the "heat" of hot peppers can cool a number of inflammatory responses, including those in burns, some nerve disorders and even possibly in arthritis.

Researchers in Thailand have found that the daily ingestion of capsicum by most of the Thai people, who use the hot pepper as a seasoning and an appetizer, may be associated with the low incidence of thromboembolic (potentially fatal blood clotting) diseases in that country. The researchers found that capsicum has a definite fibrinolytic activity, meaning that it can, to some degree, break down blood clots through an enzymatic mechanism. Significantly greater fibrinolytic activity was detected in Thais who consume capsicum several times a day than among Americans living in Thailand who consumed primarily American-style meals and little or no capsicum. These researchers noted lower-than-average incidence of thromboembolism among New Guineans, East Africans, South African Bantus, Nigerians, Melanesians, Koreans and Indians. All of these people favor hot, spicy foods.

Now an additional medical use has been found for the hot stuff. A topical cream containing capsicum has been marketed as a prescription drug called Zostrix. It helps cool the pain of several nerve disorders affecting the skin, such as shingles and postherpetic neuralgia. Capsicum or more specifically its active ingredient capsaicin has the ability of blocking something called substance P, which is involved in inflammation and pain sensations. This blocking effect makes capsicum a long-lasting anesthetic. And this explains why that old folk remedy— applying a drop or two of capsicum to the gums around an aching tooth—works.

Capsicum's pain-killing effects can be very dramatic. The pain that develops in the wake of an attack of shingles (herpes zoster) can be extreme. Until recently there was no really effective treatment for the postherpetic pain. But with capsicum cream, applied topically to the painful areas, a number of patients with this disorder have experienced substantial relief. In fact, in one study of patients whose postherpetic pain was chronic and unyielding to all other treatments, nine of twelve who stayed in the study for its duration got either complete or very significant relief with no pain recurrence for up to a year.

That study led to a larger, double-blind, placebo-controlled study that produced equally good results. Now thousands of postherpetic pain sufferers are using the cream, usually applying it three or four times daily. About 20 percent experience burning sensations from the capsicum itself. This usually occurs only during the first few days of application.

There's some evidence that capsicum cream may also be helpful in treating, among other conditions, diabetic neuropathy and the pain that occurs after amputation or mastectomy. There are clinical reports of 50–80 percent pain reduction among patients with diabetic neuropathy who have been treated with the cream. Controlled studies are underway. It may also be helpful for other painful peripheral neuropathies such as those that occur in AIDS patients.

Since substance P is involved in the pain and inflammation of rheumatoid arthritis, burns and a number of bowel diseases, it is possible that capsicum preparations may eventually prove useful in the treatment of those, as well.

If you think you have a condition that might be helped by Zostrix, consult your physician about a prescription. Or you might consider trying such over-the-counter capsicum-containing products as Heet lotion and Sloan's liniment. For internal use, I encourage cooking or seasoning with fresh, dried, powdered red peppers. As the Thai research demonstrated, it doesn't take tremendous amounts to get the anti-clotting effects. Too much red pepper (e.g., if you were to eat large numbers of them all at once) might actually damage nerves and permanently destroy some of your taste sensations. Given the hotness of these peppers, most people don't need to be encouraged to be moderate with them. Many have to be prodded to use them at all.

Fears that red peppers might cause or aggravate duodenal ulcers appear to have been exaggerated. In one study, 3 grams of red chili powder (about the same amount consumed daily by the typical person in India) were given to patients with duodenal ulcers for a month without adverse effects. Still, if you have an ulcer, consult your doctor before adding a lot of red pepper to your diet. Also, if you are taking anticoagulants or have a bleeding problem (slow clotting time), do not take capsicum without your doctor's approval. A final tip: If the pepper that you have eaten is too hot and begins burning you up, eating a banana will quickly cool you down.

CASCARA SAGRADA
("Sacred" Laxative)

Cascara sagrada, the English translation of which means "sacred bark," is known botanically as *Rhamnus purshiana*. It is used in a laxative which is derived from the dried bark of cascara sagrada; to be effective it is said that the bark must be collected at least one year before use.

The active principles in cascara are anthraquinone glycosides. Cascara is an anthraquinone laxative with a mild action. The anthraquinone glycosides are split (hydrolyzed) in the colon by bacteria, liberating active anthraquinones which then stimulate the colon. It is usually used at night, thus providing overnight relief (six to eight hours after ingested) from mild constipation.

Cascara sagrada bark is typically administered as an elixir, or in tablets or capsules, because of its unpleasant taste. Neither cascara nor any other laxative should be taken on a regular basis. Those who develop watery diarrhea from cascara should discontinue its use. Cascara could cause red discoloration in alkaline urine.

CATNIP
(Humans Like It, Too)

Catnip (*Nepeta cataria*) is an herb belonging to the mint family. Although most people think of catnip as an herb that is irresistible only to cats (and that includes lions and tigers), catnip has been used for years in folk medicine and as a tea. In fact, catnip tea was used in England before the introduction of modern Chinese tea.

Catnip is reputed to be good for a wide range of human disorders. Some find that hot catnip tea, taken at bedtime, helps them sleep better. Catnip contains nepetalactone, which is somewhat similar in chemical structure to the valepotriates thought to be the sedative components of valerian (see valerian). Some report that catnip is useful for settling mild stomach upsets. It is a relatively safe herb. Smoking its leaves, which a few report produces a mild marijuana effect, is not advised.

CHAMOMILE
(For Insomnia and Indigestion)

Chamomile tea is very popular in the United States. Many who use it say that they find it soothing and calming. Chamomile has been used in herbal medicine since the early Roman days and is commonly used worldwide. There are two kinds of chamomile (sometimes spelled camomile). Roman chamomile and chamomile are the common names used for the plant *Anthemis nobilis*. German chamomile, matricaria and manzanilla are common names for the plant *Matricaria chamomilla*.

Roman chamomile flowers have been used as an aromatic bitter (an appetite stimulant). Large doses can cause nausea and vomiting. A tea prepared from the flowers is sometimes helpful for indigestion. Those who are allergic to ragweed, asters or chrysanthemums may develop allergic rhinitis (inflammation of the nose, nasal congestion and sneezing) or contact dermatitis from the use of Roman chamomile.

German chamomile flowers have also been used as a bitter, and a tea prepared from the flowers is occasionally helpful for indigestion. Large doses can cause nausea and vomiting. German chamomile tea does have a sedative effect for many. A report in the medical literature stated that ten out of twelve subjects who were given German chamomile tea fell into a deep sleep lasting one and a half hours; this sleep began approximately ten minutes after drinking the tea. Costa Ricans use German chamomile tea for the treatment of insomnia and for dieting, claiming that the tea helps curb their appetite. It is likely that they are using higher doses, which can cause nausea. Clinical studies on the sedative, hypnotic and appetite-suppressing effects of German chamomile are warranted. A chemical, alpha bisabolol, has been isolated from the oil of *Matricaria chamomilla* and found to have anti-inflammatory activity in the rat. Recently researchers at the University of Trieste (Italy) found that topical application of chamomile in mice produced a much greater decrease in inflammation when compared with hydrocortisone.

Those who develop allergic responses (sneezing, nasal congestion, wheezing, eczema) from German chamomile should stop using it. Tincture of chamomile, which is sometimes used as a sleeping aid, is reported to cause diarrhea if overused.

CHAPARRAL
(Good for the Female Mosquito)

Chaparral and the desert creosote bush are the common names for the dwarf evergreen *Larreatridentata*. It is native to the desert areas of the Southwestern United States. Native Americans had many uses for chaparral, for example, the bark was used to make a reddish dyestuff and the wood for smoking game.

American Indians have used the leaves and stems of the plant to treat cancers, arthritis, bruises, eczema, rheumatism, snake bites, venereal diseases and wounds. Many claims but no scientific trials. Chaparral does contain the chemical nordihydroguaiaretic acid (NDGA), which has antioxidant and antiseptic properties. NDGA has been used in the food industry as a preservative. Recently NDGA has been demonstrated to increase the average lifespan of female mosquitoes. Whether this has any application to humans is another question. One thing is for sure, we must keep mosquitoes away from chaparral!

NDGA has been reported to produce lesions in the lymph nodes and kidneys of animals. Chaparral itself may cause a contact dermatitis. That is, some people's skin may become inflamed if they touch it. Chaparral is used by some as part of a detoxification program. There really is no compelling reason for anyone to use it based on the available data.

CHICKWEED
(Rich in Vitamin C)

Chickweed (*Stellaric media*) is, in fact, a weed, one that is found all over the world. Some use it as a vegetable or as a salad green. Chickweed has also been used in folk medicine.

Therapeutic claims abound. Chickweed is a folk remedy, said to be good for asthma, cancer, blood disorders, constipation, eczema, fever, hemorrhoids, infections, inflammation, obesity, tuberculosis, bruises, nose bleeds, abscesses and boils. Homeopathic physicians use it for the treatment of gout and arthritis. There is no evidence to back any of this up. It's best to use it as a vegetable or in your salad. It *is* rich in vitamin C.

COMFREY/ALLANTOIN
(Potentially Potent Stuff)

Comfrey is a very popular herb and has been used for hundreds of years as a folk remedy. The most commonly used comfrey comes from the plant *Symphytum officinale*. Russian comfrey comes from a related plant, *Symphytum peregrinum*. Comfrey is rich in protein, and some use it as a vegetable or in their salads.

Comfrey is reputed to be good for a wide range of maladies. The most consistent claims have been for its effectiveness in the treatment of gastrointestinal problems, such as peptic ulcer disease and gastritis, and for the treatment of skin ulcers when applied topically. The healing properties of comfrey for skin ulcers were reported at the turn of the century in some medical journals. For example, a 1912 study reported in the *British Medical Journal* indicated that topical application of comfrey was effective in the treatment of rodent ulcers of the skin. Rodent ulcers are usually caused by basal cell carcinomas, a common skin cancer. Comfrey taken internally has been claimed to heal fractures (hence one of comfrey's nicknames, knitbone).

Comfrey is rich in *allantoin,* which is thought to confer on the herb whatever healing properties it may have. Allantoin has been found to be useful in the treatment of wounds and *is* an ingredient in several wound-healing preparations. It is thought to work as an epithelialization stimulant, a cell proliferant and a chemical debrider. The successful use of maggots in the treatment of chronic ulcers and non-healing wounds is now thought to be due to the allantoin present in the excretions of the maggots. There are reports that allantoin is also effective in the treatment of psoriasis. Further research on the role of allantoin in the treatment of skin disorders is warranted.

Liver tumors have been reported in rats fed high doses of comfrey. Suspected carcinogenic agents present in comfrey are pyrrolizidine alkaloids (PA). Animals consuming high doses of comfrey for long periods of time are reported to suffer liver disease as well as reproductive damage. Russian comfrey is generally higher in PA than common comfrey. Because of the potential adverse effects of comfrey, it is no longer available in Germany, and in 1987 Canada banned the sale of certain types of comfrey leaf. It is, however, still widely available in the United States. Comfrey has been said to be an excellent source of vitamin B_{12}, which does not appear to be true. Comfrey ointments may be useful in the treatment of wounds because of the high allantoin content. The topical (external) use of comfrey should be safe, since the alkaloids require the liver for conversion to toxic metabolites. However, because of the herb's toxicity, I would recommend not using it internally at all.

CRUCIFEROUS VEGETABLES
(Cancer Fighters)

Once again, your mother was right when she told you: "Eat your vegetables; they're good for you." Evidence is mounting that the cruciferous vegetables, in particular, are good for you, especially in terms of protecting against cancer. This family of vegetables includes cabbage, broccoli, brussels sprouts and cauliflower.

There's so much excitement over these vegetables these days that the American Cancer Society has been running full-page ads in magazines with pictures of broccoli and other foods under the headline: "A defense against cancer can be cooked up in your kitchen." The ads identify the cruciferous vegetables as those "that may help reduce the risk of gastrointestinal and respiratory tract cancer," as well as colorectal cancer.

Actually there was some very exciting, now largely forgotten, research done several decades ago that hinted at what was to come. Two researchers published a study in 1950 showing some of the effects diet can have on the body's response to X-rays. They reported that guinea pigs exposed to whole-body X-radiation had lower mortality and incidence of hemorrhage when prefed on cabbage than when prefed on beets. This study shows how dramatically times have changed; rather than conclude that there could be something *protective* against radiation in cabbage, these researchers accounted for what they were observing by concluding that there must be something in beets that became highly toxic in irradiated animals. The notion that a "simple" food like cabbage could protect against something as potent as radiation was just too unheard of to be taken seriously at that time.

About ten years later, however, two other researchers came across the intriguing 1950 report and decided to investigate further. They again exposed guinea pigs to whole-body X-radiation after first having fed them for two weeks on varying diets. *All* of the control animals, which were fed rations of oats and wheat bran, died within fifteen days of irradiation. Animals that got oats and wheat bran supplemented with raw cabbage, on the other hand, fared far better. In seven separate trials, the cabbage-fed animals had an average reduced death rate of 52 percent.

Broccoli, another member of the cabbage family, was found, in an additional two trials, to be even more protective against radiation damage. In still two more trials, both pre- and post-irradiation feeding of cabbage were found to have statistically significant protective effects. The best results, however, were obtained when cabbage was given both before and after irradiation.

Only now are we beginning to identify some of the substances in cruciferous vegetables that contribute to these protective effects. They include such chemicals as aromatic isothiocyanates and indoles, both of which have now been shown to have anti-cancer effects. In addition, many vegetables and some fruits contain such other known anti-cancer substances as coumarins, flavonoids and beta-carotene, among others.

Studies are again being conducted with the cruciferous vegetables. Several test-tube and animal studies have shown definite anti-cancer effects. More work needs to be done, but, in the meantime, almost all of us can benefit from heeding mother's advice to "eat those vegetables."

DAMIANA
(Aphrodisiac?)

There is a picture in a Mexican book on herbs of the damiana plant next to a nude woman. Those familiar with damiana typically think of it as an aphrodisiac. Damiana, or *Turnera diffusa,* is native to Mexico and the southwestern United States. Mexicans make tea from the leaves and produce a liqueur unique to Mexico called Damiana.

Damiana is a major herbal remedy in Mexican medical folklore. It has been used for the treatment of impotence, sterility, diabetes, kidney disease, bladder infections, asthma, bronchitis, chronic fatigue and anxiety. Does it work? Many Mexicans I have spoken with say, "mas o menos" (more or less) when referring to its role as an aphrodisiac. Some find that it "calms their nerves" and may even help them sleep better. It is a relatively safe, bitter-tasting herb.

DANDELION
(Hardy Folk Remedy)

The dandelion (*Taraxacum officinale*) is native to most of the world. It is a very hardy plant, one which some believe will be among the few to survive all of the herbicides we have dumped on the planet. Dandelion is used as a food as well as a popular folk remedy.

Dandelion, like many of the other herbs discussed in this section, has been used at one time or another to treat a broad spectrum of maladies. The roots were used as a bitter in the Lydia M. Pinkham tonic. Dandelion roots have also been used as mild laxatives and diuretics. Many who use it claim that it is an appetite stimulant, mild diuretic and mild laxative. It is a safe herb and unlikely to cause any adverse side effects.

DEVIL'S CLAW
(Anti-inflammatory?)

Devil's claw (*Harpagophytum procumbens*) has been used as an herbal tea ingredient in Europe, a folk remedy in Africa and recently has entered the health food marketplace in the United States.

Africans have used the herb to treat skin cancer, fever, malaria and indigestion. In Europe, the tea is recommended for arthritis, diabetes, allergies, senility and more. There are no clinical studies to refute or verify any of this, but extracts of the plant *do* appear to have anti-inflammatory activity in experimental animals. These studies should be pursued. Devil's claw root tubers are sold in health food stores in the United States. This product does not appear to have any adverse effects, but whether it has any beneficial effects remains to be seen.

ECHINACEA
(Immune Stimulant)

One of the more exciting herbs, from the point of view of real therapeutic potential, is echinacea or *Echinacea angustifolia* and *purpurea*. Echinacea was used by the Native Americans, particularly the Plains Indians, more than 100 years ago as an antiseptic, an analgesic (pain killer) and for treatment of snakebites. Today, there is evidence that echinacea, or more specifically substances derived from it, have significant immune-stimulating activity.

Several reports indicate that the immune-stimulating property of echinacea is due to a polysaccharide. Macrophages are key players in the immune system. They are actively involved in the destruction of bacteria, viruses, other infectious agents and cancer cells. They produce some of their effects by the generation of free oxygen radicals and the production of a protein called interleukin-1. Any substance which activates macrophages could have considerable significance in the treatment of such diseases as cancer and AIDS. A report in the December 1984 issue of *Infection and Immunity* demonstrated that a polysaccharide fraction derived from *Echinacea purpurea* significantly increased the killing effect of macrophages on tumor cells. The polysaccharide also increased the production of free oxygen radicals and interleukin-1. The echinacea polysaccharide had no effect on T-lymphocytes (involved in cellular immunity) and only a modest effect on B-lymphocytes (involved in humoral immunity-making antibodies). Another report indicated that echinacea enhances natural killer cell activity, another important component in the immune system.

There may be other substances in echinacea besides the polysaccharides that have immune-enhancing effects. Recently, some smaller molecules have been isolated that may fit this category. Research must be continued in this very important area.

Note that the favorable immune-stimulating effects discussed above were obtained using extracts of echinacea, not from use of the herb itself. There is some contradictory, but unconfirmed, evidence suggesting that echinacea might actually depress T4 helper cell activity in *some* people. Anyone who is immune deficient should use echinacea only while being monitored by a physician so that the effect of the herb on the immune system can be reliably evaluated.

EPHEDRA/MA-HUANG
(Stimulant)

Ephedrine is widely used these days, to a large degree for its stimulant properties. Ephedrine, as well as pseudoephedrine and norpseudoephedrine, is found in all of the *Ephedra* species. Use of ephedra goes back a long way in Chinese traditional medicine, by the Pakistanis and others. The Chinese species is *Ephedra sinica* or ma-huang. Pakistani ephedra is *Ephedra gerardiana*. American ephedra, which contains norpseudoephedrine, thought to be an even more potent central nervous stimulant than ephedrine, is *Ephedra nevadensis,* also known as "Mormon tea" and "whorehouse tea."

In Chinese traditional medicine, ephedra is used as an anti-asthmatic, a diuretic and for the treatment of allergies, among other disorders. Other folk medicines use it in similar ways.

Ephedrine has pronounced stimulating effects on the central nervous system. It has a more prolonged though less potent action than adrenaline. It can cause blood pressure elevation and increased heartbeat. It also dilates the bronchioles and is thus helpful in the treatment of asthma. It is also used in the treatment of narcolepsy, nasal congestion and symptomatic treatment of allergies. Some use it to try to burn off fat and lose weight. There are several problems with ephedrine. Its effect wears off fairly quickly, and higher doses are needed to produce the same effect. This can lead to overuse.

There are now better drugs, with fewer side effects, to treat asthma, allergies and congestion. Large doses of ephedrine cause headache, nervousness, nausea, palpitations, dizziness, difficulty in urination, insomnia and chest pain. Pseudoephedrine is widely available in over-the-counter decongestants. There is one report that *Ephedra sinica* contains a substance that inhibits the growth of Influenza B virus. This should be pursued.

EUPHORBIA
(Toxic to Kidneys)

Euphorbia is now available in the United States and is claimed to be beneficial in the treatment of asthma, hay fever and sinusitis. The herb that is used, also known as snake weed, is from the plant *Euphorbia pilulifera*. The dried plant has been used as a folk remedy for many years. It may have an expectorant action (clears secretions from the respiratory tract) and as such could be helpful in the symptomatic treatment of the above ailments. However, there is little evidence showing that the herb is effective in this manner. Another species of euphorbia, *Euphorbia resinifera,* is an emetic and powerful laxative. This herb should not be used because of its violent action and tendency to produce kidney problems.

EYEBRIGHT
(But Don't Put It in Your Eyes)

Eyebright or red eyebright are the common names for the plant *Euphrasia officinale,* which is native to Europe and western Asia. As the name implies, it is supposed to be helpful in the treatment of problems of the eye. In fact, herbal folklore has it that it can treat all the maladies of the eye and even restore sight to the blind!

Eyebright does have some astringent properties, and tinctures of the herb have been reported to help with one eye problem—conjunctivitis—in some. Homeopathic physicians use eyebright for colds, hay fever, as well as for conjunctivitis. Unfortunately, there are many reports that application of drops of the tincture in the eye can cause itching, redness, swelling and other adverse symptoms. Application of eyebright to the eye is definitely not advised.

FENNEL
(Beware of the Oils)

Fennel and finocchio are the common names for the plant *Foeniculum vulgare,* a member of the carrot family. Fennel is used for culinary purposes, and the roots and seeds are used as herbal remedies. The seeds, which have a licorice-like taste, are used to flavor candies, pickles, breads, liqueurs, vinegars and pastries. Finocchio is used as a vegetable, often in salads.

The list of therapeutic claims for fennel is very long—without clinical evidence for almost any of them. Fennel seeds may help expel excess gas from the body. Fennel oil has been found to cause a number of adverse effects, including respiratory problems, water on the lungs (pulmonary edema), seizures and hallucinations. Those who use fennel as an herbal remedy should stick with the seeds and *stay away from the oils.*

FENUGREEK
(Good Culinary Spice)

Fenugreek (*Trigonella foenum-graecum*) is one of the oldest medicinal plants, dating back to the ancient Egyptians and Hippocrates. The women of the harem were said to eat roasted fenugreek seeds to make them more shapely, while the lord of the harem ate them as an aphrodisiac. Fenugreek seeds are used in curries and soups.

The list of beneficial properties claimed for fenugreek (mainly the seeds) is a long one but without supporting evidence. Some believe that consumption of fenugreek seeds helps clear mucous congestion. It is a good culinary spice and is used, incidentally, to flavor imitation maple syrup. The seeds of fenugreek have been reported to improve sugar control in experimental animals. This requires further investigation.

FEVERFEW
(For Migraines and Arthritis)

Feverfew (*Tanacetum parthenium*) is a common flowering plant that has been used for centuries to alleviate headaches and joint pain. Modern day research is confirming that feverfew is quite effective in treating migraine headaches and may also be useful in alleviating some of the miseries of arthritis.

Also known as bachelor's button, feverfew seems to have some unique anti-inflammatory properties. The leaves of the plant contain substances that inhibit some of the secretions of blood platelets and white blood cells. Serotonin, secreted by blood platelets, constricts blood vessels and may thus contribute to migraine. Some of the white cells secrete substances believed to contribute to the kind of inflammatory processes seen in arthritis and possibly some other autoimmune disorders. Feverfew restricts these secretions.

The feverfew migraine work looks particularly promising. There have been a number of good studies now showing positive effects. In one of the most recent of these studies, taking daily supplements of ground-up feverfew leaves (about 80 milligrams daily) resulted in a 24 percent reduction in the number of migraines and the headaches that did occur were milder and resulted in less vomiting. This was a placebo-controlled study. Some other studies have reported even better results.

There are several feverfew products on the market. Be aware that their potency may vary considerably.

FORSKOLIN
(Future Drug?)

Coleus forskohili is a plant that has been extensively used in Ayurvedic medicine (traditional Indian medicine) for centuries. It is used to treat diseases of the lungs, such as asthma, of the heart and of the brain. Historically, some of the most important substances used in modern medicine have been derived from herbs. Forskolin, or a derivative of it, could become another such substance. Forskolin is extracted from the roots of *Coleus forskohili.*

Forskolin has very potent bronchodilating activity. It relaxes smooth muscle of airways and inhibits the release of inflammatory agents. Theoretically, this means that it would be an excellent candidate for use in allergic asthmatic conditions. The downside is that forskolin is short acting and may produce some adverse cardiovascular effects. A more selective longer-acting derivative could have great importance in the treatment of allergic asthma. Another potential application of forskolin is in the treatment of glaucoma. It has been shown to lower intraocular pressure in humans, if applied topically. Studies on the beneficial effects of the herb itself are lacking.

FO-TI
(Fountain of Youth?)

Fo-ti is another immigrant from the Chinese herbal marketplace. Fo-ti, also known as hoshouwu in China, comes from the plant *Polygonum multiflorum.* Fo-ti is considered by many Chinese to have magical powers.

Fo-ti has its widest use as a tonic, that is, as an energizer. It is also said to keep the hair black, to be useful for treating insomnia, constipation, fever and cancer. Fo-ti is one of the herbs that the Chinese use to maintain youthfulness. Great claims, but seriously wanting in evidence. It is a relatively safe herb.

GARLIC AND ONIONS
(Protection Against Heart Disease, Cancer and Infection)

Evidence continues to mount that garlic (*Allium sativum*) and onions (*Allium cepa*) have formidable medicinal properties. They help protect against heart disease and cancer and have some remarkable antibiotic effects. This may come as "news" to some, but, in fact, garlic and onions have been used therapeutically for thousands of years. Members of the lily family, they are some of the oldest cultivated plants known. They were used by the ancient Egyptians, Greeks, Romans, Indians and Chinese, among others, to treat worms, tumors, headaches, weakness/fatigue, wounds, sores and infections. Athletes at the first Olympics used garlic as an energizer.

In the modern era, Louis Pasteur demonstrated garlic's anti-bacterial properties in 1858. Albert Schweitzer treated amoebic dysentery with garlic. In two world wars, garlic was used as an antibiotic to prevent wounds from becoming infected. It is credited, in that context, with saving thousands of lives. More recent research has demonstrated that garlic juice and its constituents can slow or kill more than sixty fungi and more than twenty types of bacteria, including some of the most virulent.

The scientific community really began to pay attention to garlic and onions about ten years ago when the results of an epidemiologic study were published comparing the health of three groups of vegetarians in India who consumed large amounts, small amounts and no amounts of garlic and onions over long periods of time. The mean fasting cholesterol levels for these three groups were, respectively, 159, 172 and 208 milligrams per 100 milliliters of serum. The diet of all three groups was strikingly similar except for the differences in garlic and onion intake. Those who abstained completely from garlic and onions, moreover, had blood that clotted more quickly than did those who consumed garlic and onions. The intakes in these groups were: at least 50 grams of garlic and 600 grams of onions weekly (heavy users); up to 10 grams of garlic and 200 grams of onions weekly (moderate users); and no garlic or onions ever (abstainers).

In a subsequent study, two groups of patients with coronary-artery disease were compared over a ten-month period. One group got garlic supplements while the other group did not. Those who got the garlic had steadily declining levels of lipoproteins associated with heart disease, while the group that didn't get garlic showed no decline in these lipoproteins.

Lau and colleagues have reviewed the world literature on garlic's effects on factors known to contribute to narrowing of the arteries (atherosclerosis). They conclude: "The positive reports appear to be overwhelming. The reviewers were surprised by the scarcity of negative reports." They reviewed a variety of animal studies, many well controlled, in which garlic clearly exhibited a statistically significant lowering effect on cholesterol. This effect, in most of these studies, was "dose-related," meaning that the higher the daily dose of garlic, the greater the reduction in cholesterol.

Onions by themselves have also been shown to help promote a healthy cardiovascular system. In one study the juice of a single yellow or white onion taken daily raised HDL (the "good cholesterol" that actually helps protect against heart disease) 30 percent in persons with abnormally low HDL. The researchers believe that onions can help such individuals reduce their risks of heart attack or strokes.

Various sulfur compounds contained in garlic and onions appear to account for their favorable effect on cardiovascular health. Some of these are known to have significant impact on the biosynthesis of fatty acids, cholesterol, triglycerides and phospholipids. Ajoene, a garlic compound, has a potent anti-clotting effect. This compound appears to be the crucial component in a number of garlic's therapeutic actions. Onions have compounds related to ajoene.

There are also compounds in both garlic and onions that have exhibited anti-tumor effects in animals. Epidemiologic studies in China show that eating a lot of garlic can protect against stomach cancer. Those who ate an average of seven garlic cloves a day had an incidence of gastric cancer *ten times lower* than those who rarely, if ever, ate garlic. The garlic, in this case, seemed to work, at least in part, by preventing dietary nitrites from converting to cancer-causing nitrosamines.

Animal cancer research with garlic goes back some years but has picked up a lot of momentum lately. One researcher recently showed that the garlic compound diallyl sulfide, given to mice prior to exposing them to a colon-cancer-inducing agent, has a potent protective effect. The garlic-treated animals got 75 percent fewer tumors than did control animals not given garlic. In a similar experiment, the garlic compound *completely* protected mice against esophageal cancer. In other animal work, sulphur compounds of garlic have inhibited stomach and skin cancers.

These compounds seem to enable the liver to detoxify cancer-causing chemicals before they can do much harm. Some of these substances may also be antioxidants. In addition, both garlic and onions contain bioflavonoids, known anti-carcinogens. More ambitious studies are underway, some at the National Cancer Institute, where scientists hope to create the first garlic-derived anti-cancer drug.

Allicin is another of the active sulfur compounds in garlic. It is the substance that gives garlic its antibiotic qualities (discussed above). The question the prudent consumer should ask is, are allicin, ajoene and these other active compounds still present in the "deodorized" garlic supplements sold in health-food stores? There is little doubt that fresh garlic and onions are, by far, the best way to get these health-giving compounds. Some of them definitely get lost in processing. The next time you buy a garlic supplement, break it open, smell it and taste it. The more it has retained the odor and taste of a freshly crushed garlic clove, the more likely it is to still have some of its active principles. There's no substitute though, for the real thing.

One final comment on garlic. Were those athletes at the first Olympic games in ancient Greece wasting their time (and fouling their breath) when they ate garlic in the hope it would impart extra energy and give them a winning edge? There have been many anecdotes related to garlic's energizing effects over the years, but this issue has been poorly researched. There is *one* report, based on seemingly sound data, which suggests that high doses of garlic might increase physical endurance, at least in rats. A group of researchers wanted to see if garlic could protect heart muscles against a toxic drug. They injected rats with the heart-damaging drug isoproterenol. One group of these rats got garlic in their diet for a week prior to the injection with the drug. Another group got the drug, too, but no garlic. The garlic-fed rats withstood the effects of the drug far better than the rats that didn't get garlic. The garlic-protected rats showed their greater physical endurance by swimming an average of 840 seconds before and 560 seconds after the drug injection. The rats that didn't get garlic could swim only an average of 480 seconds before and only 78 seconds after injection. At autopsy, far fewer lesions were found in the heart muscles of the garlic-supplemented rats than in the muscles of the control rats.

GINGER
(Motion Sickness Remedy)

In 1988 a major herb conference was held in Thailand. This was due, in large part, to the fact that Princess Chulabhorn, the youngest of three daughters of the King of Thailand, has a strong interest in herbs. In fact, her doctoral studies analyzed a Thai species of ginger. Ginger (*Zingiber officinale*) is native to tropical Asia and is cultivated in other tropical areas such as Jamaica. It has been used as a flavoring, a condiment and a folk remedy.

Ginger tea is supposed to promote cleansing of the body through perspiration and is also said to be an appetite stimulator, a carminative (agent which expels gas from the intestines) and helpful in the symptomatic treatment of colds, if given at their outset. It has been used in China and other countries for many years as a tonic.

Ginger does appear to have carminative properties and may help with abdominal discomfort due to "gas." A report appearing in the English medical journal *Lancet* in 1982 concluded that powdered ginger helped with motion sickness. Topically applied ginger has been reported to help in the treatment of burns and may also have antibacterial activity. Thai ginger contains a fraction which is active as a bronchodilator and may have application in the treatment of asthma. A volatile oil obtained from Thai ginger has anti-inflammatory activity.

The whole ginger plant, however, has been found to cause liver damage in animals. It is interesting to note that an alcoholic beverage prepared from Jamaican ginger, popular in some parts of the U.S. in the 1930s, caused a serious neurologic problem called "the Jake Walk." Those who collect blues music of that period are probably aware of the many references to "the Jake Walk blues."

Ginger does appear to have some pharmacologically active substances and we wish the princess of Thailand well in her continued studies of the herb.

GINKGO
(Real Miracles from the World's Oldest Tree)

Mel Brooks plays the 1,000- or 2,000-year-old man, but there actually is a life form on the planet which is more than 3,000 years old. No, it's not Mel Brooks or anything that even vaguely resembles him. It is a tree, a giant tree with a trunk that measures about fifty feet in diameter and which stands at the Dinglin Temple near Juxian, Shandong, China. This is the ginkgo tree, known in the botanical literature as *Ginkgo biloba*. This tree family has existed in its present form for thousands of centuries and was once friends with the dinosaurs. The ginkgo, to understate considerably, is a survivor. It is remarkably resistant to pests and fungi and can continue to reproduce up to an age of over 1,000 years. The ginkgo appears to produce some substances which may help *us* live healthier and longer lives, as well.

Extracts of the ginkgo leaf have been used in China for more than 5,000 years for the treatment of coughs, allergies, asthma, bronchitis and disorders of the lungs and heart. It is used in Ayurvedic medicine (traditional Indian medicine) as a constituent of an elixir called Soma. A concentrated extract of ginkgo, called Tebonin, is available in Europe and Mexico and is used for the treatment of circulatory disorders, such as peripheral vascular disease, cerebral insufficiency and varicose veins. There now exists good documentation for the effectiveness of ginkgo extracts in the treatment of these problems. More recently some active components of the tree have been isolated, identified, characterized and synthesized.

Cerebral insufficiency refers to the condition of decreased circulation to the brain. It occurs with increasing frequency as people get older and is due to atherosclerosis ("hardening") of the arteries that feed the brain. Symptoms of cerebral insufficiency include dizziness, problems with concentration, memory loss, disorientation, forgetfulness and impairment of intelligence and judgment, among others. Strokes occur when the arteries become so obstructed that blood can no longer pass through them. Animal and human studies using a concentrated extract of *Ginkgo biloba* leaves have been found to restore regional cerebral blood flow following induced or spontaneously appearing embolic (blood clot) phenomena. These extracts appear to improve energy metabolism and electrical activity in the brains of animals suffering from decreased cerebral perfusion (blood flow through the brain). In humans, these extracts have been demonstrated to increase brain perfusion as well as to increase oxygen and glucose consumption of the brain.

A long-term study of the use of ginkgo extract in the treatment of chronic cerebral insufficiency in over 100 geriatric patients has been reported. Some of the symptoms of cerebral insufficiency such as dizziness, short-term memory loss and other signs of mental deterioration were found to significantly improve following treatment with the extract. This study, although very suggestive of a positive therapeutic role for the ginkgo extract in the treatment of cerebral insufficiency, can be criticized for not being a double-blind one. *No* side-effects of the extract were noted during this long-term study.

A placebo-controlled, double-blind trial on the effect of ginkgo extract in a group of elderly subjects was reported in a German medical journal in 1985. The results showed that chronic ingestion of the extract improved mental performance in those who displayed deteriorated mental performance to begin with. This was correlated with improvement in their EEG (electroencephalogram) recordings. Nonspecific EEG abnormalities are not uncommon in the elderly with mental deterioration. Hardly any improvement was noted in the elderly with normal performance to begin with after receiving the ginkgo extract.

Ginkgo extract thus appears to increase oxygenation of brain tissue in the elderly suffering from cerebral insufficiency. Can the extract improve brain tissue oxygenation in young, healthy people subjected to conditions of low oxygen (hypoxia)? If it did, it would be of interest to mountain climbers, those living at high altitudes, those with emphysema and other chronic lung disorders. A paper in a German medical journal reported on the effects of *Ginkgo biloba* extract on eight healthy, young men who were subjected to conditions of hypoxia. The study was randomized, double-blind, placebo-controlled and crossover in design. Neurologic responses of the subjects receiving the extract were significantly better than those receiving placebo under these conditions. This is a very significant finding and should be followed up with a larger study.

In atherosclerotic peripheral vascular disease, there is decreased flow of blood going to the extremities. This is due to "hardening" of the arteries that feed the limbs. The lower limbs are more commonly affected by the condition, and the most common symptom of the disorder is called intermittent claudication. Intermittent claudication is defined as severe pain in the lower extremities, particularly the calves, which comes on with walking and is relieved with rest. Those with severe intermittent claudication often cannot walk more than a few steps before the pain begins. Another report, again in the German medical literature, reported on the use of *Ginkgo biloba* extract in patients with atherosclerotic peripheral vascular disease. The study was performed over a period of six months, and was a double-blind, randomized, clinical trial which was placebo-controlled. At the end of the six-month trial, those receiving the ginkgo extract were found to be able to walk significantly longer distances without pain than those receiving placebo. This correlated well with objective measurements which showed improved circulation.

Ginkgo biloba leaves and fruits contain, among other things, bioflavonoids, flavoglycosides (bioflavonoids containing a sugar residue within the structure), proanthrocyanidines (substances closely related to bioflavonoids) and a collection of unusual polycyclic structures called ginkgolides which are, chemically, polylacetones. It has been thought that these substances produce their therapeutic actions by acting as antioxidants (scavengers of toxic free oxygen radicals) and by inhibiting platelet aggregation. More recently, the evidence points to the ginkgolides as being the major therapeutic factors and specifically the ginkgolide called ginkgolide B. Announcement of the synthesis of ginkgolide B by Harvard University chemistry professor Elias Corey and colleagues was made in the *New York Times* (March 1, 1988) with the headline "Ancient Tree Yields Secrets of Potent Healing Substance." The article states that "ginkgolide B could eventually [have] widespread use in treating asthma, toxic shock, Alzheimer's disease and various circulatory disorders. The ginkgo compound is also being studied as a possibly safer substitute for drugs now given to recipients of transplanted organs to prevent the body from rejecting them."

If ginkgolide B is the active therapeutic agent of *Ginkgo biloba*, as it now appears to be, it seems to work by interfering with a chemical made in the body called platelet-activating factor. This substance is implicated in platelet aggregation, graft rejection, asthma and even toxic shock. Researchers at Georgetown University have found that ginkgolide B prolonged the survival of grafted hearts in rats without the undesirable side effects that are observed with drugs such as cyclosporin, which are presently used to prevent the rejection of transplanted organs.

The future of ginkgolide B is enormously promising. However, it will take years before this substance will be available as a drug. Concentrated *Ginkgo biloba* extracts are available in Europe and Mexico and are used for the treatment of circulatory disorders. Tebonin is available in Europe and Mexico, Tanakan in France and Rokan in Germany. Those who have access to these products should discuss their use with their physicians. These substances are relatively free of side effects. Those who desire to use these substances for the treatment of circulatory disorders (under medical guidance, of course) should be aware that it may take several months of constant use before any noticeable benefits are obtained. Ginkgo extracts are now available in health food stores in the United States, but they are low in active ingredients.

GINSENG
(Inscrutable "Panacea")

Panax ginseng was aptly named, for the roots of this shrub have been said to be a panacea (*panax*), a cure-all, good for everything from conquering cancer to stimulating sexual desire. Russian cosmonauts have been directed to chew the herb to fend off infections. Chinese and North Vietnamese soldiers have regularly included the herb in their combat provisions. It has been reported that both Chairman Mao and Henry Kissinger used it. Countless thousands of others certainly use it and some of its many cousins, especially Siberian ginseng (*Eleutherococcus senticosus*) and American ginseng, *Panax quinquefolius*.

Soviet researchers have been particularly keen on ginseng and have claimed their studies show the herb and its extracts can boost immunity, inhibit cancer, increase energy and physical stamina and have variable effects on blood pressure and blood sugar. At a recent international conference devoted to ginseng research, other investigators presented numerous reports on the herb's effects in animals and humans. On the issue of energy and physical stamina, results were mixed. A U.S. Army study found no effect. A Swiss study noted improved physical performance among those taking ginseng. A long-term Russian study discerned numerous benefits, including reduced blood pressure and diminished angina pain, as well as greater resistance to infection. Two Korean studies reported better adaptation to stress and quicker recovery from surgery.

In one of the few double-blind, placebo-controlled studies of ginseng, the herb was found to increase ability to do mental arithmetic among thirty-two healthy volunteers. In other studies, results have been obtained that suggest that ginseng might boost the detoxifying activity of the liver, may help accelerate alcohol clearance in the blood and may help protect against radiation. Some immune parameters were reported enhanced in a few individuals infected with HIV, the AIDS virus. This work needs follow-up.

Certainly all of these studies are intriguing, but, as noted, most lacked controls and few have been convincingly confirmed. Many of the studies contradict each other. Some show reductions in blood pressure, while others suggest ginseng can dangerously elevate blood pressure. A large part of the problem has to with a lack of quality control in ginseng products, which vary tremendously in potency and purity. One recent study of numerous ginseng products found *50 to 70 percent* of them to be diluted or adulterated.

In general, better results seem to be obtained with Siberian ginseng. It seems to have fewer adverse side effects and somewhat more predictable actions. *Panax ginseng* has an estrogen component that may prove troublesome in some. There is less of the estrogen-like activity in Siberian ginseng. The most that can be said for any of the ginseng herbs themselves is that they yield mixed results. *Extracts* of ginseng, on the other hand, have more consistent effects, including some that are immune stimulating, some that enhance glucose tolerance, some that seem to be antioxidant and some that appear to inhibit blood clotting.

Ginseng contains a complex mix of chemicals, including polysaccharides, glycosides and many other potentially active substances. Dosages used in different parts of the world vary enormously. Some warn that heavy use of ginseng (the so-called ginseng abuse syndrome) can give rise to elevated blood pressure, skin eruptions, diarrhea, swelling of tissues, sleep disorders, nervousness, weakness and tremor. One researcher said he observed many of these symptoms in individuals taking 3 grams or more of oral ginseng daily. A few others have reported masculinizing effects in women and feminizing effects in men taking large doses for long periods.

GOLDENSEAL
(Potentially Useful Derivatives)

Goldenseal is one of the most popular herbs in the United States. Goldenseal, also known as hydrastis, comes from the North American plant *Hydrastis canadensis*. Native Americans have used it as both a clothing dye and a medicinal herb.

Goldenseal has been called by some a "cure-all," by others "worthless." It has been used topically to treat acne and eczema. The Cherokee Indians used it for eye and skin ailments. Goldenseal has served as a bitter tonic and astringent and has been used as a douche for uterine bleeding and for the topical treatment of hemorrhoids and cold sores. In fact, it *does* appear to help check excessive uterine hemorrhage. However, it has been reported that the herb produces ulcerations, sometimes severe, on mucous membranes and this should preclude its use as a douche.

One of the chemical substances isolated from goldenseal is berberine. Berberine and its sulfate, berberine sulfate, have been demonstrated to have anti-cancer activity *in vitro* and also have been shown to have anti-bacterial, anti-fungal and immunostimulatory activity, as well. But, there is no documentation that goldenseal itself has any of these activities. Further, the amount of these pharmacologically active substances varies considerably from one sample of herb to another. Therefore, even if it were shown that goldenseal containing high amounts of berberine did display some anti-tumor activity, for example, this is no guarantee that the goldenseal that you obtain at your local distributor would have similar activity. As with all of the herbs, much more research is needed to determine therapeutic potential.

Goldenseal mixed with red pepper has been used as a remedy for chronic alcoholism. The results are purely anecdotal. Recently, a "detox" tea made from comfrey, goldenseal, orange peel, mullein and spearmint has been used to help addicts kick their cocaine, heroin, and methadone habits. This certainly would be great *if* it worked. Without scientific testing we can't say one way or the other. Besides, one of the ingredients, comfrey, may be quite toxic.

High doses of goldenseal may cause nausea, vomiting, a decrease in the white blood count and feelings of pins and needles in the hands and feet. Goldenseal is interesting and needs more study. Some of goldenseal's *derivatives* may eventually prove quite useful.

GOTU KOLA
(Energy Tonic)

Gotu kola, also known as fo ti tieng (not to be confused with fo-ti), is another popular herb in the United States. Gotu kola (known botanically as *Centella asiatica*) is almost always included in the "energy" formulas that can be purchased in most health food stores and at the checkout counters of some supermarkets. Gotu kola has been used as a tonic for a long time, and many claim an energizing effect from its use. A popular book on nutritional supplements states that the herb contains caffeine. This isn't true. The author of that book has confused gotu kola with a completely different herb, *Cola nitida,* which *does* contain caffeine.

Gotu kola is a staple of Chinese traditional medicine as well as Ayurvedic medicine, where it is known as brahmi. It has been reputed to treat leprosy, tuberculosis, uterine cancer, wounds, arthritis, syphilis, stuttering and hemorrhoids. In Chinese traditional medicine, it is considered to be a "fountain of youth" herb, that is, one that can increase longevity. Its major use is as a tonic.

There are reports that substances obtained from the herb may have medicinal benefits. A researcher in Sri Lanka reported in 1988 that a polysaccharide from gotu kola displayed immunomodulating activity. The plant, in fresh form, has been used for the treatment of chronic wounds, and one study showed that seventeen out of twenty-two patients had healing of their chronic skin ulcers when treated with an extract of gotu kola rich in glycosides. Further research along these lines is warranted.

One of the glycosides contained in the herb, asiaticoside, has been reported to be carcinogenic to animals. Data on the safety, as well as the effectiveness, of the herb are needed.

HAWTHORN
(Heart Tonic?)

Hawthorn (*Crataegus oxyacantha*) has been used as both food and folk remedy. The fruits, which are edible, are often made into marmalade. The major health benefit claim is that hawthorn is a tonic for the heart. That is, it is supposed to increase the heart's pumping action. It has been used as a remedy for heart disease, high blood pressure and angina (heart pain).

Hawthorn does contain many bioflavonoids, some of which are flavonoid glycosides which are thought to work in a similar way to digitoxin. Some of these substances may have a vasodilating effect that could be helpful in the treatment of angina. It is important that further research be done on these substances to determine their benefits and their safety. The cardioactive substances are found in the roots, leaves and flowers of hawthorn. Although the herb may be helpful in cardiovascular disease, anyone having such problems should not substitute hawthorn for the medicines prescribed by their physicians. Those with cardiovascular disease who wish to try the herb should only do so under their physicians' guidance.

HERBAL ANALGESIC OINTMENTS AND OILS
(Painkillers)

Four herbal products are commonly used in many ointments and liniments that appear to have analgesic (pain-killing) properties for some soft tissue problems, such as tendinitis, fibrositis, bursitis and neuralgia. Cajuput oil is derived from the leaves and twigs of *Melaleuca cajuputi* and *Melaleuca leucadendron*. Camphor comes from the wood of *Cinnamomum camphora,* and menthol comes from the *Mentha* species. Clove oil is derived from the dried flower-buds of *Syzygium aromaticum*. A popular analgesic ointment from China called Tiger Balm contains all four of these ingredients. Clove oil is a common domestic remedy for the treatment of toothaches.

HERBAL FIBER

Water-soluble dietary fiber is derived from several different plants. Since fiber has application in both therapeutic and preventive medicine, plant-derived fibers can be considered herbs. For example, guar gum is derived from seeds of the guar plant, or *Cyamopsis tietragonolba,* psyillium seed from the Indian plant *Plantago ovata,* plantain seed from *Plantago major* and glucomannan from the root of the Japanese Konjac plant, *Amorphophallus konjac*. Please refer to the section on Dietary Fiber for additional information.

HORSETAIL GRASS
(Tales of Herbal Alchemy)

Horsetail grass, equisetum and field horsetail are common names for the plant *Equisetum arvense*. Horsetail is a member of one of the oldest plant families in the world. It has been used as both a food and a folk remedy. As a folk remedy its use goes back to the 16th century.

Horsetail has been used for the treatment of cancer, bladder and kidney problems, gonorrhea, gout, rheumatism and tuberculosis. There is no evidence of its benefits for any of these ailments. It does have a mild diuretic effect.

Horsetail has a high silicon content and many of its reputed effects are said to be due to the silicon. In fact, because of the high silicon content, the herb is used for polishing and scouring. Silicon is supposed to keep blood vessels, bones, and nails healthy. The role of silicon in human health has still to get established (see section on Silicon). One of the most fanciful ideas about silicon going around is that the body is capable of transmuting this element to other minerals, especially calcium. If this were true, consumption of horsetail would, in effect, turn us into something akin to nuclear weapons!

JUNIPER
(For Flatulence and Colic)

Juniper (*Juniperus communis*) has been used as a flavoring agent, food and folk remedy. The principal flavoring agent in gin comes from volatile oil in its berries. Oils and extracts of the herb are used in many foods and as a fragrance in soaps and perfumes. The Native Americans used juniper in their medicine, but herbal medicinal use dates to the early Greeks and Arabs.

Juniper has been used as a folk remedy for many diseases. The berries, wood and oil of the herb have all been used in herbal treatments. Juniper oil has been used in the treatment of flatulence and colic; it is also a mild diuretic. Excessive doses, however, may cause kidney irritation and should not be used by those with kidney ailments. Juniper should not be used during pregnancy, either, because it may increase contractions of the uterus. Juniper oil can cause inflammation of the skin. Those who take juniper and note excessive urination or irritation of the kidneys or bladder should stop using it.

Kava Kava
(Mood Modifier?)

Kava kava (*Piper methysticum*) is native to the South Pacific islands and was used in Polynesian religious rites. A fermented liquor prepared from the roots was drunk during the rites and was said to produce a peaceful state with heightened sexuality and finally a very restful sleep. The liquor was also reputed to have mild hallucinogenic properties. Kava kava root itself, or a tea made from it, appears to reduce anxiety, fatigue and has a mild diuretic action.

There is a case report in the *Journal of the American Medical Association* (1976) which discusses a man who, after drinking several cups of kava kava tea daily for a period of six months, experienced loss of balance and appetite, a chronic intoxicated feeling, diarrhea and skin problems. He stopped the tea and after twelve months nearly all of his symptoms had resolved. Regular or heavy use of kava kava is not encouraged.

Licorice
(Of Great Medical Interest)

Licorice is best known to us as a candy, even though most "licorice" sold in stores does not contain real licorice. Real licorice comes from the dried unpeeled roots and lower stems of the plant *Glycyrrhiza glabra,* a member of the legume family, which also includes peas and beans. Licorice is one of the most important of the Chinese traditional medicines. It has been used in China, where it is known as Kan-tsao, for at least 3,000 years for the treatment of peptic ulcers, sore throats, coughs and boils. Licorice is one of the major Chinese tonics and is reputed to invigorate the functions of the heart and the spleen. It is also used as an antidote for drug poisoning.

Some of the substances isolated from licorice are of enormous medical interest. Carbenoxolone, the first successful drug for the treatment of duodenal and gastric ulcers, is a derivative of glycyrrhetinic acid, one of the active principles of licorice. A gel containing this drug has been found to be useful in the treatment of painful mouth ulcers and venereal ulcers. The licorice derivative appears to have an anti-inflammatory action in these conditions.

Glycyrrhizin is an extract of the licorice root and has been reported to be beneficial in the treatment of chronic viral hepatitis and herpes zoster. A 1987 report in the journal *Antiviral Research* demonstrated that glycyrrhizin had anti-viral activity against the herpes zoster ("shingles") virus, varicella-zoster, *in vitro*. Another report showed that glycyrrhizin was active against other viruses *in vitro,* including herpes simplex I, polio type 1, vaccinia (causes cow pox), and other animal viruses. Most recently, glycyrrhizin has been found to inhibit the human immunodeficiency virus (HIV), which is the major participant in AIDS. A sulfated form of glycyrrhizin, glycyrrhizin sulfate, appears to be an even more potent inhibitor of the virus. Clinical trials are urgently needed.

Glycyrrhizin and glycyrrhetinic acid (derived from glycyrrhizin by removing its "sugar" component) have been reported to inhibit the growth of melanoma cells *in vitro.* Glycyrrhetinic acid has inhibited the activity of two powerful tumor promoters in mice. Clinical cancer trials are warranted.

As if all of the above were not enough, glycyrrhizin has also exhibited anti-depressant effects. Further, a 1987 report from the Hebrew University in Jerusalem indicated that glycyrrhizin could retard tooth decay by inhibiting the enzyme that helps bacteria stick to the teeth. In summary, glycyrrhizin and its derivatives have impressive anti-viral activity, anti-ulcer activity, anti-inflammatory activity and may also have anti-depressant properties, among other things.

Licorice itself is a demulcent (soothes mucous membranes) and expectorant. It can be helpful for the symptomatic treatment of sore throats and cough. It also has been found beneficial in the treatment of Addison's disease. There are reports of adverse effects in those who consume large amounts of licorice for prolonged periods of time. For example, a fifty-three-year-old previously healthy man was hospitalized for congestive heart failure after eating one and a half pounds of real licorice over the course of a week. A fifty-eight-year-old woman suffered a cardiac arrest secondary to disturbances in her potassium and magnesium chemistry after eating four pounds of real licorice per week for some time. Those who should restrict their intake of real licorice include individuals with congestive heart failure, kidney and liver disease, the elderly and those taking digitalis-type medications. These adverse effects are associated with licorice's aldosterone-like activity.

LIGUSTRUM
(Immune Tonic)

The fruit of *Ligustrum lucidium,* an evergreen shrub that grows in many Oriental countries, is said to have medicinal properties similar to those of astragalus (discussed earlier in this section). Ligustrum has demonstrated immune-enhancing effects in test-tube experiments and is being used in this country by some AIDS patients, among others, often in combination with astragalus and some other herbs.

In China, ligustrum has been used for centuries to treat fatigue, infections, heart disease, body aches, dizziness and ringing in the ears. It is also used to try to retard aging and is said to be useful in cases of premature graying of hair. The typical daily Chinese dose is 6–15 grams of a decoction made with the black berries of the shrub. Active ingredients include syringin and a terpene compound. Both of these substances have favorable immune-modulating effects in test-tube experiments.

MELALEUCA
(For Skin Problems)

Melaleuca is one of the latest entries in the American health food marketplace. *Melaleuca alternifola* is a shrub-like tree that is native to a small region of New South Wales, Australia. Tea tree oil, more commonly known as oil of melaleuca, is obtained by steam distillation of the tree.

The aborigines of Australia brewed the oil into a tea which they used for various disorders. Some studies in Australia in the early 1920s suggested that oil of melaleuca had antiseptic and anti-fungal activity. It was used topically by the Australian troops during WW II to treat burns, insect bites and bacterial and fungal infections of the skin. Oil of melaleuca was introduced into the U.S. in 1986 for use as a topical agent in the treatment of such problems as athletes foot, jock itch, minor cuts, burns, sunburn, insect bites, cold sores, itching, fungal infections of the skin and as a moisturizer. There are many testimonials about the effectiveness of oil of melaleuca, but clinical studies are lacking. No adverse effects of its use have been reported to date.

MARSHMALLOW
(Soft and Soothing)

Marshmallow (*Althaea officinalis*) is an herb native to Europe. The root of the herb is mucilaginous and has been used in confectionery foods and in folk medicine. Incidentally, the candy called marshmallow typically does not contain the herb. However, marshmallows with real marshmallow *are* available but usually only at better candy stores.

Marshmallow is demulcent (soothes irritated tissue, particularly mucous membranes) and emollient (soothing to the skin and mucous membranes) and once was used in the form of an infusion or syrup for sore throat and mouth and gum pain. Some pharmacies still sell althaea syrup.

MEXICAN WILD YAM
(Source of the Birth Control Pill)

The Mexican wild yam, or barbasco, occupies an important place in medical history. Until the 1940s, the sex steroids were very expensive. The reason for this was that they had to be extracted from animals, and it took a lot of animals to make even a small amount of these substances. At the time, steroids were not believed to exist in plants. Then, in 1940, Russell Marker traveled to the south of Mexico and was the first to isolate steroids from the black root of a member of the *Dioscorea* species called cabeza de negro ("head of black") by the Mexican Indians.

Marker isolated diosgenin from the cabeza de negro; from this, progesterone and testosterone could be synthesized. Later it was found that a related plant, the Mexican wild yam, had even higher amounts of diosgenin. This yam became the source for the original birth-control pill. Mexican wild yam also contains dihydroepiandrosterone or DHEA (see analysis elsewhere). Testosterone itself is not known to exist in any plant.

MILK THISTLE
(Powerfully Protective Against Liver Toxins)

Milk thistle (*Silybum marianum*) has been used as a folk remedy for many centuries for the treatment of liver problems. Recently research has demonstrated that extracts of milk thistle do indeed protect against some very nasty liver toxins. The active principles of the herb have been identified and their mode of action is being clarified.

Amanita phalloides is one of the most poisonous mushrooms in the world. Ingestion of this mushroom leads to death 30–40 percent of the time. The toxins of the mushroom phalloidin and amanitin, are particularly destructive to the liver. Yet extracts of milk thistle can protect the liver from phalloidin. The active ingredient of the herb is a bioflavonoid mixture called silymarin, the principal component of which is silybin. In some animal experiments, when silymarin was given before poisoning by the mushroom, it was found to be 100 percent effective in preventing its toxicity. Silymarin was similarly found to be completely effective in animals if given within ten minutes after exposure to the poison. And when given within twenty-four hours it still prevented death and greatly reduced the amount of liver damage.

Silymarin also protects against the liver toxicity of the solvent carbon tetrachloride and ethanol (alcohol) in animals. Silymarin has been used in the treatment of hepatic disorders in humans. A report in the German medical literature stated that liver function in patients with chronic hepatitis improved after three months of therapy with silymarin. A later study reported on the use of 420 milligrams of silymarin daily in patients with cirrhosis of the liver. Of twenty followed up for six to thirty-six months, ten were definitely improved and four had deteriorated. Anecdotes abound regarding the successful use of milk thistle extracts in the treatment of various liver ailments. The studies discussed above suggest that silymarin may be useful in the treatment of liver diseases. Studies are certainly warranted to evaluate the possible effectiveness of silymarin in the treatment of viral and alcoholic hepatitis, cirrhosis and chronic forms of hepatitis.

Silymarin and its principal component silybin appear to function as antioxidants, protecting cell membranes from free-radical-mediated oxidative damage. This type of damage is known as lipid peroxidation. Most liver toxins, including alcohol and carbon tetrachloride produce many of their damaging effects by free radical mechanisms. It has been shown that silymarin, as well as silybin, protect red blood cell membranes against lipid peroxidation and hemolysis (breaking down of the red blood cells) induced by certain red blood cell poisons. A hemolytic anemia caused by certain drugs and some food substances is not uncommon. This condition is referred to as glucose 6 phosphate dehydrogenase or G6PD deficiency. It would be worthwhile to know if silymarin and silybin have protective effects in this disorder as well as other types of hemolytic anemias.

Milk thistle is presently available in health food stores in the United States. Some of these products contain up to 80 per cent silymarin. Those with liver problems who wish to use milk thistle should be monitored by a physician to determine the products' effectiveness. These products are relatively free of adverse effects.

MISTLETOE/ISCADOR
(Unique Immune Modulator?)

An extract of the mistletoe *Viscum album* called Iscador is under study for its immune-modulating properties. Iscador has been proposed for the treatment of some cancers and even for AIDS. Produced in Switzerland, it has, in fact, been used in some European countries for some time to treat cancer.

There is no doubt that Iscador can halt the growth of some cancers in the test tube, and it has been shown, in several studies, to stimulate immunity and inhibit tumor growth in animals.

One group of researchers, remarking on the "unusual effects [of Iscador] on the immune system," reported dramatically increased thymus gland weight in animals given six injections of the drug. The thymus gland is crucial in immunity. This effect persisted for a long period, as did several signs of enhanced immunity. These investigators also found that Iscador could significantly accelerate regeneration of red blood cells after X-radiation. They concluded that the production of thymic cells (involved in immunity) stimulated by injections of Iscador "is far greater than that reported for any other known substance."

Mistletoe, despite its toxicity, has been used medicinally for hundreds of years. Rudolph Steiner introduced Iscador, a fermentation product of the plant juice that was said to be less toxic, as a European cancer therapy in the 1920s. It is still used today. Its supporters have not claimed that it is a cure for cancer but that it can help slow the growth of cancer and may be decisive in saving or prolonging lives when combined with surgery and other cancer treatments. Greater emphasis has been placed on using Iscador as a cancer preventive or as a therapy to be used in precancerous conditions.

Lack of controlled human studies has properly engendered considerable skepticism about Iscador's efficacy in cancer. But more recent work with this substance suggests that it may, indeed, have immune-modulating and possibly some anti-cancer effects. Certainly there is enough good quality evidence to warrant more ambitious investigations.

It would help if we knew more about what is in Iscador. It appears to have bacterial, especially lactobacilli, components, as well as polysaccharides. Alkaloids have been isolated that appear to have the ability to destroy cancer cells.

MULLEIN
(Good for Cough?)

Mullein flowers from the *Verbascum* plants are widely used in Europe for the treatment of cough, bronchitis, and other pulmonary complaints. They are usually used as an infusion. Mullein is now available in health food stores in the United States. No therapeutic value has ever been demonstrated. It may have a mild demulcent effect (soothes irritated mucous membranes).

MYRRH
(Soothes Mouth and Throat Ulcers)

Those who are familiar with the Bible have heard of myrrh. Myrrh was valued for its aromatic quality and was often mixed with labdanum to produce a perfume. Myrrh was also used in incense. Myrrh gum obtained from *Commiphora molmol,* a tree native to East Africa and Arabia, is also a veteran folk remedy.

Myrrh is an astringent (has a drying effect) in mucous membranes. A tincture of myrrh, which is prepared by dissolving the gum in alcohol, is used in mouthwashes and gargles for symptomatic treatment of mouth and throat ulcers.

NETTLE
(Rich in Vitamin E)

Nettle, common nettle, greater nettle and stinging nettle are the common names for the plant which is known botanically as *Urtica dioica.*

The plant is found all over the world. The sting refers to tiny hairs on the leaves and stems which inject a skin irritant when touched. Histamine is a component of the irritant substance. The sting is lost when the plant is dried or cooked. Nettle has been used as a vegetable, in hair and scalp preparations and as a folk remedy.

Nettle has been used in folk medicine to treat cancer, liver disease, constipation, asthma, worms, arthritis, gout, tuberculosis and gonorrhea, all with highly doubtful effectiveness. Nettle is rich in protein, minerals and vitamins, especially vitamin E (one of the richest sources of the vitamin) and some use it as a dietary supplement. It is a mild diuretic.

Adverse effects from drinking nettle tea have been reported including upset stomach, burning sensations in the skin, difficulty in urination and bloating.

OATS
(Feel Your Oats/Kick Your Habit!)

Oats are one of the latest nutritional rages. You can't watch television for long without seeing at least one commercial on oats, and supermarkets seem increasingly stocked with oat bran products. This trend has to do mainly with the known cholesterol-lowering effects of oat bran. But the story is even more interesting. Some claim oats have anti-depressant and aphrodisiac properties, and *there is evidence that oats can help people kick drug habits.*

A decoction of common oats (*Avena sativa*) has been used in Ayurvedic medicine to successfully treat opium addition. It was noted along the way that several of these opium addicts also lost interest in smoking cigarettes after using an alcoholic extract of the oat plant. A paper appeared in *Nature* on an experiment with chronic cigarette smokers who were given an extract of fresh *Avena sativa*. This study was placebo-controlled, and it was found that after one month there was a significant decrease in the number of cigarettes smoked by those using the oat extract when compared with those on placebo. A diminished craving was definitely noted, *and* the effect continued even two months after the oat extract ceased to be given. A subsequent study in mice suggested that the oat extract contains a substance that is antagonistic to morphine. Continued research in this area is clearly needed.

The claimed anti-depressant and aphrodisiac properties of oats have never been convincingly demonstrated.

PARSLEY
(Aid to Digestion)

Parsley (*Petroselinum crispum*) is a member of the carrot family and is widely used as a garnish, often to mask the odors of restaurant food. Estimates are that about 90 percent of parsley used as garnish is never eaten and gets thrown away. Parsley, however, makes for some very tasty and nutritious salads. For example, parsley mixed with bulgur wheat produces a Middle Eastern salad called tabuleh. Parsley and sun-dried tomatoes likewise make an interesting salad. Parsley is also part of folk medicine.

Parsley seeds have been used as a carminative (helps expel gas from the intestines) and as an aid to digestion. The root has a mild diuretic property. Parsley is used as a breath freshener. Claims that parsley can help with amenorrhea, dysmenorrhea, arthritis, cancer and diseases of the liver are without foundation. Extracts of parsley (the essential oils and resin) in large doses have been reported to produce lowering of blood pressure, giddiness, deafness and liver and neurologic disorders. Parsley itself appears free of adverse effects.

PAU D'ARCO
(Anti-Cancer/Anti-Candida?)

Pau d'arco (*Tabebuia impetiginosa*) excited great interest when a headline in a major foreign newspaper declared: "Positive Cases Prove Discovery of a Cure for Cancer." Herbal teas made from the bark of pau d'arco, also known as lapacho, ipe roxo and taheebo, has long been used in South American folk medicine to treat cancer, infections and malaria. Unfortunately, the headline was not based on anything new or scientifically convincing. The Brazilian press has talked about pau d'arco's alleged cancer-fighting abilities for fifty years.

Lapachol, a chemical isolated from the herb, *has* been found to have anti-cancer activity in test-tube experiments, but the National Cancer Institute decided not to continue investigating lapachol when it failed to show anti-tumor activity in living animals afflicted with leukemia. Further research is warranted to determine if lapachol or derivatives of lapachol have anti-cancer activity against other types of cancer. There still are no good clinical studies on the use of pau d'arco itself in the treatment of cancer.

Some are using tea made from pau d'arco bark to treat *Candida* infections and claim favorable results. There is a substance in the herb, xyliodone, which *does* display anti-*Candida* activity, but no one has determined that this works in humans who use the herb. Lapachol has shown anti-malarial activity in animals. Again, this doesn't mean the herb itself will be helpful in treating malaria, and, so far, no one has shown that it is.

Pau d'arco bark appears relatively safe, but whether it has any real medicinal benefits remains to be seen. At high oral doses, lapachol may cause nausea, vomiting and a tendency to bleeding.

QUININE
(Good for Malaria and Night Cramps)

The bark of the *cinchona* tree has given us some of the most important drugs in modern medicine. The cinchona bark itself was used in folk remedies to treat fevers, malaria, cancer, diarrhea, colds, amebiasis, typhoid, dysentery, among others.

The major active components of the bark are quinine and quinidine. Quinine is most famous as an anti-malarial agent. It is also excellent for the treatment of nocturnal leg cramps (night cramps). Quinine sulfate is available as an over-the-counter item. This medicine, taken at 200 to 300 milligrams at bedtime, expels these cramps in many. In some cases, the cramps disappear for long periods of time after taking quinine sulfate every night for about a week or two. Medical supervision is desirable. Quinidine sulfate is used in the treatment of some types of electric disturbance of the heart.

Chronic use of large doses of quinine or quinidine can cause abdominal pain, headache, nausea, ringing in the ears, skin rashes and loss of consciousness (so-called quinine syncope). A few are very sensitive to quinine and may develop lowering of the blood count. This is reversible when the quinine is withdrawn. Eight grams of quinine taken all at once can kill you.

Quinine derivatives have been used to treat skin conditions. For example, a product called bag balm (available in pharmacies), which has as its active ingredient 8-hydroxyquinoline sulfate, is used as an antiseptic and to treat chapped teats of cows. It is also useful for the treatment of scratches, abrasions, sunburn and chapped hands in humans.

RED CLOVER
(Expectorant, Sedative, Good for Asthma?)

Red clover, also known as wild clover and cowgrass and botanically as *Trifolium pratense,* is a very popular plant in folk medicine. It is supposed to be good for a long list of ailments, but evidence for its efficacy is lacking. The Chinese use the tea as an expectorant; the Russians recommend it for the treatment of asthma, and in Europe the flowers are used as a sedative. Some enjoy red clover tea for its own sake, others claim it has a tonic effect. No adverse effects have been reported in those using the herb.

RED RASPBERRY
(Good for Nausea?)

Red raspberry (*Rubus idaeus*) is especially known for its delicious fruit. The leaves of the plant are commonly used to make a tea which is said to be useful in treating nausea. No adverse effects have been reported.

SAINT JOHN'S WORT
(Antimicrobial/Anti-Depressant)

Saint John's wort is the common name for a family made up of about two hundred species of herbs, the best known of which is called *Hypericum perforatum.* St. John's wort had never been, prior to 1988, a major star in the world of medicinal herbs. In fact, because it grows as an aggressive weed, many have considered it to be quite a nuisance. *Hypericum* infestation of the pasture and range lands of California led to serious financial losses in 1930. Economic loss from the effects of this weed is now slight because of a certain beetle which took a liking to it and now keeps its growth under control.

St. John's wort leaped into the medicinal herb arena in late 1988 following the appearance of a report in the prestigious scientific journal *Proceedings of the National Academy of Sciences.* Researchers from New York University Medical Center and The Weizmann Institute of Science reported that two substances from the herb, hypericin and pseudohypericin, displayed anti-viral activity against some retroviruses. These substances were effective at amounts which have low toxicity. Retroviruses include the human immunodeficiency virus (HIV), and the authors suggested that these herbal products could be useful in the treatment of AIDS.

St. John's wort has been used as a folk remedy for hundreds of years as a treatment for infectious diseases including colds, syphilis, tuberculosis, dysentery, whooping cough and worms. Aqueous extracts have been shown to inhibit the growth of *Mycobacterium tuberculosis* (the bacterium which is the most common cause of tuberculosis), as well as the bacteria staphylococci, shigella and *Escherichia coli.* Robert Nagourney, Alan Kapuler and I have shown (manuscript in preparation) that extracts of St. John's wort inhibit the growth of some strains of *Staphylococcus aureus,* enterococcus and *Pseudomonas aeruginosa* that are highly resistant to antibiotics. Extracts of the herb have also been reported to have anti-viral activity against herpes simplex virus, influenza virus and hepatitis B virus. It just may be that this nasty weed has some remarkable broad-spectrum activity against many different types of infectious agents. More research is needed.

Hypericum has been used as a folk remedy for the treatment of depression, anxiety, mania, hypochondriasis, fatigue, hysteria and insomnia. There is documentation that extracts of the herb do have anti-depressant effects. For example, a 1984 report in a leading German medical journal demonstrated significant improvement in depression, anxiety and insomnia in nine people who received oral extracts of St. John's wort. Side effects did not occur. Further research of this issue is definitely warranted.

It is reasonable to ask at this point, why hasn't this herb, which appears to have an enormous therapeutic potential, been given more serious consideration by medical researchers? The answer to the question must take into account its known toxicity. In fact, it is one of the herbs that the FDA does not allow to be sold for human consumption.

What is the nature of its toxicity? St. John's wort is a primary photo-sensitizer for cattle, sheep, horses and goats. It makes these animals highly susceptible to damage from the sun's rays. The exact location and, to some degree, the nature of sun-caused skin damage in these animals depends largely upon the species or breed of animal. Black-skinned animals are rarely affected. Animals suffering from an acute case of photosensitization develop intense itching of the skin and may rub the affected areas until they are raw. In addition, severe inflammation of the mucosa of the eyes and mouth may occur and this can lead to such complications as blindness and refusal of food, with subsequent starvation and death. Other symptoms of photosensitization include increased heart rate and respiratory rate, diarrhea and fever.

There is evidence that the photosensitizing substance in St. John's wort is the fluorescent pigment hypericin. Purified hypericin, when given orally, can produce photosensitization in rats. It is the reaction of this substance with the ultraviolet rays of the sun that causes the problem. The photosensitization reaction is known as hypericism or St. John's wort poisoning. Photosensitization reactions have not been described in humans participating in studies using *Hypericum* extracts. It is likely that these subjects were not receiving doses high enough to cause the reaction. The photosensitizing dose for humans is not known. It is important to determine this dose in further research.

Hypericin and pseudohypericin appear to be the active therapeutic components of St. John's wort. Hypericin yields from the herb vary from 0.0095 to 0.466 percent. Other substances found in the herb include protein, fat, tannin, vitamins A and C, carotenoids, rutin and pectin. The presence of hypericin and pseudohypericin distinguish St. John's wort from other herbs.

Hypericin and pseudohypericin are promising candidates for the treatment of HIV disease, including ARC and AIDS, as noted above. The mechanism of viral inhibition by these substances is not known, but their chemical structures suggest that they could interact with the membranes of these viruses, leading to their increased fluidization. Fluidization of the HIV membrane would essentially inactivate the virus. More studies related to the effects of these substances in AIDS urgently need to be done. Meanwhile, some with ARC and AIDS and others who are positive for the HIV virus are experimenting with teas and extracts from St. John's wort. There are several problems with this approach. The effective dose of hypericin or pseudohypericin for the treatment of these conditions is not known, there is great variability in the amount of these substances found in different preparations of the herb and the ingestion of a large amount of St. John's wort could lead to very toxic reactions. Those who do experiment with this herb should stay out of the sunlight or use sunscreens with an SPF (sun protective factor) of at least 15 if they are exposed to sunlight.

SARSAPARILLA
(Builds Muscle?/Fights Leprosy?)

Sarsaparilla has been used as a flavoring agent for such things as root beer and other beverages, candies and medicines. It is also a folk remedy used by many people around the world. There are several species of sarsaparilla used in folk medicine. For example, Mexican sarsaparilla is *Smilax aristolochiifolia,* another species of sarsaparilla is *Smilax ornata.*

The rise in popularity of sarsaparilla, particularly Mexican sarsaparilla, is mainly due to the erroneous belief among some body-builders that the root of the plant contains testosterone. Although the *Smilax* species do contain plant sterols, it has never been established that these sterols are metabolized by the human body in any way that increases muscle mass. They certainly do not contain testosterone. In fact, no plant is presently known to contain testosterone.

Sarsaparilla has been used in Morocco to treat leprosy. Extracts of sarsaparilla (*Smilax ornata*) were reported to be effective adjuncts to dapsone, the standard therapy for leprosy. This should be pursued as it may affect other infectious diseases, as well.

SCHIZANDRA
(In Search of Miracles)

Schizandra (*Schizandra chinensis*) is a Chinese herb some regard as miraculous in its medicinal effects. The fruit of schizandra, which is called wu-wei-tzu in China, has been used in Chinese traditional medicine as an astringent for the treatment of dry cough, asthma, night sweats, nocturnal seminal emissions and chronic diarrhea. It is also used as a tonic for the treatment of chronic fatigue. In China, from 3–20 grams (one-tenth to seven-tenths of an ounce) of the fruit is used to prepare a decoction for the above purposes. Its "miracles," alas, are entirely anecdotal.

Substances have been isolated from schizandra which appear to have protective effects against liver toxins in mice. And there are reports that extracts of the herb are beneficial in the treatment of various liver disorders in experimental animals. Immunomodulating substances have also been isolated from the herb, some of which have cortisone-like effects. Schizandra may prove to have some role in modern medicine yet, but it's doubtful that it will be a miraculous one.

SENNA
(Laxative)

Senna is an ancient herbal remedy that continues to be widely used in modern medicine. The two varieties of senna that are commonly used are *Cassia senna,* known as Alexandrian or Khartoum senna, and *Cassia angustifolia,* known as Tinnevelly or Indian senna. Alexandrian senna is preferred because of its milder action.

Senna is a laxative. The active principles are anthraquinone glycosides known as sennoside A and sennoside B. Cascara is also an anthraquinone laxative (see cascara); however, it is much milder than senna. The anthraquinone glycosides are broken down in the colon, liberating the anthraquinones, which stimulate the colon. The laxative action takes place from six to ten hours after administration, and, therefore, senna is usually given at bedtime.

Many preparations of senna, derived from the fruit or leaves of the plant, are available. Senokot is a standardized preparation of senna fruit available as tablets, syrup or granules. Since senna is a powerful laxative it is frequently combined with other herbs to make it milder. A popular senna laxative, Swiss Kriss, contains senna leaves mixed with licorice, anise, fennel, dandelion, juniper berries, lemon and parsley.

Senna laxatives should never be taken on a regular basis. Neither should any other laxative. Regular use can seriously disrupt colon function. Those with bulimia and anorexia nervosa often abuse senna laxatives. This can lead to some severe medical problems. Senna anthraquinones may impart a red color to the urine or feces if they are alkaline. Nursing mothers who use senna pass it on to their infants, though the infants' bowel functions do not appear to be affected. Sublaxative doses of senna (in the form of senokot) have been reported to have a spasmolytic effect, decreasing intestinal spasms.

SKULLCAP
(Sedative)

Skullcap used in America—sometimes called Virginia skullcap—comes from the plant *Scutellaria lateriflora.* The major use of skullcap has been as a sedative for "nervousness."

The Chinese use another variety of the plant, *Scutellaria baikalensis,* or Chinese skullcap, for "nervousness" and rheumatism, among other disorders. Bioflavonoids have been isolated from Chinese skullcap; these have anti-inflammatory and anti-allergic effects.

The benefits attributed to skullcap are purely anecdotal. On the other hand, the herb itself is relatively safe. However, large doses of a tincture of the herb have been reported to cause confusion, giddiness, stupor, twitching and other neurologic symptoms.

SLIPPERY ELM
(Demulcent and Emollient)

Slippery elm (*Ulmus fulva,* also known as *Ulmus rubra* because of the reddish color of its bark) is a tree native to North America. Slippery elm bark has been used in foods and is part of American herbal folklore.

Slippery elm bark was once an official drug of the U.S. pharmacopeia. It contains mucilage and was used as a demulcent. A demulcent soothes irritated tissues, especially mucous membranes, and a slippery elm bark infusion has been used for the symptomatic treatment of sore throat. Poultices made from the powdered bark have been used for skin diseases and wounds because of its soothing (emollient) effect. Some may be allergic to the pollen. It is otherwise a relatively safe herb.

TRIPHALA
(The Chicken Soup of Ayurvedic Medicine)

If there is anything akin to chicken soup in Ayurvedic medicine (traditional Indian medicine), it is triphala. Triphala is a preparation made up of three different herbs each in equal amounts. The herbs are amalki, or *Emplica officinales;* haritaki, or *Terminala chebula;* and bibhitaki, or *Terminala belerica.* Triphala has been used for nearly every ailment by the Ayurvedic practitioners.

Triphala is supposed to be helpful for the treatment of heart disease, diabetes and constipation. Triphala has now come to the United States and is claimed to regulate bowel function if taken on a continuous basis. Haritaki, also known as myrobalin, and bibhitaki are rich in the astringent tannin and have been used in India for the treatment of diarrhea as well as (in the form of ointments or suppositories) for the treatment of hemorrhoids. Triphala is relatively free of adverse effects, but its therapeutic value, if any, remains to be proven.

UVA URSI
(For Urinary Tract Infections)

Uva ursi, also known as bearberry, is the evergreen plant *Arctostaphylos uva-ursi.* The dried leaves of the plant have been used for hundreds of years as a folk remedy. Its major use has been in the treatment of lower urinary tract infections (bladder and urethra) and as a mild diuretic.

Uva ursi does contain the chemical arbutin, which breaks down in the body to hydroquinone, a substance that serves as a urinary antiseptic. Large doses or prolonged use of hydroquinone can have adverse effects, including nausea and vomiting, ringing in the ears and delirium. Uva ursi should not be used by children (may cause liver damage) or pregnant women (may cause abnormal uterine contractions). The herb should never be used for prolonged periods of time or in high doses, and it is prudent for those who use it to do so under a physician's supervision.

VALERIAN
(Sedative/Anti-Anxiety Agent)

Most of the medications used to treat insomnia disrupt natural sleep rhythms and become psychologically addictive. Natural sedatives, free of these side effects, are constantly being sought. For some L-tryptophan (see discussion elsewhere) filled the bill. Others claim that valerian root has a calming effect and helps them fall asleep more easily.

Valerian root (from the plant *Valeriana officinalis*) has been used as a folk remedy for several disorders including insomnia, hysteria, palpitations, nervousness, menstrual problems and as a sedative for "nervous" stomach.

Valerian root contains chemicals called valepotriates; these are said to be the source of its sedative effects. Mixtures of valepotriates are available in Europe.

Some studies have shown that extracts of valerian root have sedative properties and improve the quality of sleep in those with insomnia, without "hangover." Other studies have been negative. For example, a 1985 study from the Netherlands showed no anxiety-reducing activity by an extract of valerian root or purified valepotriates. However, the study *did* show that didrovaltrate, a valepotriate, as well as valeranon, an essential oil component from the herb, produced a pronounced smooth-muscle relaxant effect on the intestine. The study concluded that certain valerian preparations may produce a calming effect indirectly through local spasmolytic activity. A 1987 study from Russia reported that valepotriates inhibited caffeine-stimulated motor activity and prolonged barbiturate-induced sleeping time in mice and rats. This translates to anti-anxiety and sedative activities. The study also showed that those substances have an anti-hypoxic effect, meaning they might protect against oxygen deprivation.

Valerian is widely used as an anti-anxiety agent and sedative. In addition, some drug-rehabilitation programs are now using valerian root teas. It is important to continue research on these substances to determine their benefits and safety. Those with impaired kidney or liver functions should not take valerian except under a physician's supervision. Valerian may interact with alcohol, certain antihistamines, muscle relaxants, psychotropic drugs and narcotics. Those taking any of these drugs should take valerian only under medical supervision. Overall, the herb is relatively safe. Generally, it is unlikely that adverse effects will result from *occasional* use of two cups of valerian tea or two capsules of valerian root (of not more than 500 milligrams each) in a twenty-four-hour period.

WALNUTS
(Good for Sweaty Feet?)

Walnuts have been used in folk medicine for thousands of years. There are three general types of walnut. The walnut that most of us are familiar with is commonly known as the English walnut, caucasian walnut, Persian walnut and botanically as *Juglans regia*. Another type is the butternut, also known as the lemon walnut, oil nut, white walnut and botanically as *Juglans cinerea*. The black walnut, or *Juglans nigra*, is the third type.

The leaves of the English walnut have been used to prepare decoctions for external use in the treatment of rheumatism, gout, gum problems, dandruff and sweaty feet. There is no pharmacologic evidence to support these claims.

The bark of the butternut is said to be effective in the treatment of worms, to help with chronic constipation and in the treatment of colds and the flu. Again, there is no evidence to substantiate these claims.

The bark of the black walnut is supposed to help control diarrhea, and a poultice made from the hulls is said to get rid of ringworm. There is no evidence that supports these claims, nor is there any evidence that black walnut hulls are helpful in expelling parasites from the body, another claim made for the herb.

WHEAT GRASS/BARLEY GRASS
(Green Power)

Wheat and barley grass products, big sellers these days despite some very high prices, are said to protect against pollutants, radiation, cancer and some other ills. These claims, though far from proved, are not without some substance.

One group of researchers has found that extracts from the roots and leaves of wheat sprouts selectively inhibit some of the adverse effects of some known cancer-causing substances—at least in laboratory studies. Chlorophyll, the pigment that gives plants their green color and is fundamental for the conversion of the sun's energy into carbohydrates, has been identified as one of the factors that inhibit the mutation-promoting effect of carcinogens requiring metabolic activation. There is some evidence chlorophyll may be an antioxidant.

The biologist Yasuo Hotta has done some promising work with an extract of lyophilized (freeze-dried) barley grass (similar to wheat grass). He found that this extract protects human fibroblasts and lung cells grown in tissue culture against cell damage from X-rays and a cancer-causing agent, 4-nitroso-quinolone. The extract must be given to the cells *before* the damaging agent is introduced for this protective function to occur. Chlorophyll does not appear to be the active factor in this case.

Hotta has also reported that germ cells of older mice are protected against damage to their DNA during one phase of cell division by an extract of barley grass. The phase in question is one in which the DNA is particularly vulnerable to damage. Vulnerability seems to increase with age. Again, chlorophyll does not seem to be the active protective agent. Hotta has identified a substance from barley grass that *does* seem to be one of the active characters. Intriguingly, it appears to have superoxide dismutase-like activity. (See discussion of superoxide dismutase elsewhere.)

One of the most popular barley grass supplements being sold currently is called Green Magma. In one clinical study, Green Magma reportedly improved certain skin conditions in 80 percent of those tested. Green Magma is quite expensive, but with some of the production shifting from Japan to the U.S. it is hoped that the cost will come down.

Some good long-term studies are needed to provide a more useful evaluation of these very promising grasses.

WHITE OAK
(For Sore Throat)

White oak (*Quercus alba*) is a tree native to North America. The bark from the tree was a popular folk medicine for Native Americans. A gargle or mouthwash made from the bark may be useful for symptomatic treatment of sore throat, owing to the herb's astringent properties.

YELLOW DOCK
(Unreliable)

Yellow dock (*Rumex crispus*) is used as both a salad green and folk remedy. As a salad green, young leaves are prepared by cooking. Tea made from the herb is used mainly as a tonic. Folk medicinal uses, largely devoid of scientific support, include treatment of sexually transmitted diseases such as syphilis, treatment of gum disease, wounds, ringworm, leprosy, skin problems and tuberculosis. Yellow dock contains tannin, which has astringent action and can be helpful for diarrhea, and anthraquinones, which have laxative action. The use of the herb to treat either diarrhea or constipation is not very reliable.

Large doses of the root extract have been reported to cause diarrhea, nausea and excessive urination.

Yohimbine
(Aphrodisiac/Diet Aid?)

Yohimbine, derived from the bark of the yohimbe tree (*Corynanthe yohimbe*), is said to be one of the few genuine aphrodisiacs in nature. This may be true—at least for some people.

In a double-blind, placebo-controlled study of forty-eight men, roughly half of whom were suffering from psychologic impotence, while the other half had impotence with a physical basis, administration of yohimbine had a significantly stimulating effect. Some 62 percent of those who got 6 milligrams of the herb daily for ten weeks reported notable improvement in sexual function, whereas only 16 percent of those getting placebo reported improvement. Improvement was measured in terms of frequency and quality (rigidity and lasting power) of erections. Even among those who were suffering from psychogenic impotence, 46 percent reported positive responses to yohimbine.

How could yohimbine favorably affect both psychologic *and* physical impotence? The substance, in technical terms, is an alkaloid that blocks presynaptic alpha-2 adrenergic receptors which, theoretically, could promote increased flow of blood into the penis while decreasing outflow. And, through activity in the brain, it is postulated that it might diminish the specific forms of anxiety and depression that contribute to psychologic erectile failure. Yohimbine, considered by some to be a "psychedelic" drug in the 1960s, has an excitatory, mood-elevating effect in some people.

Animal work is suggestive of a genuine aphrodisiac component in yohimbine. A real aphrodisiac peps up the sex drive not only of those with drooping desires but also those with normal libido. This is exactly what yohimbine has been shown to do in experiments with male rats. Whether the rats were sexually normal and experienced, sexually naive and inexperienced or sexually inactive, yohimbine increased their sexual arousal and activity markedly—within twenty minutes of injections of low doses.

Yohimbine is generally taken in tablet form (orally) in humans. It is available by prescription only. The usual dose for sexual problems is one 5.4-milligram tablet three times a day for up to ten weeks. If sweating, nausea or vomiting occur, the dose is cut to one-half tablet three times a day, gradually building up to the full dose. The drug should not be used by those with ulcers, kidney or heart disease. Nor should it be used when taking the antihypertensive medication cloni-dine or any tranquilizer, anti-depressant or other mood-modifying drug.

It has generally been thought that yohimbine has no application in women (and the drug should never be used during pregnancy), but recently a Polish study suggested that the substance might help some women lose weight. The twenty-four women studied were 73 percent overweight in terms of the standard Metropolitan Life Insurance Company tables. When given placebos the women lost an average of 3.9 pounds per week; when given yohimbine, the average loss was 5.3 pounds per week. The yohimbine increased weight loss by 36 percent. The researchers believe that yohimbine stimulates lipolysis and thus helps keep fat from accumulating.

Yohimbine—a fascinating herb that deserves more research.

TEN

Other Supplements

This chapter analyzes a number of food supplements that cannot be characterized as vitamins, minerals, lipids, amino acids, nucleic acids or herbs. The supplements included are:

Acidophilus/Yogurt/Kefir
Bioflavonoids/Propolis/Disodium Chromoglycate
Brewer's Yeast/Skin Respiratory Factor/Glucan
Coenzyme Q_{10}
Dietary Fiber
Enzymes (Wobe-Mugos, etc.)
L-carnitine
Lipoic Acid
Mushrooms: Shiitake and Rei-shi
PABA
Pangamic Acid/DMG
Royal Jelly

Seaweeds
Spirulina and Chlorella
Succinates and Cytochromes
Wheat Germ and Octacosanol

ACIDOPHILUS, YOGURT, KEFIR, ETC.
(Health Culture)

Yogurt, kefir and some other health food items are milk fermented by the bacterium *Lactobacillus acidophilus* (and other bacteria). Acidophilus and various of its products are said, without documentation, to lower cholesterol levels, clear the skin, extend life span and enhance immunity. Acidophilus is useful in the maintenance of intestinal and vaginal ecologic balance. People taking oral antibiotics over long periods of time may benefit from oral acidophilus or intravaginal acidophilus. Acidophilus helps keep alive those harmless or useful microorganisms that if eliminated might be replaced by potentially harmful pathogens. Many doctors recommend acidophilus for the purpose of preventing, for example, yeast infections of the vagina. (Do not use acidophilus intravaginally, however, without directions to do so from your doctor.) Recently, it was reported that a cup of yogurt daily reduced the incidence of vaginitis threefold in a study of women with a history of recurrent vaginal candida infections. There are many anecdotel reports that people feel better, in general, when they regularly consume products that contain acidophilus. The often heard claims that cultures (no pun intended) in which yogurt is a primary staple of daily diet produce an excessive number of happy ancients are unproved. There is no reason, however, to discourage the consumption of these products. One report shows yogurt to be a well-tolerated source of milk for lactase-deficient persons.

Make sure that the yogurt you eat contains *Lactobacillus acidophilus.* If you can't be sure whether a yogurt contains the bacteria, you might consider making your own yogurt.

BIOFLAVONOIDS, PROPOLIS AND SODIUM CHROMOGLYCATE
(Making a Strong Comeback)

Bioflavonoids are widely found in food plants where they impart color to flowers, leaves and stems. There are at least five hundred naturally occurring varieties. Bioflavonoids were named "vitamin P" many years ago by the late Hungarian researcher Albert Szent-Gyorgyi, who won the Nobel Prize in Medicine for, among other thing, his discovery of vitamin C. It was in the course of isolating vitamin C that Szent-Gyorgyi came across the bioflavonoids. He had a friend with bleeding gums and thought this condition might have something to do with a vitamin C deficiency. He gave the man some of his early, *impure* vitamin C preparation and, sure enough, the man's bleeding gums cleared up.

Later on, confronted by a recurrence of the bleeding gums, Szent-Gyorgyi decided to try again—this time with *pure* vitamin C. He expected to observe an even more dramatic result. No such luck. The man's gums went right on bleeding. Szent-Gyorgyi re-examined his earlier preparation and decided that the effective impurity was one of the bioflavonoids. He tried these by themselves and reported that they worked. He named these substances "vitamin P." The bioflavonoids thus first came into use primarily as protectors of capillaries, the tiniest blood vessels in the body. The bioflavonoids were said to strengthen or preserve the structural integrity of these vessels, preventing bleeding disorders related to numerous maladies.

The bioflavonoids or "vitamin P" did not completely fulfill the definition of a vitamin and no deficiency states, at least in the United States, were identified for them. However, many physicians began prescribing bioflavonoids, encouraged by dozens of positive studies. Then, in 1968, the Food and Drug Administration, relying primarily upon a review of the bioflavonoid literature conducted by a panel of the National Academy of Sciences/National Research Council, withdrew the bioflavonoid drugs from the marketplace, declaring that they were ineffective in humans "for any condition" whatsoever. The more than fifty drug companies, including many of the pharmaceutical giants, that had been manufacturing bioflavonoid preparations for prescription use were obliged to halt production—at least for distribution in the U.S.

Overall, this was a curious episode, to say the least. The *Medical Letter,* in an article called "Requiem for Flavonoid Drugs," Feb. 9, 1968, voiced its support for the FDA action but acknowledged that "many of the authors who investigated these drugs and found them effective were as competent as most of the authors whose reports on drugs now appear in medical journals, and their studies were of about the same quality as many of the studies now being reported." The *Medical Letter* was trying to say that even competent researchers make mistakes. True enough. But, looking back, one has to wonder if the dozens of independent researchers whose findings tended to confirm one another shouldn't be considered more trustworthy than the conclusions of a single review panel. Review panels also make mistakes, and, as we shall see in a moment, recent studies of these substances strongly suggest that they can have important roles in medical therapeutics. But first, let's look back at some of the earlier studies.

One of the more interesting of these was reported by Griffith in 1955. He used the bioflavonoid rutin at daily doses of 200 to 600 milligrams to treat capillary fragility, and the easy bruising associated with it, in patients who also had hypertension. He noted, after ten years of observation, a significantly lower death rate in those receiving rutin than in those not receiving it. It has been postulated that this could have been due to a decrease in cerebral hemorrhage, a leading cause of death in hypertensives, in those treated with rutin. Other pre-1968 studies showed increased capillary strength in those given bioflavonoids, and one placebo-controlled report demonstrated a significant decrease in mid-menstrual cycle bleeding in women getting citrus bioflavonoids.

The 1968 FDA directive stopped physicians from prescribing bioflavonoids but did nothing to prevent the consumer from purchasing them at health food stores, usually in combination with vitamin C. The claim is that vitamin C cannot be fully or properly utilized by the human body except in the presence of bioflavonoids. This—rather than the old claims concerning capillary protection—is the major reason that most consumers are using supplemental bioflavonoids today. There is evidence that bioflavonoids, which *do* have antioxidant properties, help sustain vitamin C's own antioxidant capacity. This, however, would only be significant in cases of vitamin C deficiency. It has also been found that vitamin C itself protects the bioflavonoid quercetin from oxidation.

There is no good evidence that bioflavonoids enhance the absorption and utilization of vitamin C in the human body. In fact, there is even one study that showed synthetic vitamin C to be better absorbed and utilized by the body than either vitamin C teamed with the bioflavonoid rutin or "natural" vitamin C in the form of orange juice.

Now let's fast-forward to the 1980s, which can be called the renaissance of the bioflavonoids. For starters, let's look at the abstract of a review article in a 1984 edition of the journal *Trends in Pharmacological Sciences:* "Naturally occurring flavonoids have potent anti-allergy, anti-inflammatory and anti-viral activity. Since they are common dietary constituents the question arises: are they natural biological response modifiers?" Given the bizarre history of the bioflavonoids this latest about-face should probably not surprise us. What, in fact, happened was that despite all the controversy surrounding these substances, there were a few scientists who continued to study them. What they are finding could again restore bioflavonoids to a prominent place in modern medicine.

In 1988, at the Second International Conference on Antiviral Research, several reports attested to the anti-viral activity of the bioflavonoids. Several derivatives of quercetin were found to have anti-viral activity against picornaviruses *in vitro*. This family includes the polioviruses, ECHO viruses, Coxsackie viruses *and* rhinoviruses. The latter are the major causes of the common cold. Quercetin had no anti-viral activity by itself but *did* when combined with—surprise—vitamin C! Quercetin is very easily oxidized, and vitamin C protects against this.

The bioflavonoids quercetin, hesperidin and catechin have been found to have anti-viral activity against herpes type I, respiratory syncytial virus and para-influenza virus *in vitro*. There are anecdotes that bioflavonoids can cure colds, but there has been no scientific documentation of this. But because of the test-tube anti-viral activity of some bioflavonoids against rhinoviruses, clinical trials to determine what effect bioflavonoids might have in the treatment and prevention of colds should be conducted.

Test-tube studies with quercetin, quercetin derivatives and bioflavonoids, using mast cells and basophils (cells involved in allergy reactions), suggest an anti-allergy role for these substances. They prevent the release of histamine and other mediators involved in allergy reactions. It is possible that they do this by stabilizing the membranes of mast cells and basophils, making them less reactive to allergens. It does not seem unlikely that the efficacy of Estivin, an old over-the-counter anti-allergy preparation, used especially by some with hay fever, is due to its bioflavonoid component. (Estivin, derived from rose petals, is very helpful for some but, ironically, causes allergic reactions in others who are sensitive to the Thimerosal used to preserve it.) More studies are needed to further investigate a bioflavonoid role in the treatment and prevention of allergies.

Several studies, performed on cells *in vitro,* show that quercetin and other bioflavonoids are potent anti-inflammatory agents. They appear to inhibit formation of inflammatory prostaglandins and leukotrienes, the release of inflammatory mediators by cellular lysosomes and lipid peroxidation. Once more, clinical trials are called for.

Still other bioflavonoid activities which have recently been demonstrated include anti-spasmodic activity (decreases smooth-muscle contractility), immunomodulation and, once again, reduction of capillary fragility.

So far, so good. There is a downside, though. Quercetin is highly mutagenic in a certain bacterial strain and has been found to cause chromosomal damage in cultured mammalian cells. Rutin and some other bioflavonoids also have these effects. On the other hand, there is no evidence that quercetin, rutin or other bioflavonoids cause cancer in animals. In fact, they may *protect* against cancer. People have been consuming bioflavonoids for many years without any evidence of increased risk of cancer. Still, clinical studies are urgently needed to resolve this issue.

The 1980s have witnessed an increased interest by scientists in the medical benefits of herbs. It turns out that many of the medicinally active substances of herbs are bioflavonoids. Active bioflavonoids from ginkgo and other medicinal herbs are discussed in another section of this book.

Bioflavonoids are being used in other countries for the treatment of various medical problems. Troxerutin, related chemically to rutin, for example, is used for the treatment of varicose veins, hemorrhoids, night cramps and other circulatory problems. It is supposed to work by reducing capillary fragility and by increasing tissue oxygenation. There are many anecdotal reports of its efficacy, but still little in the way of clinical studies.

Propolis had been a popular item in the health stores for the past few years. It is claimed to have immune-enhancing and energy-boosting abilities, among other things. Propolis is a resinous material that bees make from plant fluids rich in bioflavonoids. Bees use propolis to close openings in their hives. The hives are thus protected from weather and are made almost sterile. Again, there are many anecdotes claiming health benefits from propolis but no studies to back them up. Be aware, too, that some preparations of propolis cause allergic responses in some individuals. These preparations apparently contain pollen.

A bioflavonoid-like substance widely used in the United States is *sodium cromoglycate*. There are several forms of the drug. Intel is used for the treatment of allergic asthma, Nasalcrom for allergic rhinitis and Opticrom for allergic eye problems. Sodium chromoglycate is a derivative of an herb that was used for centuries in Egyptian medicine. Some report that dissolving one to two capsules of the substance in warm water and taking this before each meal significantly helps them with their food sensitivities. Controlled studies are needed to confirm this.

Bioflavonoids occur in fruits, vegetables, nuts, seeds, leaves, flowers and bark. Rutin is found in buckwheat. These substances have been found to have potent healing properties within plants themselves. The typical American gets about a gram of bioflavonoids a day via diet. If you want to increase your intake eat more fruits, vegetables, nuts and seeds.

BREWER'S YEAST/SKIN RESPIRATORY FACTOR/GLUCAN
(Nutritional Treasure Trove)

Just about every ailment imaginable can be cured by *brewer's yeast,* according to some. There are many who say they couldn't get through the day without a tablespoon of brewer's yeast mixed with tomato juice. Recently there have been negative claims, as well. Some say yeast is the cause of a multitude of problems ranging from chronic fatigue, memory disorders, immunodeficiency, endocrine abnormalities, irritable bowel syndrome, allergies, cancer and much more. It's time that we got all of this sorted out.

In the first place, there is great variation in yeasts. Brewer's yeast is quite different from the yeast that often causes vaginal infections and which is blamed for so many medical woes, *Candida albicans.*

Many claim that any form of yeast can promote candidiasis, but there is no evidence at all that ingestion of brewer's yeast increases susceptibility to or exacerbates *Candida* infections.

The brewer's yeast that is sold in health food stores is the same type of yeast that is used in the brewing process. Brewer's yeast is an excellent source of several nutrients including thiamine (vitamin B_1), riboflavin (vitamin B_2), nicotinic acid, pyridoxine (vitamin B_6), pantothenic acid, biotin and folic acid, as well as some minerals and trace minerals, especially chromium and selenium. It also contains about

8–10 percent nucleic acid, which may have an immune-enhancing effect (see nucleic acids). A similar type of yeast, torula yeast, differs in that it is a poor source of chromium and selenium. It is possible that there are substances in yeast that do make people feel better, that do make skin healthier, and so on. It is certainly time to do some decent studies with standardized brewer's yeast to see what yeast really can do.

A few substances have been isolated from brewer's and baker's yeast (same as brewer's yeast but used differently) which do have medicinal value. One of these is called the *skin respiratory factor* (SRF), sometimes known as live-yeast-cell derivative. SRF has been used in a proprietary hemorrhoid product, Preparation H, for over forty years. It appears to work as a wound-healing agent. Chemical identity of SRF is still unclear. Some believe it to be a derivative of picolinic acid (similar to nicotinic acid), but this is uncertain. SRF has been shown to have biologic activities associated with increased oxygen consumption by fibroblasts (cells involved in wound repair), such as wound epithelialization, collagen formation and early angiogenesis (formation of new blood vessels).

Over the years there have been some anecdotal reports that Preparation H (the active ingredient of which is SRF) is very good for treating skin problems, even wrinkles. It has also been reported, anecdotally, that topical application of Preparation H is beneficial for the treatment of varicose veins.

The first official report showing that SRF would be beneficial for wound healing came from the University of California, San Francisco, School of Medicine. The authors demonstrated that SRF increased collagen production in excised human skin fragments (in the test tube) and increased oxygen uptake of human fibroblasts. They also showed that SRF was beneficial to wound healing in the skins of rats and rabbits.

A more recent report showed that application of SRF to skin-graft donor sites in burn patients produced signs of significantly earlier healing. SRF appears to be a promising substance for wound and burn healing. Further research is warranted with this substance and the identification of its active ingredient should be sought. Brewer's yeast taken orally is said to be good for the skin. Possibly SRF has something to do with this effect, if it is real.

Another derivative of brewer's yeast, *glucan,* has been reported by scientists at the Weizmann Institute of Science in Israel to significantly affect the wound-healing process in mice. Glucan is a polysaccharide. It appears that glucan activates macrophages, which, in turn, promote growth of fibroblasts and capillaries, thus accelerating wound repair.

Brewer's yeast may turn out to be a treasure trove of health-giving substances. More research will tell the rest of the story.

COENZYME Q_{10}
(Rx for Heart Failure)

Coenzyme Q_{10} is part of the system across which electrons flow in the mitochondria of cells in the process of energy production and, as such, is biologically very important. There is a relationship between coenzyme Q_{10} (CoQ_{10}) and vitamin E, which, nonetheless, have many distinct functions. Deficiency states may occur.

Preliminary studies suggest that CoQ_{10} may have a number of potentially valuable therapeutic actions, including enhanced immunity, but most of the interest to date has focused on its possible impact on cardiovascular disease. Some of these studies have detected CoQ_{10}-induced improvement of heart-muscle metabolism and effectiveness in the treatment of coronary insufficiency and congestive heart failure.

Researchers at the Methodist Hospital in Indianapolis and at the Institute for Bio-Medical Research at the University of Texas have treated heart-failure patients with CoQ_{10} with considerable success. CoQ_{10} is said by these researchers to enhance the pumping capacity of the heart and to eliminate the often major side effects associated with conventional heart-failure drugs. Heart-failure patients were said to have a relative deficiency of CoQ_{10} in their hearts and to be responsive to daily oral supplements of CoQ_{10}, which, it is reported, increases the production of energy in heart-muscle cells. Some 91 percent of the patients studied showed improvement within thirty days of beginning CoQ_{10} supplementation. Certainly more investigation of this intriguing vitamin-like nutrient is warranted.

DIETARY FIBER
(Good News for Those with Heart Disease, High Cholesterol, Diabetes, Weight Problems and More)

During the early part of the century, fiber, or "roughage" as it was more commonly known, was thought by some to be beneficial to intestinal health. Then followed a long period, lasting until about 1970, when fiber was discussed as "unassimilable carbohydrates" that could be irritating to the intestine. That's all changed again, and the medical and nutritional literature now abounds with evidence of the substantial and often surprising health benefits of dietary fiber.

This evidence suggests that fiber may protect against some forms of cancer, may reduce the risk of coronary heart disease and help control obesity and diabetes, among other things. There is no question any more of the major importance of dietary fiber as a food constituent.

Dietary fiber, for the most part, is composed of the edible plant polysaccharides that typically help form the structure of plant-cell walls. While it is true that fiber is neither digested nor absorbed in the small intestine, it *is* digested in the *large* intestine, and some of its digested products do get into the body and appear to significantly reduce the production of cholesterol.

Cereals, vegetables and fruits are important sources of fiber. Up until the early 1970s, foods were increasingly being processed to rid them of fiber; even today dietary intake of fiber is much lower in the United States than it was a hundred years ago.

There are several different types of dietary fiber; some are good for lowering cholesterol and improving sugar control in diabetics. Others are better at preventing and treating constipation, hemorrhoids and other lower gastrointestinal problems. This variety has created confusion among consumers.

The best way to categorize fiber is as *insoluble* fiber and *soluble* fiber. Insoluble fiber does not dissolve in water, while soluble fiber forms a highly viscous solution when dissolved in water. Insoluble dietary fiber is found in whole grains and brans of wheat, rye, rice and corn and in cellulose. Soluble dietary fiber is found in fruits, dried peas and beans, barley, oats, gums (guar, xanthan, locust bean), mucilages (psyllium) and pectins. Generally, insoluble fiber (e.g., wheat bran) is better for lower intestine health (bowel regularity, etc.) and soluble fiber is better for lowering cholesterol and aiding in diabetes and obesity.

Fiber-consciousness began growing soon after Burkitt, an English surgeon, published his suggestion in 1969 that the low incidence of cancer of the colon and rectum among those living in tropical parts of Africa might well be due to their high intake of dietary fiber. Burkitt's data commanded attention, particularly in the United States and Europe, where the incidence of colon and rectum cancer was high and rising and where the intake of dietary fiber was low and getting lower.

Soon after Burkitt's report appeared in 1969, another English researcher further upset orthodox thinking about fiber when he reported that symptoms of diverticular disease of the colon (diverticulosis: small herniations through the wall of the large intestine) could be treated with considerable success by a diet high in fiber. This flew in the face of the then prevailing—but usually unsatisfactory—treatment for this disorder with bland *low-fiber* diet.

The preferred treatment for the symptoms of diverticulosis, the incidence of which increases with age, is now 15 to 30 grams daily of supplementary fiber, mainly of the *insoluble* variety, usually in the form of coarse wheat bran (which also takes care of constipation and hemorrhoids). It is *probable* that increasing intake of dietary insoluble fiber will also help *prevent* the development of this disorder.

Occasionally, it should be noted, the sac-like herniations (diverticula) become inflamed. This condition is called *diverticulitis* (as opposed to *diverticulosis,* in which inflammation is absent) and is usually associated with fever and severe abdominal pain. It is mandatory that this condition be managed by a physician, and, in contrast to diverticulosis, a bland *low-fiber* diet *is* prescribed for diverticulitis. The reason for this is that, when the large intestine or a portion of it is inflamed, you want to decrease, not increase, intestinal motility to aid in the healing process (sort of put it to rest for awhile).

Claims that dietary fiber protects against cancers of the colon and rectum, though supported by some epidemiologic evidence, still remain unproved. The data are strong enough, however, that the National Cancer Institute recommends a high-fiber, low-fat diet to help prevent some forms of cancer. It is known that many foods contain traces of cancer-causing chemicals that are more likely to do damage the longer they stay in the intestine. Some researchers postulate that, by reducing the amount of time food stays in the intestine and by diluting fecal constituents, the high-fiber diet reduces the risks of colon and rectal cancers. In short, increased insoluble fiber intake may help quickly rid our systems of cancer-causing substances known to be present in our diets. A recent four-year chemoprevention trial (randomized, double-blind, placebo-controlled) demonstrated a decrease in the number of rectal polyps in patients with familial adenomotous polyposis as the amount of dietary fiber increased. This disorder is a precursor of colorectal cancer.

Perhaps the most important and exciting feature of *soluble* fiber is that it lowers serum cholesterol levels. There are now at least seven well designed and well executed studies demonstrating that rolled oats or oat bran significantly lower total cholesterol and LDL-cholesterol levels. In the first reported study (1963), twenty-one subjects were given 140 grams daily of rolled oats, and an 11 percent decrease in serum cholesterol was observed after three weeks. Two studies were reported in 1981. In one, 125 grams daily of rolled oats were given to ten subjects, and an 8 percent decrease in cholesterol was found after three weeks. In the other, 94 grams of oat bran were given to eight subjects, and a 13 percent decrease in cholesterol and a 14 percent decrease in LDL-cholesterol were noted after ten days.

Two studies reported in 1984 again confirmed the cholesterol-lowering virtues of oats. Ten subjects were fed 100 grams a day of oat bran (one bowl of hot cereal and five oat bran muffins) in one study, and a 19 percent decrease in cholesterol and a 23 percent decrease in LDL-cholesterol were observed after three weeks. The same authors reported that feeding subjects four ounces of dried beans daily (as cooked pinto and navy beans or as a bean soup) for the same time produced a 23 percent lowering of cholesterol and a 24 percent lowering of LDL. In the other study reported that year, twelve subjects given 50 grams daily of oat bran had a 12 percent drop in cholesterol after six weeks.

Another good study was reported in 1986. In one, 41 grams of oat bran or 145 grams of dried beans were consumed by ten subjects respectively for one-half year, with a 26 percent lowering of cholesterol in each case. No further lowering was noted in a few subjects who continued on these diets for almost two years. The most recent study (1988) also reported on the effect of oat bran in subjects with *normal* (to begin with) cholesterol levels. Researchers at the University of California, Irvine, School of Medicine found a 5.3 percent drop in cholesterol, an 8.3 percent reduction in triglycerides and an 8.7 percent decline in LDL in nineteen young, healthy medical students who ate 34 grams of oat bran muffins daily for one month. No changes were found in subjects consuming wheat or wheat and oat bran muffins. The authors conclude "these findings suggest that oat bran taken daily can significantly lower serum cholesterol and triglyceride levels in a young, healthy population."

Very interesting and very important. There can be little doubt that oat bran lowers cholesterol. A review of all the studies so far indicates that those with *elevated* cholesterol levels appear more responsive than those with normal levels, but even those with normal levels can profit from increasing their oat bran intake. Oat bran is mainly composed of the soluble fiber beta-D glucosan. This forms a highly viscous solution when dissolved in water or milk, and the gelatinous texture of oatmeal is due to this gum.

The percentage decrease in cholesterol per gram of oat bran can be calculated approximately. Percentage decrease = 0.156 × grams of oat bran per day + 1. One rounded tablespoon of oat bran contains about 5 grams of fiber and about 15 grams of oat bran. About one-third of oat bran is fiber. One oat bran muffin typically contains about 15–17 grams of oat bran. Therefore, two oat bran muffins daily can lower cholesterol levels about 6.3 percent over a period of a few weeks in most cases, four oat bran muffins 11.6 percent, etc. Each oat bran muffin contains about 200 calories. You can get about 50 grams in one bowl of oat bran cereal. This could lower cholesterol by about 9 percent and has fewer calories than the muffins. The cholesterol-lowering effect can be seen as early as two weeks.

Other soluble fiber can lower cholesterol, as well. Four ounces of dried beans (navy, pinto, etc.), for example, can have the same cholesterol-lowering effect as 3.5 ounces of oat bran. Five grams of grapefruit pectin three times daily (from grapefruits and grapefruit peels) have been reported to lower cholesterol by 7.6 percent and LDL by 10.8 percent. Psyllium, derived from the husks of psyllium seeds, is a soluble mucilloid fiber; 3.4 grams of psyllium taken three times daily lowers cholesterol by 14.8 percent and LDL by 20.2 percent after eight weeks. Guar gum also lowers cholesterol.

How do these soluble fibers work in lowering cholesterol? They are converted (through bacterial action) in the large intestine to short-chain fatty acids. These fatty acids, in turn, inhibit cholesterol synthesis and lower cholesterol levels in rats, and it is likely that they work similarly in humans. In addition, the fibers may directly bind to cholesterol in the intestine, carrying it out of the body. Soluble fiber is, in addition, effective in improving glucose tolerance. It has been demonstrated that insulin-requiring diabetics needed lower amounts of insulin when they were placed on high-fiber diets (mainly of the soluble variety). Since then there have been some confirmatory reports of this phenomenon. Guar gum given 10 grams twice daily with food improved glucose tolerance in diabetics in a couple of studies. Xanthan gum given at 12 grams daily was also seen to improve glucose toler-ance in diabetics, and psyllium powder, 3.6 grams three times daily with meals, significantly improved glucose tolerance in a few studies.

Soluble fiber appears to slow the digestion and absorption of car-bohydrates and may thus decrease the rise in blood levels of sugar following meals. The available data in support of a role for dietary soluble fiber in the treatment of diabetes are strong enough that the National Diabetes Association of the U.S., Canada, Great Britain and Australia have all endorsed high-fiber diets as an aid in diabetic control.

As if the cholesterol-lowering effect and improvement of glucose tolerance by soluble fiber were not enough, there are now quite a few reports showing that diets rich in soluble fiber, as well as soluble fiber supplements such as guar gum, psyllium and others, help decrease appetite and thus help with weight control. Mixing up 3.6 grams of psyllium powder (without sugar) in a glass of water or tomato juice and drinking it before meals makes many feel full before they start eating.

Since different types of fiber (insoluble, soluble) do different things, it is important that we eat a variety of all fibers. The typical American diet contains, on the average, 10–15 grams of fiber daily. Even the most conservative nutritionists believe that is much too little. Some believe that an intake of from 20–40 grams would be healthier, but healthier yet would be an intake of from 40–60 grams daily.

Foods with a lot of insoluble fiber include brans from wheat, rice and corn. There are a number of cereal and bread products on the market rich in these substances. Foods rich in soluble fiber are dried beans, fruit, oat bran and barley, also gums (guar, xanthan, locust bean), mucilages (psyllium) and fruit pectins. Look at labels. More and more manufacturers are listing fiber content of foods. Some are dif-ferentiating between soluble and insoluble. Try to consume different types of fiber to reap the varying benefits.

Fiber is often present in plant foods along with phytic acid and sometimes oxalic acid. Fiber and these substances can bind to minerals (calcium, zinc, iron, etc.). Fiber itself may bind to beta-carotene and vitamin B_2. It is still not clear if long-term, high-fiber diets cause min-eral or vitamin deficiencies, but it would be prudent if you increase your fiber intake substantially to also increase your mineral and vita-min intake. This can be done by eating foods rich in these minerals and by taking a vitamin/mineral supplement.

Insoluble fiber increases bowel motility and may thus cause loose bowel movements, cramps, bloating and gas in some individuals. In fact, abdominal distress is not uncommon among those who make large, abrupt additions of fiber to their diets. Soluble fiber is less likely to cause loose bowel movements, but can cause bloating and a feeling of fullness (good for those wanting to lose weight). The best approach is to increase fiber intake gradually.

There are a few situations in which a *decrease* in fiber intake is at least temporarily necessary. These include the disease diverticulitis, radiation therapy (especially to the abdominal and pelvic regions), enteric fistulae, and short bowel syndrome. Fiber may bind to digestive enzymes, so those with malabsorption problems who notice increased diarrhea and floating stools should either increase intake of digestive enzymes or decrease fiber intake under their physician's supervision.

For most of us, though, *more* fiber is the key—one that can unlock remarkable health benefits.

ENZYMES (INCLUDING WOBE MUGOS)
(Can You "Dissolve" What Ails You?)

Digestive enzymes have been touted for some time as internal cleansers and even as anti-cancer agents. The pancreatic enzymes have found legitimate use, for some time now, in pancreatic insufficiency and a number of malabsorption syndromes, in which the body's ability to digest and utilize various nutrients is seriously impaired. People with cystic fibrosis, for example, suffer from these syndromes and are helped by oral enzyme preparations.

There is no evidence that *most* people, as some have claimed, suffer, to varying degrees, from an inability to digest food properly and thus can benefit from enzyme supplementation. Recently, however, a group of researchers has come up with a far more sophisticated reason why some people may benefit from these supplements.

German researchers have conducted studies in animals and humans showing that "immune complexes" can be significantly cleared from the body with the use of a preparation of enzymes they call Wobe-Mugos. This preparation consists of pancreatic enzymes and bromelain (enzymes obtained from pineapple). They have reported sometimes dramatic results in such diseases as rheumatoid arthritis, multiple sclerosis and systemic lupus erythematosus.

Immune complexes, in simplest terms, are combinations of antibodies and antigens. When the body's other immune defense systems fail to rid the body of these complexes, an inflammatory process begins that can lead to serious disease, often of the autoimmune variety, such as rheumatoid arthritis.

The German researchers, as well as some now in the U.S. and elsewhere, have conducted studies both in the test tube and in animals and humans that, reportedly, demonstrate the ability of Wobe-Mugos and related enzyme preparations to dissolve and clear these complexes.

Some of these researchers have hypothesized that these enzymes might prove beneficial even in AIDS, which, increasingly, does appear to have a significant autoimmune component. At this time there is no evidence at all, however, that these enzymes are useful in AIDS.

This work is certainly intriguing and deserves follow-up by others. For now, however, I do not recommend supplementation with enzymes except under a doctor's supervision and for appropriate and established indications.

L-CARNITINE
(More Help for the Heart)

Chemically, carnitine is a quaternary amine (the same chemical family that includes choline) and exists as two stereoisomers (structures that are mirror images of each other) called L-carnitine (the active form found in our tissue) and D-carnitine (biologically inactive form). An equal mixture of the two forms is called DL-carnitine. L-carnitine is synthesized in the human body, chiefly in the liver and kidneys, from essential amino acids, lysine and methionine. Three vitamins, niacin, B_6 and C, as well as iron, are involved in this synthesis.

It is now established that L-carnitine is essential for the maintenance of good health in humans. L-carnitine is absolutely necessary for the transport of long-chain fatty acids into the mitochondria, the metabolic furnaces of the cells. Fatty acids are the major sources for production of energy in the heart and skeletal muscles, structures that are particularly vulnerable to L-carnitine deficiency. A number of L-carnitine-deficiency states have now been identified, several of which are genetic in origin. Symptoms of such deficiencies include muscle weakness, severe confusion and angina ("heart pain").

There are a few groups at particular risk of L-carnitine deficiency. These include chronic kidney failure patients on hemodialysis and patients with liver failure. Even some healthy subgroups have additional needs for dietary L-carnitine. These include strict vegetarians, newborns, pregnant women and women who are nursing infants.

It has only recently been recognized that dietary L-carnitine is essential for optimal health. The future looks bright for this substance so long as medical science continues to investigate it.

Claims for this substance include: 1) Protects against cardiovascular disease; 2) protects against muscle disease (and helps build muscle and stamina); 3) protects against liver disease; 4) protects against diabetes; 5) protects against kidney disease; 6) aids in dieting.

Clinical trials have demonstrated positive effects of L-carnitine supplementation in patients suffering from various forms of cardiovascular disease. One group, for example, demonstrated significantly improved tolerance to exercise in patients suffering from coronary artery disease who were given intravenous L-carnitine. Others have also demonstrated increased tolerance to exercise among L-carnitine-treated patients with coronary artery disease. In another study, two matched groups of patients suffering from angina pectoris (the severe chest pain that often accompanies insufficient flow of blood and oxygen to the heart muscle) were given two different forms of carnitine. Notable improvement was observed in both groups during the first thirty days in which oral carnitine was provided. Between thirty and sixty days, however, *further* improvement was observed in the group receiving L-carnitine (50 milligrams per kilogram of body weight daily) but *not* in the group receiving DL-carnitine (100 milligrams per kilogram of body weight daily).

It was reported some time ago that supplemental carnitine can significantly reduce total blood lipids (fats and fat-like substances), a finding confirmed in recent years by Japanese researchers who reported that giving 900 milligrams per day of oral L-carnitine could notably reduce levels of blood triglycerides, which are among the lipids implicated in cardiovascular disease. Oral L-carnitine, in this trial, was as effective as intravenous L-carnitine. The lowering effect continued so long as L-carnitine was supplied; triglyceride levels rose again when carnitine was withdrawn. No effect was noted on cholesterol. However, in another study, 1 gram of oral L-carnitine administered daily over a period of ten to fifteen weeks produced a substantial increase in high-density lipoprotein (HDL) cholesterol in two normal men. HDL is the "good" cholesterol, the part that is *protective* against coronary artery disease.

Research to date thus suggests a potentially important role for L-carnitine in the treatment and possibly the prevention of some forms of cardiovascular disease. There is no evidence at present, however, to suggest that persons with *normal* carnitine levels and normal fatty-acid metabolism will benefit from non-dietary carnitine supplementation. Further research is warranted. Recently L-carnitine supplementation has been shown, in a well designed study, to increase walking distance in patients with intermittent claudication due to peripheral vascular disease.

As for claims regarding muscle and stamina, patients with some forms of muscle-weakening diseases, most of which are hereditary, have been shown to have carnitine deficiencies that in some instances respond to carnitine supplementation. Claims that carnitine can help build muscle and increase physical endurance have led to the use of this substance by some athletes and body-builders. It is possible that normal individuals may derive some energy-enhancing benefits from carnitine supplements, but there is no proof that this is the case.

Nor is there much evidence that carnitine is directly protective against liver disease. Carnitine deficiencies, however, may disturb the normal processes of liver metabolism of lipoproteins, contributing to potentially dangerous elevations in blood levels of triglycerides and cholesterol. (See discussion of cardiovascular disease above.)

Concerning diabetes, though abnormalities of carnitine metabolism have been reported in diabetics, there is no proof that supplemental carnitine will prevent diabetes.

The claim that carnitine protects against kidney disease apparently arises from reports that the now often noted carnitine deficiency of kidney patients undergoing hemodialysis could be prevented via oral carnitine supplementation. There is no evidence, however, that such supplements will benefit *normal* individuals who seek to prevent the development of kidney disorders.

It has been hypothesized that carnitine might be a useful supplement for those who are on low-calorie diets, that carnitine, by enhancing the efficiency of fatty-acid oxidation (increasing the burn rate of calories stored as fat), may make low-calorie diets easier to tolerate by reducing feelings of hunger and weakness that result from less efficient oxidation of fats. This is an intriguing idea worthy of some investigation.

On the negative side, it must be noted that symptoms of myasthenia (progressive weakness of certain muscle groups without evidence of atrophy or wasting) have been reported in kidney patients being maintained for prolonged periods of time on hemodialysis and supplemental DL-carnitine. Symptoms disappeared upon withdrawal of the DL-carnitine. When, at a later date, these same patients were given the L-form of carnitine (L-carnitine), the myasthenia symptoms did *not* return. These findings suggest that supplements should be in the form of L-carnitine and *not* in the form of DL-carnitine.

The dietary intake of L-carnitine for optimal health is unknown. In fact, the amount of L-carnitine in the average Western diet remains undefined. An unpublished analysis of hospitalized patients in the United States showed dietary intake of between 2 milligrams and 300 milligrams daily while on hospital diet. No recommendation can be made until more—and better—information is at hand.

Dietary sources richest in L-carnitine are red meats (lamb and beef in particular). Dairy products contain some L-carnitine. Vegetables, fruits and certain cereals contain little or no L-carnitine. (Avocados have some; so does the fermented soybean product tempeh.) Supplements are available in both the DL form and the L form. If you use carnitine supplements use *only* the L-carnitine.

Remember that the DL form of carnitine has been shown to cause a myasthenia-type syndrome in some patients. The L-carnitine form, on the other hand, has *not* produced negative side effects, even in some individuals taking 1.6 grams daily for more than one year.

LIPOIC ACID
(The Next "Meta-Vitamin" Superstar?)

Lipoic acid or thioctic acid is a cofactor in two important energy-producing reactions in the body. It is sometimes called a "meta-vitamin" or "conditional vitamin." Usually the body makes enough of it, but under certain conditions deficiencies could occur and then supplementation might be useful. In experimental animal work, lipoic acid has been found to be helpful in the treatment of some aspects of diabetes, including some of the neurologic complications of that disease.

In other animal work, lipoic acid has prevented atherosclerosis and has demonstrated immune-enhancing effects. Lipoic acid, at this writing, is not yet available as a supplement in the United States, though I've heard of plans to market it here in the near future. It is certainly an interesting substance that should be further researched. It could become the next meta-vitamin superstar, following in the path of L-carnitine and coenzyme Q_{10}.

MUSHROOMS: SHIITAKE AND REI-SHI
(Immune Boosters/Anti-Cancer Agents)

Not too many years ago mushrooms suggested psychedelic phenomena. Today, people are more interested in certain mushrooms' possible immune-enhancing and anti-viral effects. Most of the interest is focused on the shiitake and Rei-shi mushrooms.

The shiitake mushroom, also known as the Japanese forest mushroom (*Lentinus edodes*) is the most popular edible mushroom in Japan. It has been much employed in the traditional medicine of Asia for thousands of years. It is reputed to be a tonic, a stimulant and an aid in the prevention of cerebral hemorrhagic strokes. Recently it has been demonstrated that extracts of the mushroom can lower cholesterol levels and have anti-tumor, anti-viral and immune-stimulating effects. Research in Japan shows that the mushroom itself can lower blood pressure in those with hypertension and can also lower cholesterol levels.

A major therapeutic component in the mushroom appears to be the polysaccharide lentinan. Lentinan is a definite immune stimulant. Among other things, it boosts interleukin-1 and interferon production. A report in the *New England Journal of Medicine* indicated that giving lentinan to two patients with probable "pre-AIDS" improved the patients general conditions and improved their immune status in certain particulars. The report concluded that "this agent may prove to be effective in AIDS." Further studies are needed. Japanese researchers report that mice with tumors respond favorably to lentinan and that mice with both immune deficiency and cancer respond positively to a diet high in the shiitake mushroom. Another report by the Japanese concluded that lentinan could inhibit even the metastases of advanced tumors in experimental animals.

Another Japanese mushroom, known as Rei-shi (*Ganoderma lucid-*

ium), is likewise reputed to have important medical benefits. The mushroom is also known as ganoderma, ling-chih-tsao and wu-ling-chih in China. It also contains a polysaccharide which has known immune-enhancing activity. It may increase T cell and macrophage activity. The mushroom itself appears to have anti-tumor properties, probably owing to the polysaccharide which has been reported to inhibit the growth of tumor cells in animals. In addition, ganoderma has been successfully used in the treatment of viral hepatitis where it seems to work as an immune enhancer. Ganoderma is also said to be beneficial in the treatment of chronic bronchitis, peptic ulcer disease, hypertension, insomnia and high cholesterol levels. And it supposedly protects the liver against certain toxins. Further research with these intriguing mushrooms should be encouraged.

PABA
(Burned Out)

There's one undisputed positive use for PABA (para-aminobenzoic acid)—as a topical sunscreen to shield the skin from the damage of ultraviolet radiation. Beyond this the claims for PABA, as a skin rejuvenator and anti-arthritis substance, are anecdotal. Other anecdotal claims persist that supplemental PABA can halt hair loss and restore color to graying or white hair, but you can also talk to many who have tried PABA for these purposes without success. I do not recommend PABA except as a topical sunscreen. Those who do take it orally should be aware that it causes nausea and diarrhea in some individuals. In addition, PABA is stored in the tissues and in continued high dosage may prove toxic to the liver. Some enthusiasts have recommended daily doses of a gram or higher; these doses could produce such adverse effects as anorexia, nausea, fever and skin rash. If for some reason you feel compelled to take PABA internally, do not take more than 30 milligrams daily in supplemental form. (Natural sources of PABA include liver, kidney, whole grains, wheat germ, brown rice, bran.) Do not take PABA if you are using any of the "sulfa drugs" (sulfonamide antibiotics); PABA will seriously diminish their effectiveness. (See analysis of Gerovital H3, next chapter, for more on PABA.)

High doses of the potassium salt of PABA called Potaba have been used for the treatment of Peyronie's disease, a disease of excessive fibrosis of the penis. There is no evidence that Potaba is effective for this disorder nor for any other disorder of excessive fibrosis such as scleroderma.

PANGAMIC ACID/DMG ("VITAMIN B-15")
(The Do-Everything "Vitamin"?)

It has been claimed, at one time or another, that pangamic acid, or "vitamin B_{15}," as it is popularly, but erroneously, known, cures nearly everything. Its credentials as a panacea are said to be based on its extreme potency as an "oxygenator" of body tissues, bringing them all up to optimal snuff, enhancing, among other things, the "brilliance" and "flash" of orgasm, increasing one's ability to do yoga, mopping up free radicals like mad, saving people from the need for amputation of gangrenous limbs, etc., etc.

It would be wonderful if pangamic acid (which is not a vitamin by any stretch of the imagination; there is no evidence whatever that the body has any dietary need of it) could do even a small fraction of the things claimed for it. Unfortunately, there is only scant evidence that it can have any therapeutic effect in *any* ailment and there are claims now that two of the active ingredients in pangamic acid may promote cancer.

Almost all of the claims made for pangamic acid or dimethylglycine (DMG), which is the hypothesized active ingredient, are based upon Soviet research. A researcher who investigated the Soviet work noted that "nearly all of these studies suffer from methodologic flaws which seriously limit their probative value. Often patient populations and diagnostic criteria are incompletely described, and comparisons between treated subjects and suitably matched controls are lacking." Another author has similarly faulted the Soviet research, noting "the methodological laxness and wild-eyed enthusiasm of Russian clinical reports." Claims that DMG has lipotropic effects (promoting optimal utilization of fats) are persistent in the literature and are not in themselves farfetched, but there are other substances, such as choline, that work better in this regard and are safer.

Studies of DMG outside the Soviet Union have generally failed to find any therapeutic value in it. One group reported that DMG is of no value in the treatment of epileptic patients with refractory seizures (the type that do not yield to standard medications). Their study was double-blind. Others have reported a significant DMG-induced enhancement of both humoral- and cell-mediated immune response, but there is no confirmation of this work. A recent investigation of DMG's reputed ability to boost energy and athletic performance found no effect whatsoever.

It is unfortunate that there has been so much hype and so many unsubstantiated claims made for DMG. It is possible that it may have some positive value, but most researchers are now loath to investigate DMG for fear of fueling even higher hopes for the substance. This fear is heightened by the possibility that DMG may have harmful side effects.

There is evidence that DMG, thought by many to be the active product of pangamic acid, may be mutagenic and thus potentially able to cause cancer. In the widely accepted test of mutagenesis, substances that turn out to be mutagenic have, according to one survey, a 90 percent probability of being carcinogenic as well. Neville Colman, M.D., of the Hematology and Nutrition Laboratory of the Bronx Veterans Administration Medical Center in New York, "concluded," according to an article in JAMA "that the main component of this vitamin B_{15} formulation is capable of reacting to form a potential carcinogen under conditions simulating those found in the human digestive tract." Other researchers have reported that diisopropylamine-dichloracetate (DIPA-DCA), the major constituent of another pangamic product, is also mutagenic. These findings, though they require confirmation by others, constitute ominous red flags.

The FDA has sought to have pangamic acid banned as an unsafe food additive. Pangamic acid may, indeed, be unsafe, but the additive argument may be doomed since it can be demonstrated that DMG, at least, is an intermediary metabolite naturally present in many foods. In any event, the intelligent consumer will steer clear of any and all products said to be "pangamic acid," "calcium pangamate," "B_{15}," DMG or anything related thereto.

My recommendation is unequivocal: *Don't* use any products labeled or related to "pangamic acid," "calcium pangamate," DMG or "B_{15}." Some of the substances included in these products may be carcinogens.

ROYAL JELLY
(Could Be Rich Stuff)

Royal jelly is a "miracle substance" for at least one entity—the queen bee. This milky-white gelatinous substance is secreted in the salivary glands of worker bees for the sole apparent purpose of stimulating the growth and development of queen bees. What it can do for humans is a far more controversial matter. The claims are exuberant; it's supposed to extend life span and, in general, reinvigorate the body. Royal jelly is rich in pantothenic acid (part of the vitamin B complex; see analysis of pantothenic acid earlier in this book), a substance essential for many metabolic processes.

Pantothenic acid, as previously discussed, has shown some evidence of being useful in the treatment of some bone and joint disorders. It was reported that relief from various of the symptoms of rheumatoid arthritis could be achieved with injections of pantothenic acid. Intriguingly, even better results were reported by these researchers when pantothenic acid was combined with royal jelly, suggesting there might be some additional therapeutic agent in the latter. Daily intramuscular injections of royal jelly alone proved ineffective, but daily injections of a mixture of royal jelly and pantothenic acid resulted in greater improvement than had been noted with pantothenic acid alone.

It has been hypothesized that the possible additional therapeutic factor in royal jelly might be a substance called 10-hydroxydec-2-enoic acid, as this is another major constituent of the jelly. One group reported that "the injection of royal jelly or of 10-hydroxydec-2-enoic acid . . . affords complete protection against transplantable mouse leukemia." I know of no follow-up to this finding, but there has been some confirmation with respect to calcium pantothenate (pantothenic acid) and various arthritic conditions. There has also been a report that 10-hydroxydec-2-enoic acid has anti-microbial properties.

At this point I cannot say that people who are spending their money on royal jelly have bees in their collective bonnets. Neither, however, can I recommend the stuff, though I *do* believe that pantothenic acid may be helpful in some cases of arthritis, as outlined in my analysis of that substance. More research on royal jelly is needed and deserved.

SEAWEEDS AND DERIVATIVES
(Anti-Cancer/Anti-Viral Potential)

The use of seaweed as food goes back thousands of years. In fact, Sze Teu wrote in 600 B.C., "Seaweed is a delicacy fit for the most honorable guest, even for the king himself." Contrary to popular belief, seaweed is not a plant. It belongs to the protoctista kingdom. Seaweed, although plant-like, is more primitive than plants and has been on the planet for a much longer time, reproduces differently from plants and unlike plants, has no free leaves, stems or roots. Seaweeds, also called algae, are divided into four groups: *Chlorophycea,* or green algae; *Phaeophycea,* or brown algae; *Rhodophyceae,* or red algae; and *Cyanophyceae,* or blue-green algae. In a strict sense, the *Cyanophyceae,* some of the oldest organisms on earth, are bacteria and include spirulina and chlorella.

Among the seaweeds often used as foods in the U.S. are hijiki, kombu, wakame and arame, all brown seaweeds or algae. Wakame is used to make miso soup, among other things. The red seaweeds often used as foods include nori, agar or agar-agar and dulse. The seaweed that comes wrapped around your sushi is nori. People who buy kelp are buying brown seaweed, while those who buy "Irish moss" are getting a red seaweed. All of these products are widely available in health food stores, oriental food outlets and an increasing number of supermarkets.

Seaweed products are widely used additives in foods, cosmetics, medicines and many industrial products. The foam of beer, for example, is due to the stabilizing effect of alginate, a seaweed product. Seaweed also has a long history in folk medicine, including traditional Chinese and Indian (Ayurvedic) medicine.

Seaweed has been used as a folk remedy for fever, eczema, wounds, gallstone and liver disease, gout, menstrual problems, kidney disease, scabies and cancer. Seaweed is still used for the prevention and treatment of goiter throughout the world. The reason is that it is very rich in iodine (see iodine section). There are close to 300 million people in the world with endemic goiter that could be cured by eating seaweed. Seaweed has been used—and very effectively—for over a thousand years, particularly the red kind, to treat intestinal worms. Products derived from seaweed have been used to treat wounds, acid reflux and heavy-metal poisoning. Recent research demonstrates that seaweed derivatives inhibit the growth of cancer and have anti-viral activity including activity against the AIDS virus. Let's look at some of the most promising of these derivatives.

Alginates:

Alginates are polysaccharides derived from brown seaweed or kelp. They have wide use as additives in the food, cosmetic and drug industries. Alginates are also used to make dental impressions. Medicinally, they are used in some antacids for the treatment of acid reflux ("heart-burn") and esophagitis. Recently a wound dressing made from calcium alginate has shown great promise in the treatment of exudative wounds, such as those found in diabetic decubitus (bed sores) and scleroder-mal ulcers. Sailors have been treating their wounds with seaweed for hundreds of years. The wound dressing will soon be available in the U.S. It may also have a beneficial effect in the treatment of burns.

Alginates bind tightly to strontium, barium, cadmium and radium. Cows are often fed alginate, which completely binds to radioactive strontium 90, allowing it to pass out of the body without any of this toxin getting absorbed. Alginates can be used to treat or prevent poisoning by these elements. Alginates also bind with lead but not as well. Alginate is a good treatment for "ouch-ouch disease." This disease (yes, that's its real name) is found in Japan and is due to poisoning by cadmium-containing water used to irrigate rice fields. A major symptom is painful joints.

Carrageenans:

Carrageenans are sulfated polysaccharides from red seaweeds, such as Irish moss. Carrageenans are widely used in the food industry and intakes of up to 5 grams daily are considered safe by the FDA. The major carrageenans are designated carrageenan kappa, carrageenan lambda and carrageenan iota. All of these have been shown to inhibit herpes simplex virus type 1 and type 2 (oral and genital forms, respec-tively) *in vitro*. Those polysaccharides also inhibit some other viruses, including retroviruses. Lambda carrageenan has been found to be a potent *in vitro* inhibitor of the AIDS virus, HIV. Other sulfated polysac-charides, such as dextran sulfate and heparin (see discussions else-where) and pentosan polysulfate, are also inhibitors of this virus. Clinical trials of the carrageenans and their effects in those with HIV infections are urgently needed. Alginic acid, on the other hand, shows *no* activity against herpes or HIV. Possibly, if alginic acid were sulfated (it is *not* sulfated in its natural state), it, too, would have these anti-viral effects.

Fucoidin:

Polysaccharide fractions from edible seaweeds have been shown to be effective in slowing or stopping growth of tumor cells in animals and also have been found to inhibit chemical carcinogenesis in rats. The main active anti-cancer component in brown seaweed is believed to be a sulfated polysaccharide called fucoidin. Further research is needed.

SPIRULINA AND CHLORELLA
(OK, But . . .)

Spirulina are blue-green bacteria (cyanobacteria) and chlorella are small green algae (chlorophyta). They are supposed to be diet aids, good for the skin, and general tonics and rejuvenators. There's nothing in the scientific literature to support the claims, save for one report which only notes that spirulina is rich in gamma-linolenic acid (GLA), the same substance that is being derived today, for the most part, from oil of evening primrose (see previous analysis). How good a source of GLA spirulina really is remains to be determined. It appears doubtful that spirulina can compete with evening primrose in this respect. Similarly another report identifies the beta-carotene in spirulina as a possible anti-cancer substance. So buy beta-carotene. It's a lot cheaper.

SUCCINATES AND CYTOCHROMES
(In Pursuit of the "Winning Edge")

These substances are, increasingly, finding their way into "energy" formulas, the claims for which are greater endurance. They are being pitched at competitive athletes looking for the "winning edge." Cytochromes are found in the final common pathway of ATP production, and succinates are intermediate metabolites in the energy-producing pathway of the cell. Both *are* vital to energy production in the body, but, unfortunately, there is no evidence that supplementing with these substances has any energy-producing effect. Neither is there any evidence that these supplements are harmful except to the pocketbook.

WHEAT GERM/WHEAT-GERM OIL/OCTACOSANOL
(Save Your Money)

Many people consume wheat germ and the oil derived from it as sources of "natural" vitamin E and octacosanol. There is no persuasive evidence suggesting that vitamin E or any other substance derived from these sources is any more effective than vitamin E purchased in capsule form. The oil in these capsules, moreover, is far less likely to be rancid than that in the wheat germ.

An unconvincing argument has been made, based upon inadequate research, that wheat-germ oil is superior to concentrated vitamin E supplements. The reason for this, it is claimed, is that the germ oil contains octacosanol, a 28 carbon alcohol. Manufacturers and promoters of wheat-germ oil now compete with one another on the basis of how much octacosanol their respective products contain. The fact is there is little in the scientific literature to indicate that octacosonal plays any significant role in human biology and health.

It is interesting and instructive to note that those who write articles touting octacosonal frequently cite a particular scientific paper, clearly implying that this paper supports their claims; in fact, however, this paper is about the catalytic reagent dicobalt octacarbonyl, which has nothing to do with octacosanol!

One final note on this subject: It now appears that earlier discoveries showing a possible beneficial role of wheat-germ oil in the treatment of muscular dystrophy may have been due to an entirely different substance, such as selenium, which it now appears may play some role in this disorder, although this remains to be clearly demonstrated.

ELEVEN

Other Substances

Though the pharmaceuticals and other chemicals discussed in this chapter are seldom thought of as "food supplements," some of them are, in fact, being treated as such. Others, including some that have not yet been approved for use in this country, are popular in "alternative" and "underground" health networks. Substances analyzed in this chapter include:

Aspirin
Bee and Flower Pollens
BHA and BHT
Charcoal
Chondroitin Sulfate
Deaner
Dextran Sulfate
DHEA

DMSO
Experimental Immunomodulators
Fruit Acids
Gerovital H3
Glandulars
Hyaluronic Acid
Hyperbaric Oxygen
Memory Enhancers
Minoxidil and Other Baldness Remedies
Oscillococcinum
Oxygen Therapies
Sanguinaria and Other Plaque Fighters
Superoxide Dismutase
Testosterone and Steroids
Thymic Therapies
Transfer Factor

ASPIRIN
(The Once and Future "Miracle" Drug)

Aspirin, the original "miracle" drug, continues to surprise all of us. Recent research suggests that aspirin is not only an effective pain killer, it may also be very useful in helping to prevent heart attacks and may even be an immune stimulant. Some very preliminary work hints at a direct anti-viral role for the little white pill, while some older research (that needs follow-up) indicates that aspirin might be helpful in the treatment of diabetes.

American Indians, among others, long ago chewed white willow bark as a pain killer. Scientists later identified salicin as the analgesic component in this bark. Others subsequently synthesized a similar substance, salicylic acid, and tried using it for pain relief. It worked but created burning pains of its own in the stomach. A trip back to the drawing board nearly 100 years ago produced the successful variation that is still with us today—acetylsalicylic acid, better known as aspirin.

Current research suggests that aspirin in high doses can have anti-inflammatory effects (useful in some cases of arthritis, for example), that, in moderate doses, it can relieve headache pain and that, in small doses, it can help prevent heart attacks.

A Harvard study investigated the effects of taking a single 325-milligram tablet of aspirin every other day. The study involved 22,000 male physicians all of whom received either this very low-dose aspirin regimen or placebo. The risk of heart attack was reduced 44 percent in those men who got the aspirin.

In other recent studies, aspirin, either taken alone, or in combination with a drug called streptokinase, dramatically reduced the death rate from heart attacks when given soon after these attacks. By itself, aspirin, given within twenty-four hours of a heart attack, reduced mortality by 21 percent.

Aspirin's efficacy in this context is due to the drug's ability to prevent (and help dissolve) blood clots. It should be noted, however, that in people with hard to control high-blood pressure, aspirin may actually *increase* the risk of hemmorhagic stroke. Such individuals should not use aspirin without their doctors' consent and supervision.

The aspirin doses that are being used to help prevent heart attacks range from one-half of a 325-milligram tablet every other day to one full 325-milligram tablet daily. Some are using one 325-milligram tablet every other day. Optimal preventive dose has not yet been established. Do not take even these small doses regularly without your doctor's consent. Gastrointestinal irritation and bleeding are not uncommon among those who take high-dose aspirin. *Long-term* use of even low-dose aspirin may lead to some of the same problems. For many, however, the benefits of aspirin will be found, in consultation with physicians, to far outweigh the relatively small risks.

Adding to a resurgence of interest in aspirin are findings that the drug may have immune-stimulating and even anti-viral effects. Some research indicates aspirin can boost production of interferon and interleukin-2, both important in immunity. There's some preliminary data suggesting that aspirin might be helpful in the treatment of some cancers, and a therapeutic role for it in AIDS is currently being sought. It *has* been shown to inhibit the influenza virus in test-tube studies.

In addition, new work hints at possible roles for aspirin in the prevention and treatment of some eye diseases, including cataracts. Other research efforts are investigating the possibility that aspirin might prevent pre-eclampsia, a form of high blood pressure that sometimes develops late in pregnancy and can cause birth defects and miscarriage. Some older work that should be further investigated suggested that aspirin might help improve glucose metabolism in diabetics.

Aspirin is certainly one of the most fascinating and useful substances available. Nearly a century after it was developed (and many centuries after its predecessors were found to be helpful), it is still creating new medical "miracles."

BEE AND FLOWER POLLEN
(Cure-Alls?)

Bee and flower pollens are said to energize the body, regulate the bowels, dispel prostate problems, regulate weight, renew the skin, ward off heart disease and arthritis, relieve stress, boost immunity, inhibit cancer, diminish allergies and so on.

Few genuinely scientific studies have been done with these substances. Those that have been done have failed to find any real use for these substances. In a double-blind, placebo-controlled study of forty-six people, those who received bee pollen in 400-milligram doses daily for seventy-five days scored no better than the controls (who received placebo) on any of the physiologic variables examined. There was no evidence of enhanced energy or physical fitness.

Flower pollen, said to be purer, has fared no better. Many people are allergic to these substances.

On the basis of unconfirmed reports that pollen can boost immunity, some AIDS patients are now using these products. There's nothing to suggest they will do any harm (unless one is allergic to them), but, unfortunately, the best evidence suggests they will do no good, either.

BHA AND BHT
(Beware)

BHA and BHT are both antioxidants that are commonly added in *minute* quantities to foods, especially oils and fats, as preservatives. (They are also used to preserve some plastics and rubber.) Recently claims have been made that these chemicals control herpes infections, combat cancer and extend life span. Some have suggested that gram and even higher daily doses of these substances are safe and effective against herpes. The best available scientific evidence does not support these claims; indeed, there is evidence indicating that the regular use

OTHER SUBSTANCES / 365

of these chemicals in supplement form may pose very substantial health hazards.

Butylated hydroxyanisole (BHA) and butylated hydroxytoluene (BHT) have both exhibited some positive, as well as negative, qualities in small and preliminary studies. It is *possible* that one or both will eventually be shown to have value in the treatment of certain disorders under some circumstances. It is certain, however, that if that happens these substances will be treated as drugs and not as innocuous "food supplements."

Both BHA and BHT are recognized antioxidants. One researcher has reported increased average life span in long-lived strains of mice given BHT supplements. Increases as great as 30 percent were noted. Another mouse study indicated that large doses of vitamin E and BHT given in combination could inhibit the accumulation of "age pigments" in cells. However, BHT was found to *decrease* the average life span of the fruit fly in one study. At present there are insufficient supporting data to assess the validity of these findings or to interpret their possible significance for humans.

As for cancer, the experimental data related to protective claims are stronger with respect to BHA than to BHT. BHA has been shown to inhibit chemically induced cancers in a number of mouse and rat animal models. BHA, in several of these investigations, has been shown to strongly increase the activity of an enzyme called glutathione S-transferase, which has the ability to detoxify many cancer-causing chemical agents. Evidence that BHT also can inhibit some cancers is in far shorter supply.

There is, in fact, a growing body of evidence suggesting that BHT can *promote* the growth of some cancers. Researchers, working with mice, showed that BHT promotes the growth of lung cancers caused by three chemical carcinogens. Other work has shown that the incidence of lung tumors increases even when BHT is not given to test animals until as late as five months after the cancer-initiating chemical is injected. BHT, therefore, does not appear to be a primary cause of these cancers but, rather, encourages and boosts the growth of cancer once it gets started. There has been confirmation of tumor-promoting effects of BHT in various strains of mice. A recent report showed that although BHT inhibited liver cancer in rats exposed to a carcinogenic agent, it promoted bladder cancer.

Claims have been made that BHT can protect against herpes and other viruses. The relevant scientific data relate to *in vitro* (test tube) inactivation by BHT of various lipid-containing viruses, including herpes simplex and cytomegalovirus. But what applies *in vitro* often does not apply *in vivo* (in the living body), and at present there is no proof that BHT can inactivate *any* virus in humans. The claims that BHT can in very large doses prevent outbreaks of herpes is purely anecdotal. And even these positive anecdotes are countered by negative ones. I personally know people who have taken large doses of BHT daily in hope of warding off herpes attacks or shortening the duration and intensity of those attacks once they developed; they report that BHT was ineffective in every respect. There is no justification for using BHT to try to prevent or treat herpes; and to do so, as outlined above, may entail some serious risk.

Apart from the cancer risks, the use of BHT poses some other perils. Allergic reactions, though admittedly isolated ones, have been reported to even the small quantities of BHT that have been added to some foods as preservatives.

We still do not have enough information to make *absolutely conclusive* judgments about these substances. But until we do—and in view of BHT's demonstrated cancer-promoting properties—the prudent consumer will keep a healthy distance from either of these potent chemicals when they are offered as food supplements.

CHARCOAL
(Catching Fire)

That's right. Charcoal is a hot "supplement" these days—and for some good reasons. It's not only a great "de-gasser," it's also showing signs of being a useful "de-cholesterolizer."

One fairly recent double-blind, placebo-controlled study found activated charcoal to be more effective that the drug simethicone when it comes to quelling flatulence, bloating and the irritable bowel syndrome. This confirmed an earlier double-blind study.

Actually, charcoal was a popular remedy for gas more than a century ago. But then, with the advent of antacids and simethicone, it fell out of fashion. Now it's being rediscovered and is available in health food stores and most pharmacies without prescription. Charcoal has been called a "rigid sponge." Its enormous surface area makes it ideal for soaking up many different substances, including gas.

That charcoal might also be good at reducing cholesterol has been suggested by a preliminary study of seven patients with hypercholesterolemia or high levels of cholesterol in the blood. When given 8 grams of activated charcoal three times daily for a month, these subjects exhibited an average 25 percent reduction in total cholesterol and an average 41 percent reduction in the particularly harmful LDL cholesterol. Meanwhile, their "good cholesterol," HDL, went up an average of 8 percent. The only side effect was black stools.

This very preliminary but also very promising study needs prompt follow-up.

Previous studies have shown that oral activated charcoal can be useful in the long-term management of kidney patients who are at particular risk of developing high cholesterol levels and atherosclerosis. High doses of charcoal (20 to 50 grams daily) have helped many kidney patients excrete wastes their failing kidneys would otherwise have difficulty handling, and reductions in cholesterol of up to 43 percent and reductions in triglycerides (blood fats) of up to 76 percent have been reported in kidney patients thus treated.

Some may wonder how one can safely take such high doses of charcoal. The reason for this is that charcoal is not absorbed by the intestine. Instead charcoal simply rides through the system, binding with cholesterol, toxins and other wastes and then passes through the body.

If there is a downside, it is that activated charcoal can also bind with and inactivate some therapeutic drugs and supplemental nutrients. Charcoal should be taken at least one hour before or after therapeutic drugs or nutritional supplements are taken. Those on prescription drugs should use charcoal only with their doctors' approval. Those who take very high doses of charcoal (e.g., 50 grams per day or higher) over long periods of time should supplement with a well-balanced vitamin/mineral formula. High doses of charcoal, in any case, should be taken only with medical supervision.

Note that charcoal is available in tablets, powder and capsules. Most people will find only the capsules palatable and, despite the relatively small amounts of charcoal in these capsules, just a few will usually help control gas. If there are particular foods you like (such as beans), but which give you trouble, you might try taking three or four capsules right after you complete your meal. If trouble still develops, take three or four more.

CHONDROITIN SULFATE
(In the Membrane-Fluidizing Family?)

Chondroitin sulfate is a sulfated polysaccharide and, as such, has properties in common with hyaluronic acid, dextran sulfate and heparin (see discussion of those substances, this section). These are probably all membrane fluidizers and, as such, may have rejuvenating effects on the cells and may disorder the membranes of some viruses, making them less infective—at least in theory. Experimentally, there is some evidence this is true, as well.

Chondroitin sulfate is found in the cartilages of most mammals, including man. Most claims made for this substance have been related to cardiovascular and bone diseases. There is some evidence that chondroitin sulfate can lower cholesterol and triglyceride concentrations in the blood and protect against blood clotting.

This is a promising substance that deserves further research. It is available as a supplement in some health food stores.

(See discussion of hyaluronic acid, this section, for news of a drug that combines chondroitin sulfate with hyaluronic acid.)

DEANER (DMAE)
(Life *Shortener?*)

"Deaner" and "Deanol" were the registered names of prescription drugs that contain dimethylaminoethanol (DMAE), thought to be a precursor of acetylcholine (see discussion of choline elsewhere in this book). Like choline, DMAE has been used to treat various disorders of the nervous system. It appears to have a beneficial role in the treatment of tardive dyskinesia and Huntington's chorea. There is no support, however, for recent claims that DMAE is a potent life extender that might benefit the general population. The life spans of some animals were reported to have been extended through DMAE supplementation, but a more recent study not only failed to confirm this but *found the opposite to be true.* Deanol-treated animals actually had *shorter* life spans than control animals that did not receive this substance. Some have noted the relationship of DMAE to Gerovital H3 (see analysis in this chapter), one of the breakdown products of which is diethylaminoethanol (DEAE), a close chemical relative. If DMAE has any efficacy at all it appears likely that this is due to its role as a choline precursor in the liver. The choline synthesized in the liver from DMAE can go to the brain via the blood and may play a role in the regulation of acetylcholine there. No such role can be conceived of for DEAE.

Deaner is no longer a prescription drug and is now sold in some health food stores. It certainly should not be used as a dietary supplement, as some "life extension" enthusiasts have suggested.

DEXTRAN SULFATE (WITH A NOTE ON HEPARIN)
(Promising AIDS Treatment?)

Dextran sulfate has been one of the hottest "underground" treatments for HIV disease. It has been used for many years in Japan, where it is an approved drug, as a reputed anti-atherosclerotic agent. When injected it is definitely an anti-coagulant. It is also used in oral preparations, but only a small amount of it gets absorbed in this form.

Studies by the Japanese that dextran sulfate can inhibit HIV infection have been confirmed by research in the U.S. This work, however, was in the test tube and not in AIDS patients themselves. Studies are underway now with those patients. There are a few positive preliminary reports and some anecdotal reports of improvement in overall well-being, in elevated T-helper cells and so on.

There are also some reports that dextran sulfate is useful in combination with the approved anti-AIDS drug AZT and that this combination allows for a lower dose of AZT without any loss of effectiveness. If this is so, it is significant because AZT, at standard doses, is often quite toxic.

The FDA is permitting AIDS patients to bring dextran sulfate to the U.S. for personal use, pending the outcome of formal trials of the substances. Many are taking oral doses up to 3 grams per day and even higher. Those with advanced (but not early) AIDS often have difficulty tolerating doses higher than 3 grams. These higher doses can cause diarrhea, bloating and cramping. A few experience these side effects at lower doses.

No one knows for sure how dextran sulfate exerts anti-viral effects. It appears to be a membrane fluidizer, and it seems likely that if it can get to the HIV virus it could disorder the membrane of the virus, possibly making it less capable of infecting cells. Since it does not get absorbed very well, any anti HIV action that it has would have to be at the level of a putative reservoir of viral activity in the gut.

Heparin, a widely used anti-coagulant, is related to dextran sulfate. The Japanese have shown that it is also active against HIV in the test tube. Some AIDS patients have tried this substance, as well, with as yet inconclusive effects. More research is needed on dextran sulfate and heparin to determine if these substances will play any role in the treatment of HIV disease. Another smaller sulfated polysaccharide, pentosan polysulfate (aka SP 54), is also being explored for its possible value in the treatment of HIV disease. This polymer will probably be more readily absorbed. Those with bleeding disorders should *not* use any of these substances.

DHEA
(Promise in Pursuit of Proof)

Dehydroepiandrosterone (DHEA) is a hormone produced by the adrenal glands. It is also found in the Mexican wild yam. There are claims that DHEA will prevent or cure cancer, inhibit weight gain, extend life span, reduce stress, fight AIDS—and so on. For a while DHEA supplements were hot sellers in health food stores, but the FDA stopped such sales, declaring that DHEA is, in effect, an experimental drug.

DHEA and DHEA analogues do, in fact, look promising in some preliminary experimental cancer work. DHEA has protected against and slowed the progression of some cancers in animal work. Human work has only recently begun. There is also some animal work suggesting that DHEA might, indeed, have some favorable impact on obesity.

Suggested mechanisms for DHEA's possible anti-cancer, anti-obesity effects include its hypothesized ability to inhibit an enzyme that is involved in the production of fat and of substances that may promote chemical carcinogenesis.

As for the anti-aging claims, those are based upon observations that as we grow older, blood levels of DHEA steadily decline. These observations are accurate but, as of this date, no one has shown that giving DHEA supplements can extend life span in humans. Some animal experiments have shown enough promise in this regard, however, that this claim should be further investigated.

One group of researchers has begun doing that. They studied 242 men between the ages of fifty and seventy-nine years over a long period of time. They found that DHEA levels decreased in these men with age. Those with histories of heart disease had particularly low levels. And lower levels, in general, were consistently associated with increased risk of death from any cause—even after adjusting for age, blood pressure, serum cholesterol level, obesity, fasting plasma glucose level, smoking and history of heart disease. This important study certainly suggests—but does not prove—that DHEA may confer some protection against several—and perhaps all—degenerative processes.

The DHEA supplements that were on the market were of unknown quality. Some were said to contain almost no DHEA. Some oral DHEA is believed to be destroyed by the liver and does not reach target tissues. Research should be done to see whether oral DHEA has any efficacy. There *are* many anecdotal reports that it is effective.

DHEA—or, more likely, one of its analogues—may turn out to be a wonder drug, but it's not there yet.

DMSO
(Aging "Wonder Drug")

DMSO, though no longer considered a "wonder drug," is still a big seller. Dimethyl sulfoxide (DMSO) has been used since the 1940s as an industrial solvent. It was introduced into therapeutic practice in the 1960s and since then has been used by tens of thousands of individuals as a treatment, applied topically, for strains, sprains, bruises and arthritis.

After once banning research on DMSO out of fear that the chemical might cause serious eye damage, the FDA later allowed investigations to continue and, in 1978, approved the use of DMSO to treat the symptoms of interstitial cystitis (fibrosis of the bladder wall, occurring primarily in women over forty). DMSO is being studied—but has not been approved—for use in a number of skin, nerve and autoimmune diseases. It is also being studied to see what effect it might have on some forms of cancer and on brain-injured patients, victims of spinal-cord injury and cerebral stroke.

Some studies have turned up negative findings but, at the same time, have not reported serious side effects, either to eyes or kidneys, following long-term, *low-dose* DMSO treatment. There is some preliminary evidence that intravenous DMSO may have some usefulness in the treatment of brain-injured individuals; but the use of DMSO for this purpose—as for most others—remains speculative pending well-controlled studies of the sort that have largely been lacking to date.

One group has reported that a 3 percent concentration of DMSO in the drinking water of a strain of mice that spontaneously develop a serious disease syndrome had significant beneficial effects. The mice studied have a gene that gives rise to tumors of the lymph nodes and autoimmune diseases resembling systemic lupus and rheumatoid arthritis. Some 90 percent of those mice given DMSO in their drinking water, commencing at ten weeks of age, were still alive at forty weeks, according to the report of these researchers, while only 50 percent of the control mice, which did not get DMSO in their water, were alive at twenty weeks. There were far fewer tumors among the forty-week-old survivors than among the twenty-week-old controls. Another set of mice— all older and already in advanced stages of disease when started on DMSO-laced drinking water at seven months of age—exhibited significant tumor-mass regression after the DMSO was introduced. Levels of autoantibodies against DNA (of the sort implicated in some autoimmune syndromes) were diminished in DMSO-treated mice. These intriguing findings need follow-up.

DMSO may have antioxidant properties, but this has not yet been established. The proposed modes of action of DMSO are almost as numerous as its claimed benefits; none of these modes has been widely accepted. This, however, has not stopped nearly a dozen states from permitting doctors to prescribe DMSO for various ailments. Certainly no one should use DMSO without a doctor's prescription and then only after asking to see the evidence that the substance is effective for the ailment in question. The DMSO that is being sold in many stores and on the street should be avoided; it is almost never of the relatively pure grade used in clinical trials. Contaminants pose a real risk.

EXPERIMENTAL IMMUNOMODULATORS
(Naltrexone, Imuthiol and Antabuse)

Naltrexone is an opiate antagonist. It is used at high doses to get people off opiate drugs. Its use in this respect is well established and that is its only indication as an approved drug in the United States. (Appetite suppression has been reported at high doses, as well, but this effect has not yet been tested for in well controlled studies.)

At much smaller doses, there is some evidence that naltrexone may have immune-modulating effects. Many with HIV disease are using it. Some claim to be benefiting. One researcher has reported an increase in T-helper cells in these patients. He has also observed a decrease in the level of a form of interferon that is associated with viral diseases. He sees that decline as one of the signs that the naltrexone may be doing some good.

The doses used in HIV patients are only 1.75 milligrams per day. It seems to work better, in this context, at this low dose than at higher doses. Since naltrexone does not come from the manufacturer in these low doses it must be specially prepared.

Naltrexone deserves further research. It could turn out to be of benefit in a number of immune disorders and viral infections.

Imuthiol is an experimental immune-enhancing drug currently being investigated in Europe and the U.S. In preliminary studies, it was shown to be capable of boosting the T-helper cells that sharply decline in numbers and effectiveness among AIDS patients and some others.

Since Imuthiol is not yet available, there has been great interest, among HIV patients in particular, in *Antabuse* (disulfiram), a drug available in the United States that gets metabolized in the body to the same substance that is the active ingredient of Imuthiol. Antabuse is approved for use in alcoholism. Taken with alcohol, it makes one very sick. This aversive effect discourages alcohol use. In alcoholism, Antabuse is used at 250-milligram daily doses. As an immune modulator, only three of these 250-milligram tablets are taken each week.

It is hoped that well controlled trials of Imuthiol and Antabuse will be completed soon.

FRUIT ACIDS
(The "Natural" Face Peel?)

Move over Retin A; you're about to face some new competition in the wrinkle-reducing department. Promising preliminary work indicates that alpha-hydroxy acids (better known as fruit acids) may eventually turn out to be as effective as Retin A in reducing fine wrinkles when applied topically. The fruit acids are found in grapes, oranges, apples, lemons, grapefruit and in sour milk and sugar cane, among others.

When fruit acids were first used to treat age spots, researchers observed a reduction in wrinkles, as well. Fine wrinkles yielded to the acids more readily, but even some moderate wrinkles were said to disappear, sometimes with as little as two months of treatment. The typical treatment involves applying the acids to the skin and washing them off after two or three minutes. These observations must still be confirmed in controlled studies.

The fruit acids appear to work in the same fashion that chemical peels do. The latter use caustic chemicals that destroy the upper layer of skin cells and stimulate new collagen production at a deeper level. It is the collagen that gives skin its youthful appearance and elasticity. The fruit acids appear to provide for a more gentle and, in a sense, a more natural approach to the cosmetic peel. They are, reportedly, far less irritating and do not produce the extreme sun sensitivity that Retin A and the standard chemical peels produce.

Clinical trials with the fruit acids are presently underway.

GEROVITAL H3 (GH3)
(Granddaddy of the "Anti-Aging" Drugs)

Gerovital H3 (GH3) is a procaine preparation first developed and promoted as an anti-aging agent by Dr. Ana Aslan, director of the Institute of Geriatrics in Bucharest, Rumania. According to the Rumanian National Tourist Office, the Aslan clinic has treated "world-renowned actors, actresses, writers and statesmen," who have had conferred upon them, in the process, "the secret of eternal vigor and youth." Well, the first part of that, at least, is true. Numerous prominent individuals still make annual and semiannual pilgrimages to Rumania in search of the fountain of youth—and to be certain that they get the "original," the "authentic" Aslan formula. Others settle for procaine products packaged in Mexico or produced in Nevada, one of the few U.S. locations where it can be legally dispensed.

As for the "eternal vigor and youth," don't get your hopes up. Claims that GH3 and its imitators can extend life span, rejuvenate skin and hair, halt and even reverse senility, increase sexual potency, overcome arthritis, protect against cardiovascular disease and nervous disorders have, without exception, proved false. Studies claiming to demonstrate these effects are few in number and inadequate in design; most are uncontrolled or poorly controlled. When adequately controlled studies *have* been conducted, they have failed to support the claims made for this substance.

GH3 is a 2 percent procaine hydrochloride solution to which minute amounts of the following have been added as "stabilizers" or "buffers": benzoic acid, potassium metabisulfite and disodium phosphate. The procaine (which is the same as the novocaine anesthetic that you get when you go to the dentist) is supposed to be the active ingredient. Procaine, however, is rapidly hydrolyzed (decomposed) once it enters the bloodstream, even after buffering or stabilizing agents are added, and there is no evidence—or even any good reason to suspect—that these additives can sustain the activity of procaine long enough to produce the claimed benefits. Of course, some have theorized that the breakdown products—primarily para-aminobenzoic acid (PABA) and diethylaminoethanol (DEAE)—are the active ingredients. The problem with this argument is that neither of these substances has been shown to possess the miraculous powers claimed for GH3 (see discussions elsewhere in this book of PABA and DMAE, which is chemically related to DEAE). Moreover, the amounts of these substances that result from the breakdown of GH3 are extremely small.

Claims, taken seriously for a time by many researchers, that GH3 is an effective anti-depressant, especially in the aged, have largely failed to be confirmed. It was claimed that procaine could inhibit the formation of a brain chemical—monoamine oxidase (MAO)—that has been associated with depression. The evidence that this is so is scant but probably still deserves some further follow-up. At best, GH3 may have mild anti-depressant activity.

There is no evidence that GH3 has any effect on aging. Adverse side effects infrequently occur and include allergic reactions, abrupt drop in blood pressure, respiratory difficulty and convulsions. Some of these reactions may be due to contaminants in some of the products, the costs of which, incidentally, are often very substantial. GH3 is not recommended.

GLANDULARS
(Snake Oil Revisited)

"Raw glandular concentrates"—usually referred to simply as "glandulars"—are being marketed by an increasing number of companies. This isn't a revival of the old "monkey-gland operation," but it's equally as silly. The argument is that aging is largely a function of failing glands; ergo, those glands can be revived and rejuvenated, at least to some extent, by eating the concentrates of various animal glands. Claims are made that glandulars can reverse everything from hypoglycemia to cancer. Glandulars are supposed to be particularly useful in propping up sagging sex drives. One company has even put out his-and-her glandular formulas for more effective sexual functioning. Some body-builders have also begun taking glandulars, buying claims that they can help build muscle. There is *no* convincing, legitimate evidence whatever that any of these claims has any substance. Nor is there any biochemical reason to even suspect that these substances would be useful. Some of them, in fact, may be harmful; it is possible that some of these organ concentrates contain some of the many toxins livestock are exposed to, such an antibiotics, growth hormones, pesticides, herbicides and fertilizers. There are often higher concentrations of these toxins in the organs than in the other tissues of these animals. Avoid glandulars.

HYALURONIC ACID
(For the Eyes and Bones)

Here is another one of those promising sulfated polysaccharides that may be useful membrane fluidizers and, as such, cell rejuvenators and, in some cases, anti-viral substances.

Recently a new drug has been approved by the FDA that combines a form of hyaluronic acid (sodium hyaluronate) with chondroitin sulfate (see discussion of that substance elsewhere). This drug (Viscoat) is injected into the eye to protect against corneal loss during cataract surgery and artificial lens implantation.

There are early indications that Viscoat may also be useful in the treatment of arthritis, acting as a long-lasting lubricant when injected into affected joints. More research will have to be done on this issue before Viscoat can be sold for this use, as well.

HYPERBARIC OXYGEN
(Space-Age Antibiotic)

If you watch much television or go to the movies, you've no doubt seen an undersea diver come up too quickly from great depth and develop "the bends." The bends—or decompression sickness—can force air bubbles into the diver's blood vessels, and these can be fatal. If the diver is lucky he or she is rushed to a "hyperbaric oxygen chamber" in which 100 percent pure oxygen is breathed under great pressure— enough pressure to safely "squeeze" the air bubbles out of the blood. Then the diver is gradually brought back to normal atmosphere.

Can oxygen administered under greater than atmospheric pressure achieve other miracles? Many seem to think so—and there is at least some evidence to back them up. Hyperbaric oxygen, which has enjoyed sporadic episodes of popularity going back many years, is definitely in vogue again. What looked like science fiction in the 1930s now looks more like space-age medicine to many.

And hyperbaric oxygen *is* medicine; it is regarded as a drug. Some now claim its "accepted indications" include acute air or gas embolism and decompression sickness (of the sort experienced in the bends), carbon monoxide and cyanide poisoning, some forms of gangrene and some problem wounds that won't heal, tissue and bone damage caused by radiation treatments and several other conditions.

In some situations, hyperbaric oxygen works by directly killing microorganisms that are keeping bone or tissue from healing. Some of these microorganisms can only live in a low-oxygen environment. The hyperbaric oxygen is also said to energize some of the immune cells that normally control infection. And, in other instances, the oxygen stimulates circulation and promotes formation of new blood vessels, encouraging healing and re-growth of tissue in the process.

Some researchers continue to regard hyperbaric oxygen as useful only in decompression sickness, but an ever-increasing number of major (and some not-so-major) medical centers are acquiring hyperbaric chambers, and clinical anecdotes related to its usefulness in diverse conditions abound. Good studies, however, are few. More well-controlled research is badly needed.

MEMORY ENHANCERS
(Hydergine, Centrophenoxine, Vasopressin, Ethoxyquin, Phosphatidylcholine, Phosphatidylserine, Ginkgo, Piracetam, Anaricetam, Vinpocetine)

Hydergine is perhaps the best known of the purported memory-enhancing drugs (aka cognition activators). It is one of the most widely used drugs worldwide, though still little-known in the U.S. Hydergine is said to retard aging of the brain, improve memory, counteract senility in some cases and, generally, keep the gray matter humming optimally.

Hydergine affects enzyme systems that are involved in the electrochemistry of nerve signals. There is evidence that Hydergine increases the level of nerve-signal transmission, especially at dopamine and serotonin receptor sites in the brain. Completely unsubstantiated claims have been made that Hydergine can increase intelligence in normal people.

There are, on the other hand, numerous double-blind studies showing that Hydergine can be helpful in chronic senile cerebral insufficiency, a form of diminished mental capacity characterized by confusion, loss of short-term memory, disorientation and depression. It is caused by the aging process, including narrowing of the blood vessels to the brain.

Patients with this disorder who get 1.5-milligram tablets of Hydergine three times per day have consistently performed substantially better on a number of subjective and objective tests related to mood, memory and cognition than have control patients receiving placebos. Usually three months of such treatment is needed before these benefits are observed. Some believe the drug must be continued indefinitely in these cases. So far no serious side effects have been noted.

Hydergine is available as a prescription drug. It is certainly an interesting substance worthy of more research, especially in the U.S.

Other reputed memory enhancers include *centrophenoxine* (not yet available in the U.S., it is said to inhibit "age pigments" that impair mental function and memory), *vasopressin* (a hormone that, anecdotally, has resulted in dramatic memory restoration in a few cases, can have serious side effects and should only be used with a doctor's prescription), *ethoxyquin* (highly experimental and not yet approved for human use), *phosphatidylcholine* and *phosphatidylserine* (both discussed earlier in the lipids section) and *ginkgo* (see herb/plant section).

Two other substances for which memory-enhancing effects have been claimed are *piracetam* (also called *Nootropil*) and the related drug *anaricetam*. Piracetam has been shown to have a positive effect on learning ability in animal experiments. It has also been shown to increase circulation to and oxygenation of the brain in other animal work. It has been used overseas to treat learning disorders in children with variable results. Anecdotally, it is reported to enhance memory in those with memory problems. Some claim it is a mental sharpener and psychic energizer.

Anaricetam is similar to piracetam but is said to be about five times more potent. It has been used in Switzerland to treat dyslexia in children, again with variable and still inconclusive results. It is also being used experimentally in the United States in some patients with the Chronic Fatigue Syndrome (CFS). It is being used in this context as a central nervous-system stimulator. There is some very preliminary indication that it might be helpful in CFS.

Many, possibly all, of these substances deserve more study. It would be interesting to see how some of them work in combination with one another. Possibly such combinations would yield better results.

Another "memory enhancer" exciting a lot of attention lately is *vinpocetine,* already being marketed in Japan, Mexico, Eastern Europe and elsewhere. Several animal and human studies have yielded positive results when the drug was used to try to curb both "normal" and age-related forgetfulness. Vinpocetine is being tested in the United States and a major drug firm plans to bring it into the market here in the near future.

MINOXIDIL AND OTHER BALDNESS REMEDIES
(Chemical Cover-Ups)

For the first time ever, there is a drug on the market approved for the use of growing hair. Its trade name is Rogaine, its chemical name minoxidil. Minoxidil was originally prescribed for oral use in treating hypertension. An unexpected side effect was hair growth in some patients. This led to the development of a topically applied solution of 2 percent minoxidil. After several years of testing, Rogaine has been approved as a prescription drug.

How effective is it? That's the question fifty million Americans with thinning or non-existent hair are asking doctors all over the country. Upjohn Company, Rogaine's manufacturer, tested the substance in 1,431 patients in twenty-seven medical centers across the United States. For the first four months of the year-long study, a double-blind, placebo-controlled protocol was used. Progress was rated both by the patients' own evaluations and by the evaluations of medical investigators.

During the four-month placebo-controlled phase of the study, 41 percent of those getting the Rogaine said they experienced no new hair growth; 32 percent reported "minimal growth;" 25 percent reported "moderate growth;" and 0.7 percent said they enjoyed "dense growth." The medical investigators, however, perceived far less growth. They reported "moderate growth" in only 8 percent and "dense growth" in 0.7 percent. Interestingly, 10 percent of those getting only a placebo reported "moderate growth," and, more interesting still, the medical investigators claimed to see new "minimal growth" in 16 percent of those getting placebos and "moderate growth" in 4 percent of the placebo group.

Despite the less than clear-cut results in the double-blind phase, by the end of the twelve-month study period 40 percent of those who had been getting Rogaine reported "moderate growth" and 8 percent claimed "dense growth." The medical investigators generally agreed, saying that 31 percent of the patients had experienced "moderate growth," while 8 percent enjoyed "dense growth."

There is no doubt that minoxidil can stimulate new hair growth in some individuals, but the results, more often than not, are far from dramatic. Moreover, you must continue to use minoxidil or you will quickly lose any new hair growth. Long-term studies are still lacking, but there is some preliminary evidence suggesting that even with continued use of minoxidil there may be new hair loss after a year.

Rogaine is an improvement over everything else that has been marketed for hair growth but it is, at best, a halfway solution to an age-old problem. Preparations containing polysorbate 60 (as used, for example, in the so-called Helsinki formula) are unlikely to be any kind of solution to the problem. Polysorbate 60, despite the many hair-raising claims made for it, failed to demonstrate any efficacy at all in a double-blind, placebo-controlled study.

Recently news of a Chinese herbal preparation called "101 Hair Regeneration Liniment" has been exciting some attention in the U.S. Its precise formulation has never been revealed but it is said to contain at least nineteen different herbs and possibly other substances. A Japanese travel agency is already setting up "baldy" tours to China to sample this new treatment, the claims for which are quite extravagant. Time will tell if "101" is genuinely useful or just another snake oil. Several other substances are also currently under investigation, but for now it looks like minoxidil is not only the drug of choice, it's the *only* drug with established, albeit weak, hair-growth potential.

How minoxidil works no one is certain, though it is known to dilate the small blood vessels, such as those found in the scalp. That, in itself, would not produce hair. There is speculation that the drug somehow stimulates hair follicle cells. It seems to work better, according to some, when it is combined with Retin A (see discussion elsewhere). The latter is said to enhance penetration and further stimulate the follicles. In one study, a 0.5 percent solution of minoxidil (which is one-fourth the 2 percent solution normally used) combined with a 0.025 percent solution of topical Retin A was said to produce hair growth results about twice as good as those reported when minoxidil is used by itself. This study needs follow-up.

OSCILLOCOCCINUM
(Flu Remedy?)

Oscillococcinum is a homeopathic remedy compounded from duck heart and liver. It is a popular treatment for influenza in Europe. Reports of its effectiveness are purely anecdotal. There is no documentation that the substance helps prevent or treat influenza.

OTHER OXYGEN "THERAPIES"
(Ozone and Hydrogen Peroxide)

Hydrogen peroxide, the same stuff that is used to bleach hair, is being sold in some places as "aerobic oxygen." Others, in the alternative-medicine underground, are actually injecting this stuff, claiming that it can impede cancer, kill viruses and bacteria and restore immunity.

Similar claims are being made for ozone, another very toxic oxygen form. Some AIDS patients are undergoing "ozone therapy."

Both these substances are very powerful free-radical generators and as such are just the opposite of the antioxidants that protect us from so many harmful substances and degenerative processes.

It is true that these substances can kill some microorganisms, but, then, so can all manner of poisons. They also kill healthy cells and can be immune suppressive.

The claims that are being made for these substances in connection with cancer, AIDS and viral infections are without foundation. These substances are potentially dangerous and I strongly recommend complete avoidance.

SANGUINARIA, CHLORHEXIDINE AND OTHER MOUTHWASHES
(Plaque Fighters?)

Sanguinaria, an extract of the bloodroot plant, is said to help remove and prevent dental plaque and is now being used in some major mouthwashes. Actually, there is no real proof that sanguinaria has any anti-plaque effect, but it does have anti-bacterial effects. It may inhibit bacterial activity that produces acids harmful to the gums.

Chlorhexidine, the active ingredient of the prescription mouthwash called Peridex, *does* prevent plaque buildup and can even reduce inflammation of gums caused by the plaque. On the downside, chlorhexidine can stain teeth, requiring more trips to the dentist for cleaning. For those with plaque-caused gum disease, however, chlorhexidine is a real boon.

That old reliable, *Listerine,* is now also recognized by the American Dental Association as useful for "helping reduce above-gumline plaque and gingivitis" or inflammation. It is the only over-the-counter mouthwash to be thus recognized. It is not as effective as the prescription-drug Peridex discussed above. Listerine helps keep new plaque from accumulating but does nothing to break down the old deposits. The active ingredients in Listerine include the volatile oils, eucalyptol, menthol, thymol and methyl salicylate.

There are many other mouthwashes on the market, including one called Plax, but none of these has shown any convincing plaque-fighting ability. Several lack even clear-cut anti-bacterial ability.

SOD AND LIPSOD
(Tomorrow's "Miracles" Today)

Superoxide dismutase, an enzyme that in its different forms is associated with copper, zinc and manganese, is a truly remarkable substance. It is one that bids well to become the stuff of some of tomorrow's *real* "miracle drugs." Indeed, it's already showing exceptional promise in the experimental treatment of a number of serious disorders. In addition, if there are real candidates for "anti-aging" drugs, superoxide dismutase (SOD) has to be counted high among them.

Before I go further, however, I must tell you that the SOD that is being sold in vitamin stores today is *not* the stuff miracles are made of. Research has convincingly demonstrated that these oral SOD products are entirely destroyed in the gut before they can get to the tissues they are supposed to benefit.

The claims that are being made for the readily available oral SOD products are actually based upon findings related to injectable and liposomal forms of SOD (available only to researchers in experimental contexts). But read on, because in the not very distant future some of these SOD substances will almost certainly become available to you, perhaps just when you need them most.

SOD is a tremendously potent antioxidant. Without SOD to protect our cells and safeguard their energy-making processes, we'd all burn up, wither and harden in short order. SOD, more than any other substance in the body, keeps our membranes fluid, our tissues and muscles supple, our cells safe from the very "fires" that burn inside them.

It's little wonder, then, that SOD is being shown, in numerous studies, highly effective in those "hardening" diseases and disorders in which skin, connective tissue, muscle and so on literally begin to lose their life. These include such disorders as rheumatoid arthritis, scleroderma and a variety of autoimmune disorders. Tissue hardened by radiation therapy has also been partially restored with SOD therapy, and heart muscle, deprived of blood and oxygen by heart attack, has also benefited dramatically from the ministrations of SOD.

Much of the pioneering work on SOD has been done by A. M. Michelson of the Institut de Biologie Physico-Chimique in Paris. Michelson and his associates, as well as Japanese and American researchers, have now documented remarkable results using various superoxide dismutases, including liposomal superoxide dismutase (LIPSOD).

LIPSOD is SOD encapsulated in a liposome (see discussion of these very promising "delivery vehicles" in lipids section of this book). Though injections of non-liposomal SOD have proved very beneficial in many cases, results with LIPSOD are even better because the liposome (injected or, in some cases, applied topically) gets more readily and widely distributed throughout the body, its organs, tissues, cells.

I have personally seen the effects of LIPSOD in both scleroderma, a serious autoimmune disease that affects both skin and viscera, and in postradiation damage. In work I did in collaboration with Michelson I saw a significant regression of very severe scleroderma in a woman who received two injections of LIPSOD weekly. Significant improvement was seen in two weeks. Treatment continued for three months. One year posttreatment the patient showed signs of recurrence, indicating the probable need for periodic maintenance therapy. The French and Japanese have reported positive results in LIPSOD-treated scleroderma patients, as well.

Research on the effects of SOD and LIPSOD in the treatment of radiation-damaged tissue is much better established. Here, again, I had opportunity to personally treat, in collaboration with Michelson, a man whose bladder had been badly damaged by cancer radiation therapy. The tissue and muscle of the bladder wall had become dry, hardened and fibrotic, with the result that this patient had so little control that he, typically, had to urinate forty to fifty times daily! Within a few weeks of beginning LIPSOD treatment, frequency of urination dropped to four to five times daily and has remained there for several months now.

In one study of the effects of LIPSOD on postradiation-treatment fibrosis in fifty patients, researchers found that even when several years had elapsed since the damage occurred, notable benefit could be obtained with just three weeks of treatment. Significant softening of fibrosis was seen in 82 percent of the patients, with an average 33 percent reduction in fibrosis size. Several fibroses completely regressed. At last report, more than a year posttreatment, these benefits have persisted without need of retreatment.

Other researchers have reported excellent results with SOD and LIPSOD in cases of Crohn's disease, Behcet's disease, Raynaud's syndrome, Kawasaki disease and unresponsive anemia. Others see a bright future for SOD in heart attack patients.

Giving SOD at the same time the heart is fully re-supplied with blood after a blocked artery has caused a heart attack can significantly reduce further free-radical damage in cardiac muscle. This may have a very significant effect on heart attack survival rates.

It appears that the therapeutic potential of SOD and LIPSOD have only begun to be explored. SOD's protective effects against all of the degenerative processes could make it a genuine anti-aging substance, affecting all parts of the body.

Animal experiments and other early investigations now underway suggest that SOD and, especially, LIPSOD may be useful in multiple sclerosis, Alzheimer's disease, Peyronie's disease, in organ transplantation and possibly even in AIDS.

TESTOSTERONE AND STEROIDS
(The Good, The Bad and The Evil)

Let's start with the bad and the evil—but be aware there's some potentially good news here, too, news suggesting a possible role for testosterone as an "anti-aging" substance in men.

There's little positive to be said about the use of anabolic steroid drugs among athletes and body-builders. Under certain circumstances, the anabolic steroids *do* build muscle/lean body mass but at a sometimes high cost to health. These drugs are now being used not only by some "power" athletes (such as football players) but also by some endurance athletes, such as runners. Even some high school and junior high school athletes are using them.

All of these drugs are, to varying degrees, both androgenic (masculinizing) and anabolic (muscle building). There are a great many of them and, typically, several are used in alternative fashion and in various combinations. These drugs have potent effects on the body's hormones and metabolism, many of them undesirable. The risks aren't as terrible as some have claimed, but they *are* significant.

Among possible side effects of these substances are psychologic disturbances (including abnormal aggression), usually reversible male infertility, altered (often diminished) sex drive, acne, sleeping problems, gynecomastia (development of female-like breasts) in men, hirsutism (hairiness) and other masculinizing effects in women and male pattern baldness in both men and women.

Those, by the way, are characterized by some as the "minor" side effects of anabolic steroids. The "major" side effects, if those aren't bad enough for you, include adverse effects on cholesterol, liver damage and increased risk of getting several cancers. The cancer risk is not high but it's there. The cholesterol elevation is far more prevalent.

It is particularly unfortunate that an increasing number of adolescents are now using anabolic steroids. They are at particularly high risk of developing serious problems, including, ironically, stunted growth. More women are also using anabolic steroids, which, in their case, can result in *irreversible* deepening of voice, hirsutism, male pattern baldness and enlargement of the clitoris.

So what good can be said of these substances? Well, in relatively short-term, carefully monitored use of some of them can be helpful in speeding the recovery of individuals who have suffered accidents or illnesses that have wasted their muscles and robbed them of vitality.

Testosterone itself, the primary male sex hormone, often declines as men age. The situation is not as dramatic as in women whose primary sex hormone (estrogen) declines very sharply at menopause. But just as women can often benefit dramatically from estrogen-replacement therapy after menopause so may some men benefit from testosterone replacement as they age.

Hormone replacement therapy is widely accepted medical practice in women. This is not true with respect to men, but perhaps it should be. There are enough hints of benefits that some serious studies should be launched to investigate this issue.

A number of men, possibly quite a significant number, suffer erectile impotence as they age, due to declining testosterone levels. If testosterone deficiencies can be demonstrated, then periodic injections of the hormone can often overcome the impotence. Depending upon the form given these injections can be spaced anywhere from two weeks to three months apart.

Impotence, however, is only one sign of possible testosterone deficiency. Other associations have been made recently with reduced levels of testosterone. One group of researchers found, for example, that elderly men with a history of heart attack tend to have significantly reduced serum testosterone. So do those older men with histories of heavy drinking. These researchers suggested that giving testosterone to men with low levels of the hormone might have cardioprotective benefits.

Interestingly, when the male sex hormone was first identified many decades ago it was considered by many doctors to be a miracle substance that could retard male aging and prolong man's prime. For a time testosterone was used not only to buck up drooping sex drive but to instill more energy, both physical and mental, in the aging. There were many clinical anecdotes claiming that testosterone could dispel even incipient senility in some men.

When it was discovered, however, that giving large doses of testosterone can promote abnormal, sometimes malignant growth in the prostate, people began backing off, and the idea of using testosterone as an anti-aging substance faded. Only recently has the idea again surfaced.

Testosterone is no panacea and there *are* risks involved in its long-term use. But the idea that it might be very beneficial in those men with clear-cut deficiencies certainly warrants investigation. Such deficiencies, moreover, may be more prevalent than was previously suspected. The use of testosterone, of course, requires a doctor's supervision. With proper monitoring, its use in *appropriate* individuals should create only minimal risks.

THYMIC THERAPIES
(AIDS to Aging)

Thymosin, a group of hormones first identified in the 1960s, are under investigation, in various forms, for everything from AIDS to aging. These are the hormones produced by the thymus gland, which is intimately involved in immunity and is known to begin deteriorating relatively early in life and to be almost non-functional in advanced age.

About fifteen years ago, researchers at the University of California School of Medicine in San Francisco used thymosin "fraction 5," an extract from the thymus glands of calves, to treat a child with a severe immune-deficiency disorder. The child made remarkable progress and today, after intermittent treatment with what is now often called thymic factor, is a healthy teenager.

This led to many further studies with many different thymic extracts. These extracts have become not only more numerous but also more pure and specific over time. Some are now being synthesized in the laboratory. Some believe that the many different thymic components that have been identified in recent years are required, at different stages, by important immune cells for full and proper development.

A small number of thymic factors have so far been tried in cancer therapy. The studies are still preliminary and results are inconclusive, although improved immune function has been observed in many of these patients. Actual tumor regression has been observed in a few studies. Other studies suggest that thymic factors may make some cancer chemotherapies and radiation therapies more effective and less destructive to the immune system. Viral infections have also been reported diminished in cancer patients treated with thymic factors.

Research on thymic factors in AIDS has produced mixed results. Studies are continuing.

That thymic preparations might be useful in autoimmune disorders is suggested by a study in which sufferers of rheumatoid arthritis, given a synthetic thymic factor, experienced significant relief. More study is needed.

Soviet researchers, meanwhile, have reported using another thymic factor in the treatment of psoriasis, a severe skin condition that is the result, many believe, of disordered immunity. The Russians reported that 79 percent of those treated enjoyed pronounced improvement and that fifty-five of seventy-eight patients treated went on to complete recovery after a month of thymic injections. In seven patients followed for two to three years posttreatment, there have been no relapses, according to this report.

These are very promising substances that need further scientific investigation. Some of these thymic factors have found their way into the alternative-medicine underground. I don't recommend use of these complex substances except under a doctor's supervision. They should be regarded as drugs and not as nutritional supplements or anti-aging substances that can be taken without medical supervision.

TRANSFER FACTOR
("Soluble Cellular Immunity")

The discoverer of transfer factor called it "soluble cellular immunity." It is an extract of healthy lymphocytes, cells of immunity, and is used in an effort to transfer cell-mediated immunity from a healthy person to an immune-compromised person. The healthy person is one who is known to be immune or resistant to the problem being treated. Many are seeking out transfer factor these days in an effort to dispel Chronic Fatigue syndrome and fight AIDS, autoimmune diseases and some cancers.

Transfer factor has been under study for many years and it is now generally accepted that it can be helpful in treating some viral and fungal infections. Just how helpful remains open to question. Even though numerous studies have been done, many of these have been small and poorly controlled. Results have often been inconclusive.

Transfer factor, used in conjunction with anti-fungal drugs, has been quite effective in the treatment of chronic candidiasis—and the immunity it conferred in some patients has persisted for several years. It has also been effective in protecting against herpes simplex and chicken pox in some.

Transfer factor may have a role as an adjunct therapy in some cancers. In one study it was shown to significantly extend the survival times of patients who underwent surgery for lung cancer.

Its roles, if any, in AIDS and Chronic Fatigue syndrome remain to be elucidated. There is some preliminary evidence that transfer factor can restore some aspect of immunity in patients with pre-AIDS who are not yet severely immune compromised. Studies are underway to assess the effects of transfer factor in Chronic Fatigue syndrome.

Transfer factor is, in several respects, a promising substance, particularly when used in conjunction with other therapies. Whether it will really live up to its name ("soluble cellular immunity") remains to be seen.

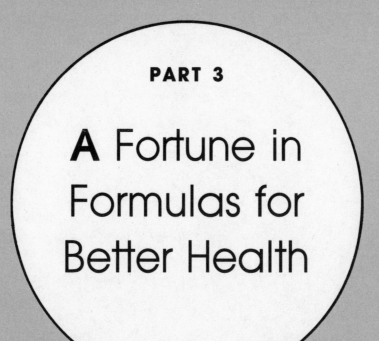

PART 3

A Fortune in Formulas for Better Health

TWELVE

The Basic Formulas

for Health

Maintenance

The following formulas are *suggestions* for people in different life situations. Use these formulas as general information to help guide you in the right direction. The use of some of these formulas requires medical monitoring. Some of the substances mentioned in certain formulas are either not available in the United States or are presently not approved for such use by the FDA. Those wishing to try these items should do so *only* under a physician's guidance and with informed consent. Cautionary notes and other specifics are included under the various formulas.

Note: I have written that the typical, supposedly "well-balanced" American diet is a disaster waiting to happen. *U.S. News and World Report* has quoted me as saying, "as a nation we are overfed and often seriously undernourished." We get plenty to eat. But we don't eat the right things and, consequently, suffer from a number of serious nutritional deficiencies. Our diets are directly associated with the number one killer, coronary artery disease, as well as certain types of cancer. In addition, a wide range of disorders including obesity, diabetes, digestive difficulties, immune deficiencies, skin problems, fatigue, headaches, body aches and many other ailments have been associated with the standard American diet, which is high in cholesterol and fats, especially of the saturated variety, low in dietary fiber, high in refined sugars and high in animal products. Those who have changed to diets low in fat and cholesterol, high in dietary fiber, fruits and vegetables are slimmer, healthier and more energetic.

Many still mistakenly believe that generally healthy people do not require micronutrient (vitamin and mineral) supplementation so long as they get a "well-balanced" diet. And, in fact, it *isn't* likely that *gross* vitamin and mineral deficiencies will occur in healthy individuals eating generally adequate diets. My research indicates, however, that it is prudent for even those individuals to take a daily vitamin and mineral supplement to ensure maximum nutritional insurance. The reasons for this were made evident in the preceding chapters. We live in times that are particularly stressful, in terms of both psychological and environmental factors.

We really do not yet know the optimal vitamin and mineral requirements for maximum health and longevity. The RDAs for the micronutrients only address the issue of *short-term* problems that occur due to deficiencies. They do *not* address the issue of *long-term* consequences of suboptimal intake. Many studies are now underway to investigate this and to determine optimal intakes of the vitamins and minerals for preventing degenerative diseases.

There is growing evidence that substances in our "well-balanced" diets contribute to cancer and other degenerative diseases. Many of the micronutrients we've been discussing help neutralize these toxic oxidants. Many of the vitamins and minerals are antioxidants that can help protect against cancer, cardiovascular diseases and osteoarthritis, among other ills. A vitamin and mineral supplement is recommended for even healthy individuals as a key element in the prevention of many of these degenerative diseases.

The following "basic formulas" are the ones I recommend for most healthy men, *pre*menopausal women, teenagers and children. The contents and amounts, as well as the recommended forms, are derived from studies reviewed in this book. These recommended amounts are approximations of what appears optimal at this time, based on the best available evidence. Future research will, no doubt, eventually yield more definitive data. The reader should review all the material in the preceding chapters related to each substance before using any of the suggested formulas. Special attention should be paid to any noted "precautions."

Note that, with a few exceptions, the vitamins and minerals are *not* recommended in megadose amounts, that is, in amounts greater than about ten times the U.S. RDA. Exceptions to this arise when vitamins are recommended in higher amounts for specific or therapeutic purposes. I believe that a properly balanced vitamin/mineral supplement usually obviates the need for megadose supplementation. For example, selenium and zinc, present in the right balance and amounts, spare the antioxidant activity of vitamin E, making intake of amounts of vitamin E much greater than 200–400 IUs daily unnecessary and unjustified. A balanced supplement is a highly efficient supplement, and that is what I have strived for here and in all of the formulas that follow.

Micronutrient amounts in the formulas are expressed in ranges. The lower numbers are for those who want to take no more than one-a-day vitamin/mineral supplement. The higher numbers are for those who wish to take more than just a one-a-day. So-called insurance formulas are available which have the higher doses. The micronutrients in the insurance formulas are contained in several tablets which are split into either two doses and taken with breakfast and dinner, or into three doses, one with each meal. Some of the antioxidant protection afforded by micronutrient supplements may take place before the supplement is absorbed into the bloodstream. This is because many of the foods we eat contain substances that cause free-radical damage. Antioxidants, taken with each meal, could help prevent this damage in the stomach and intestine.

In all the formulas pay attention to milligrams (mg) and micrograms (mcg). There's a *big* difference. There are 1,000 micrograms in one milligram.

Basic Formula for Adult Men

Note: The basic formula for men omits iron, since even a marginal iron deficiency in men who consume more than 2,000 calories daily suggests a disease process that requires medical investigation. Adult males on weight-loss diets, however, *should* take supplementary iron

TABLE 3   BASIC FORMULA FOR MEN

Vitamins	Recommended Form(s)	Amount
Vitamin A	beta-carotene	3–15 mg (5,000–25,000 IUs)
Vitamin B_1	thiamine	1.5–10 mg
Vitamin B_2	riboflavin	1.7–10 mg
Niacinamide	niacinamide	20–200 mg
Pantothenic acid	calcium pantothenate	10–50 mg
Vitamin B_6	pyridoxine	2–20 mg
Vitamin B_{12}	hydroxycobalamin or cyanocobalamin	6–30 mcg
Biotin	biotin	100–300 mcg
Folic acid	folic acid	200–400 mcg
Vitamin C (ascorbic acid)	calcium ascorbate, sodium ascorbate, or ascorbic acid*	60–600 mg
Vitamin D	ergocalciferol (vitamin D_2) or chole-calciferol (vitamin D_3)	200–400 IUs
Vitamin E	d-alpha-tocopheryl acetate or d-alpha tocopheryl succinate	30–200 IUs

* Some find ascorbic acid irritating to their stomachs.

(see Weight Loss Formula), as should adult men who are endurance athletes (see Athletic Formula), as these individuals are more vulnerable to iron deficiency.

Basic Formula for Women (Premenopausal Women Not on the Pill)

Note: The micronutritional formula I recommend for this group is similar to the Basic Formula for Men, with the exception of iron. Since premenopausal women have a monthly blood loss, as well as a lower iron reserve than men, it is prudent for them to take an iron supplement, especially if they have heavier than normal menstrual flow or if they are fitted with IUDs (intrauterine devices), which may predispose them to additional blood loss.

The best form of iron is found in meat and is called heme iron. Liver

TABLE 3   BASIC FORMULA FOR MEN (Continued)

Minerals	Recommended Form(s)	Amount
Calcium	calcium citrate preferred/lactate, gluconate, glubionate, carbonate acceptable forms	200–1,000 mg
Copper	copper gluconate	1–2 mg
Chromium	high chromium yeast or chromium picolinate preferred/ chromic acetate acceptable	50–200 mcg
Magnesium	magnesium gluconate preferred oxide, sulfate acceptable	200–400 mg
Manganese	manganese gluconate	5–10 mg
Molybdenum	sodium molybdate	50–100 mcg
Selenium	high selenium yeast or L-selenomethionine	50–200 mcg
Zinc	zinc gluconate, zinc picolinate	10–15 mg
Iodine	potassium iodide or from kelp	75–150 mcg

is a good source of heme iron, and liver extracts and pills used to be big favorites for the treatment of anemias. They are rarely recommended these days, however, because of the great variability of their content, among other problems. Iron supplements contain a different form of iron, one which is not as readily absorbed. Ideally, supplementary iron should be taken by itself or with vitamin C *between meals* for maximum absorption. Available iron supplements include ferrous fumarate, ferrous sulfate, ferrous gluconate and carbonyl iron, also known as micronized elemental iron. Carbonyl iron is a good delivery form of iron but requires hydrocholoric acid for its absorption and therefore needs to be taken with meals. The other iron supplements mentioned are best absorbed on an empty stomach. They do get absorbed, but to a lesser extent, with food. Ferrous sulfate is a popular iron supplement, but some find it irritating to the gastrointestinal tract and prefer ferrous fumarate, which is usually less irritating. Women who take iron in a multivitamin/multimineral preparation should be aware that calcium, and particularly calcium phosphate, decreases the absorbability of iron. Vitamin C, on the other hand, increases it.

Women who require iron supplements for the correction of iron-deficiency anemia should be under a physician's care. They usually require iron in amounts of at least 50 milligrams daily to correct their problem. Those who take iron for nutritional insurance reasons should not take any more than 10–18 milligrams daily.

The Formula

Same as the Basic Formula for Men except: Add iron in the form of fumarate, sulfate, or carbonyl iron (elemental micronized iron), in the amount of 10–15 milligrams daily. Those who use carbonyl iron, which is now available in some multivitamin/multimineral pills, should take it with food.

Basic Formula for Teenagers

Note: Many teenagers have suboptimal intakes of several vitamins and minerals. Some reports indicate that intake of a few vitamins and minerals is actually well below the RDAs in this group. It is no secret that many teenagers have very bad diets. It would be prudent for teenagers to take at least a one-a-day multivitamin/multimineral preparation.

The Formula

Same as the Basic Formula for Men. Add iron (ferrous fumarate or carbonyl iron) at 10–15 milligrams daily; especially recommended for teenage women.

Basic Formula for Children (from age four to teenage years)

Note: Children are *most vulnerable* to nutritional deficiencies, since they are in their most active growth period. Many children eat diets consisting largely of highly sweetened foods and beverages. Most children can benefit from a micronutrient supplement.

The Formula

A one-a-day vitamin/mineral product containing the low-end doses of the Basic Formula for Men. Iron is usually listed on most of the food items that children eat. If the child is not getting much iron, then a supplement of 10 milligrams of iron in the form of ferrous fumarate or iron carbonyl makes sense. Make sure this is acceptable to the child's pediatrician. Children with iron deficiency or iron-deficiency anemia require medical treatment.

THIRTEEN

Special Formulas for

Women

Formula for Women Using Oral Contraceptives

Note: There is evidence that women who use oral contraceptives have greater requirements for vitamin B_6 (pyridoxine) and folic acid. Oral contraceptives appear to interfere with these vitamins. The mood changes (such as depression) that many women who use oral contraceptives experience have been attributed to decreased synthesis of the neurotransmitter serotonin. This decreased synthesis may be a consequence of decreased vitamin B_6 status.

The formula I recommend here is the same as the Basic Formula for Women except that, in addition to the iron which is added in that formula, I also recommended a total daily B_6 intake of 20 milligrams.

The Formula

Same as Basic Formula for Women except: Bring vitamin B_6 intake to 20 milligrams daily.

Formula for Pregnant Women

Note: Pregnant women are known to have special requirements for many of the micronutrients, particularly folic acid and iron. In the case of iron, it is highly unlikely that pregnant women can obtain iron from the foods they eat in sufficient quantities to prevent iron deficiency. It is thus recommended that pregnant women take *30 to 60 milligrams of supplementary iron daily.* Some pregnant women may require more than this. Every pregnant woman should be carefully evaluated by her obstetrician to determine the amount of iron needed to prevent deficiency.

Acceptable forms of iron are ferrous sulfate, ferrous fumarate and carbonyl iron. Carbonyl iron needs to be taken with meals because its absorption requires stomach acid secretion. Ferrous sulfate and ferrous fumarate are best absorbed on an empty stomach and, ideally, should be taken about one hour before a meal. Many women, however, suffer gastric irritation when they take iron on an empty stomach. Ferrous sulfate is usually more irritating in this respect than ferrous fumarate. If switching to the fumarate form doesn't alleviate this irritation, then take your iron with meals.

Iron contained in a multivitamin/multimineral preparation that includes calcium, particularly in the form of calcium phosphate, may lead to decreased absorption of iron. On the other hand, vitamin C (ascorbic acid) enhances iron's absorption.

Pregnant women also have increased requirements of folic acid, magnesium and calcium. It is likely that they have increased requirements for such micronutrients as zinc as well. Occasionally children are born with vitamin K and biotin deficiencies. It is unlikely that these conditions are due to vitamin K and biotin deficiencies of the pregnant woman. Addition of vitamin K to the Formula for Pregnant Women however, will not hurt and *may* help prevent these deficiencies in the newborn. Vitamin K deficiency leads to bleeding disorders.

This formula should be used only after discussion with your obstetrician. You will note that the ranges of some of the vitamins are set lower than the basic formulas for men and women. The probability of any adverse effects from these vitamins on the fetus is extremely low even at the higher doses of the above formulas, but, to err on the side of caution, the upper dose limits are lowered here. Compare your supplement formula with the following formula to determine if yours is adequate. There are some good formulas available. Typically, the pregnant woman takes the formula (without iron) *with meals* and takes iron separately on an empty stomach. Some formulas are low in calcium and magnesium and these minerals can be taken as individual supplements along with the formula for pregnant women.

Formula for Postmenopausal Women

Note: Osteoporosis, a bone disease characterized by decreased bone density, increased brittleness of bone and loss of bone calcium, is not uncommon in postmenopausal women. There is evidence that supple-

TABLE 4 THE FORMULA FOR PREGNANT WOMEN

Vitamins	Amount
Vitamin A (as beta-carotene)	3–6 mg (5,000–10,000 IUs)
Vitamin B_1	1.5–5mg
Vitamin B_2	1.7–5 mg
Niacinamide	20–50 mg
Pantothenic acid	10–50 mg
Vitamin B_6	2–5 mg
Vitamin B_{12}	6–30 mcg
Biotin	100–300 mcg
Folic acid	400–800 mcg
Vitamin C	70–250 mg
Vitamin D	200–400 IUs
Vitamin E	30–100 IUs
Vitamin K (as K_1 or phytonadione)	50–100 mcg

Minerals	Amount
Calcium	600–1200 mg
Copper	1–2 mg
Chromium	50–200 mcg
Iron (as ferrous sulfate, ferrous fumarate, or carbonyl iron)	30–60 mg
Magnesium	200–400 mg
Manganese	2.5–5 mg
Molybdenum	50–100 mcg
Selenium	50–200 mcg
Zinc	10–15 mg
Iodine	75–150 mcg

(See Basic Formulas for Men and Women for recommended form of each nutrient)

mentary calcium may help in the prevention of this disease. More recently, there is some evidence that the trace mineral boron and vitamin K may also help.

The worst aspect of osteoporosis is that it puts women at risk for life-threatening bone fractures. Estrogen and progesterone replacement therapy appears to make the biggest impact on the prevention of osteoporosis and fractures in postmenopausal women. Evidence suggests that adequate calcium intake throughout a woman's lifetime is more likely to prevent osteoporosis than if started at the time of menopause. Fluoride supplementation looks promising as another preventive measure. (See fluoride section for additional information.) Exercise is also important in osteoporosis prevention. Walking twenty to thirty minutes at least three times a week while getting your heart rate up to 60–70 percent of your maximum heart rate is not only a very good form of exercise but also one that you are more likely to stick to. Maximum heart rate can be calculated by subtracting your age from 220.

Many postmenopausal women feel cold even though they have completely normal circulation and completely normal function of thyroid glands. It turns out that even mild iron deficiency without the presence of anemia may account for this. Iron supplementation frequently corrects this symptom.

Calcium carbonate is the most widely used calcium supplement. Calcium absorption from this form depends, however, on stomach acidity and, therefore, should be taken with meals and not on an empty stomach. Many postmenopausal women *do* take calcium carbonate on an empty stomach, and this may be one of the reasons that the effects of calcium on postmenopausal osteoporosis protection appear so variable. Calcium citrate does *not* require stomach acidity for its absorption and can thus be taken on an empty stomach. Some postmenopausal women produce less hydrochloric acid than normal, and many people take drugs (such as cimetidine and ranitidine) which decrease hydrochloric acid production. For those people, calcium citrate is the better choice. The citrate part of the molecule may have the added benefit of preventing formation of calcium kidney stones.

Postmenopausal women with high concentrations of calcium in the blood should *avoid* calcium supplementation. Postmenopausal women with kidney failure should not take magnesium supplements.

The Formula

Same as the Basic Formula for Women except:

1) Total calcium intake for women taking estrogen-replacement therapy should be 1,000 mg daily and, for those not taking estrogens, 1,500 mg daily. I recommend *calcium citrate* for the reasons given above.

2) Add 3 mg of boron in the form of sodium borate.

3) Add 50–100 mcg of vitamin K.

4) Remember that exercise is a very important ingredient of this formula (see Note above).

5) See precautions above.

Formula for Women with Premenstrual Syndrome (PMS)

Note: Premenstrual syndrome, or PMS, occurs commonly, is very little understood and controversy abounds as to its proper treatment. PMS refers to cyclic symptoms experienced by women during their reproductive years. These symptoms may include anxiety, irritability, depression, mood swings, fatigue, food cravings (especially for sweets), weight gain, bloating, breast tenderness, dizziness and headache. These symptoms typically begin about seven to ten days prior to menstrual bleeding (the "period") and usually resolve with the onset of bleeding.

The use of nutritional supplements is sometimes useful in the treatment of PMS symptoms. I have often had success in treating PMS by using specific nutrients for specific symptoms. L-tyrosine appears helpful for depression and fatigue, perhaps the most disabling symptoms of PMS. Vitamin E often relieves breast tenderness. Phosphatidylcholine is sometimes useful in controlling some mood and memory problems. Vitamin B_6 has been reported to occasionally relieve some PMS symptoms, especially the emotional ones. Scattered reports suggest that L-carnitine may help with bloating. Magnesium and zinc may also help with some PMS symptoms.

Gamma-linolenic acid, found in evening primrose oil, spirulina (blue-green bacteria), among others, is only *rarely* helpful in PMS. Drug treatment has also been used for PMS. Oral and intravaginal progesterone have occasionally been helpful but, overall, have not been found to be reliable in the treatment of PMS. Anti-depressant medications are sometimes useful. Exercise, dietary changes and stress-relieving measures are often the most useful treatments.

The Formula

Same as the Basic Formula for Women except:

1) Vitamin B_6 (pyridoxine) can be increased to a total of 20–50 mg daily during the symptomatic time. Doses higher than 50 mg daily for prolonged periods are not recommended because of the possibility of neurologic side effects (see vitamin B_6). Those who do take higher doses should be under a physician's supervision.

2) Vitamin E can be increased to a total of 400 IUs daily for breast tenderness.

3) L-tyrosine may be helpful for PMS-associated depression and fatigue. Capsules of 500 mg can be taken on an empty stomach an hour before each meal for a total of 1,500 mg daily. Some women may need higher amounts of L-tyrosine, up to 2,000 mg before each meal, for a beneficial effect. Those who need doses higher than 1,500 mg daily should be under a physician's supervision. Do not use L-tyrosine if you are taking an MAO (monoamine oxidase) inhibitor type of anti-depressant (e.g., Nardil or Parnate). If you have high blood pressure, do not use L-tyrosine except under medical supervision.

4) Phosphatidylcholine may be helpful for PMS-associated hypomanic moods or memory problems. Doses of from 1 to 10 grams daily are unlikely to have adverse side effects. Start with the lower dose. In place of phosphatidylcholine, you may want to try choline at doses of 100 to 1,000 milligrams daily. Again, start at the lower dose first. If you find that taking phosphatidylcholine or choline increases your depression, stop taking it.

5) L-carnitine at doses of 2,000 mg daily may help relieve the bloated feeling often associated with PMS. It appears to have a mild diuretic action at this dose.

FOURTEEN

Miscellaneous

Formulas

Formula for Cholesterol Control

Note: One of the more positive things the 1980s will be remembered for is the dawning of the era of cholesterol-consciousness. There is no longer any doubt that an abnormally high cholesterol level is a major risk factor for coronary artery disease, the number one killer of adults in the country. Lowering cholesterol level reduces the risk. In fact, a major study on cholesterol and coronary artery disease conducted by the National Heart, Lung and Blood Institute reported, among other things, that a 1 percent reduction in cholesterol level leads to a 2 percent reduction in coronary artery disease and its deadly consequences.

We are also now in a better position to say what acceptable cholesterol levels should be. The lowest risk of coronary artery disease is associated with serum cholesterol levels less than 180 mg per deciliter. For adults, a cholesterol level of less than 200 is desirable (less than 180 even more so), and for children and teenagers, a cholesterol level of less than 180 is the goal. Cholesterol is divided into HDL cholesterol (HDL = high density lipoprotein) and LDL cholesterol (LDL = low density lipoprotein). HDL cholesterol is "good" or protective cholesterol, while LDL cholesterol is "bad" or non-protective cholesterol. LDL cholesterol should be below 126. HDL cholesterol is desirable above 40 in men (the higher the better) and above 50 in women. Cholesterol levels in adults between 200–240 are considered borderline high, and above 240 they are considered to be very high and highly undesirable. Cholesterol levels should be checked after fasting (no food after midnight); blood should be drawn the first thing in the morning. For the sake of accuracy, it is often wise to have the blood analyzed *twice*.

What can you do if you have elevated cholesterol? In the first place, you should begin eating a healthier diet. The best diet for maximum cardiovascular health should be one that contains no more than 20 percent fat in calories, with about equal amounts of polyunsaturated, monounsaturated and saturated fats, no more than 100 mg of cholesterol daily, 65 percent carbohydrates (mainly of the complex variety), 45–60 grams of dietary fiber, protein mainly from plant and fish sources, and little or no red meat. In addition, minimize intake of dairy products and coconut and palm oils. This is *not* the typical American diet. Caloric intake should be restricted to prevent obesity, although with the above low-fat, high-dietary-fiber diet, obesity is much less likely to be a problem. Exercise is very important, particularly aerobic exercise, which can help raise the good cholesterol (HDL) while lowering total cholesterol.

If an improved diet and exercise still leave you with an unacceptable cholesterol level, I would recommend supplements before I would recommend cholesterol-lowering prescription drugs. Soluble dietary fiber has been documented to lower cholesterol levels. Eating one cup of oat bran cereal daily or three to four oat bran muffins daily can lower your cholesterol level up to 10 percent within a month. Or you can blend one tablespoon of pectin (unsweetened) or one tablespoon of psyllium seed husks into water or orange juice and take this two or three times daily with meals. Beans are also a good source of soluble dietary fiber.

If you need to go to the next step, try nicotinic acid. *This is a tricky one because of possible adverse side effects and should be tried only under medical supervision.* For a cholesterol-lowering effect, we are talking megadose amounts of nicotinic acid. Side effects of nicotinic acid include the notorious "niacin flush," a burning, itching, reddening, tingling sensation, usually in the face, neck, arms and upper chest, which may persist for half an hour or even longer, causing some people fright and others discomfort. The flush is *not* dangerous but is bothersome to many. It can be dampened by taking an aspirin tablet (325 milligrams) about a half hour before taking the nicotinic acid, and the flush usually becomes less intense with continued use of nicotinic acid. Other side effects may include palpitations, impaired glucose tolerance, aggravation of peptic ulcers, elevation of uric acid levels, elevation of liver function tests and, rarely, hepatitis.

Nicotinic acid is usually started at 100 mg three times a day with meals and then increased by 100 mg every few days until one is taking a total of 1,500–3,000 mg (1.5–3 grams) daily. These doses can lower cholesterol levels considerably. Recently long-acting forms of nicotinic acid have become available. These forms have lower incidences of most of the above side effects including the "niacin flush." One can start by taking one 250-mg tablet with food and then, if the only side effect noted is a mild flush, immediately begin taking 250 mg three times daily with meals for one week. Next go up to 500 mg three times daily with meals. Have your cholesterol level checked after four weeks, and, if it requires lowering even further, increase the dose to 1,000 mg three times daily with meals. Nicotinic acid should always be taken with meals and *no one should take these megadoses without medical supervision.*

A few studies have indicated that supplementary *chromium* may increase the helpful HDL cholesterol. A recent study (randomized, double-blind, placebo-controlled) demonstrated that a form of chromium called chromium picolinate, taken at 200 mcg daily, lowered cholesterol by about 5 percent after several weeks. This was statistically significant.

Activated charcoal, most commonly used in medicine to detoxify patients who have taken overdoses of drugs, can also lower cholesterol levels. The problems with it are that it is messy to work with and can stain your teeth, clothes, cups, glasses, utensils and stool (not the kind you sit on) black. You can get it out of your teeth, clothing and kitchenware fairly easily, but it is still a nuisance. When it is blended in orange juice, it is tasteless, but the orange juice looks like motor oil. It's easy to joke about it, but the fact is that it does work and if taken correctly (see Formula below), is very low in adverse side effects.

One study and a few anecdotal reports suggest that *L-carnitine*, taken at 1 gram daily for several weeks, increases HDL cholesterol. There is no real documentation, however, that supplementary L-carnitine can lower cholesterol levels.

On the other hand, there *are* a few studies indicating that *pantethine*, at doses of 600 to 1,200 mg daily, lowers cholesterol levels after several weeks. No adverse effects have been reported at these doses.

A now well-known study of the Greenland Eskimos sought to discover how they could be so cardiovascularly fit given their high fat intake. It turned out that their diet of whale blubber contains a lot of omega-3 polyunsaturated fatty acids, now popularly known as *fish oils*. Fish oil supplements have been shown to lower LDL cholesterol levels in those people who have elevated fasting triglycerides (much greater than 140 mg per deciliter). There is little evidence that they lower cholesterol in those with normal triglyceride levels.

The Formula

Except for the first four items, the following should be done in a step-by-step fashion. *Make sure that you are being monitored by a physician while doing this.*

1) Diet. See above comments.

2) Exercise. Regular aerobic exercise is a very important part of the formula. Exercise can be a brisk walk for twenty to thirty minutes at least three times a week. Get your heart rate to about 60 to 70 percent of your maximum heart rate. Maximum heart rate = 220 minus your age. Measure your pulse at your wrist or neck. If you have a cardiac problem, check with your physician before starting on any exercise program. If you are just starting a program, work your way up slowly and enjoyably.

3) Choose the appropriate vitamin/mineral regimen (review the various formulas). Add to this regimen chromium in the form of chromium picolinate at 200 mcg daily if you are not already taking that much. Keep chromium at a total of 200 mcg daily.

4) Eat one cup of oat bran cereal or three to four oat bran muffins daily. Alternatives include a three to four-ounce serving of beans, or a tablespoon of pectin or one tablespoon of psyllium husks in water or orange juice two to three times daily with meals.

5) Nicotinic acid. *Requires physician supervision.* Try long-acting nicotinic acid. Start with 250 mg three times a day with meals for one

week. Then increase to 500 mg three times daily with meals. Have your cholesterol level checked after being on this dose for four weeks. Increase to 1,000 mg three times daily, if required. See above Note for side effects and other cautionary notes.

6) Pantethine. Usually comes in 300-mg capsules. You can try one three times a day with meals for four to five weeks. Have your cholesterol level checked. If there is no noticeable difference you can discontinue it.

7) Fish oils. This is for those who have high cholesterol and high triglyceride levels. Recommended dose is 2,000–3,000 mg daily of eicosapentaenoic acid, or EPA. Check the label of your product to determine the amount of EPA in each capsule. There is much variation in EPA-containing products. The milligram amount of the capsule typically refers to EPA *plus* other substances. That is why you have to check specifically on the amount of EPA in the capsule. Take for four to five weeks. Then have your physician check your cholesterol, triglyceride, LDL cholesterol and HDL cholesterol levels to determine if the supplement is beneficial.

8) Activated charcoal. If you want to try this one, the recommended dose is 8 grams three times daily with meals. That's about one ounce a day. Blend in orange juice. Do not take at the same time as you take any medications, because the medications can bind to the activated charcoal and never get into the body. Best to take about an hour before eating. If taking medications, use charcoal only under the careful supervision of your physician. Have your cholesterol checked after taking this for about four or five weeks to see if it's having any beneficial effect. Not many people remain on this substance for any great length of time.

Formula for Cardiovascular Protection

Note: Elevated cholesterol is not the only factor involved in cardiovascular disease. The factors include platelet adhesiveness, spasm of the muscle of the wall of the artery, free oxygen radical damage to tissue, immunologic alterations and possibly a chronic viral infection of the diseased vessel.

Just as we can lower cholesterol (see Formula for Cholesterol Control), so can we do things to counteract some of these other factors. There are a number of ways, for example, to decrease platelet adhesiveness or stickiness, a factor in blood clots. The same type of diet that is good for cholesterol control is also good to keep platelets fluid. High-fat diets, especially of the saturated variety, decrease platelet fluidity and increase adhesiveness. Just the opposite is true with low-fat diets. Certain foods, in particular, increase platelet fluidity, such as fish, garlic, onions and hot chili peppers. Fish contain omega-3 fatty acids; hot chili peppers contain capsaicin; and garlic and onions contain other platelet fluidizing substances. Certain vitamins and minerals also decrease platelet adhesiveness, especially vitamin E and selenium. There is evidence that supplementary pantethine, at doses of 600 to 1,200 mg daily, decreases platelet stickiness. And let's not forget aspirin. One 325-mg aspirin every other day, or half of one every day, can significantly decrease the adhesiveness of platelets.

Magnesium appears to be very important in the regulation of muscular contraction of blood vessels. Spasms in the muscles of an artery that feeds the heart can result in angina (heart pain) or in heart attack, and when the muscle of an artery that feeds the brain goes into spasm the result can be a stroke. Spasms of these arteries are more likely to occur when the vessels are already partially obstructed by cholesterol and other fatty deposits. Drugs called calcium channel blockers are widely used in cardiology to help prevent these spasms. Magnesium, manganese and possibly calcium are natural calcium channel blockers. There is increasing evidence that supplementary magnesium is beneficial in the treatment of coronary artery disease.

The disruption of blood flow that occurs in atherosclerotic arteries leads to increased production of toxic free oxygen radicals, and, in turn, these cause tissue damage in the heart and brain. Most of the antioxidant defense systems have their origins in dietary vitamins and minerals, including beta-carotene, vitamins C and E, selenium, zinc, copper and manganese. It is essential that intake of these micronutrients is adequate in a cardioprotective formula.

The Formula

1) Review and follow the Formula for Cholesterol Control, which includes specifics on diet, exercise and use of supplements.

2) Include garlic, onions and hot chili peppers in your diet. As with exercise, if you have never used these food items, you need to add them gradually to your diet. This is particularly true of hot chili peppers. Start with a little at a time.

3) Magnesium. The recommended intake of magnesium for those at risk for coronary artery disease or stroke, or those who have already suffered these ills, is 400 mg daily.

4) Aspirin. It is prudent for those at risk for coronary artery disease or stroke to take a 325-mg aspirin tablet once every other day or half of one tablet every day. Those who have a history of high blood pressure or history of peptic ulcer disease should not do this except with their physician's consent and supervision. It is advisable for those who have coronary artery disease, atherosclerotic cerebral vascular disease, atherosclerotic peripheral vascular disease, and those who have suffered heart attacks or strokes (except of the hemorrhagic kind), to take a 325-mg aspirin once every other day or half of one every day with their physician's consent. This is also advised for those who have had bypass surgery.

5) See sections on pantethine and the omega-3 fish oils, which are other substances that can decrease platelet adhesiveness.

Formula for Cancer Protection

Note: There is steadily increasing evidence coming from epidemiologic studies, laboratory investigations and clinical intervention trials that diet has a very important effect on cancer. On the one hand, there are foods associated with *increased* incidence of certain types of cancer, while on the other hand, there are foods that appear to *protect* against a cancer. Foods that *increase* cancer risk are foods high in fat, particularly of the saturated variety, foods that are salted, pickled, or smoked and foods containing nitrites or which are nitrite-cured. Obesity itself may increase the risk of cancer in some. Foods that may *decrease* the risk of cancer include the cruciferous vegetables, cabbage, brussels sprouts, kohlrabi (cabbage turnip), broccoli and cauliflower, as well as foods rich in vitamin A and C such as fresh fruits, dark green leafy vegetables, sweet potatoes, carrots, pumpkin and winter squash and foods rich in dietary fiber such as whole-grain cereals, vegetables, beans and fruits. Other foods such as the shiitake mushroom and seaweeds appear to have immune-enhancing, as well as anti-cancer, properties.

Several naturally occurring substances have been isolated from the foods that appear to confer protection against cancers. Aromatic isothiocyanates and indoles, for example, are found in the cruciferous vegetables; selenium in grains from selenium-rich soil, nuts (especially Brazil nuts), shellfish and edible mushrooms; vitamin C (ascorbic acid) in citrus fruits and some vegetables; beta-carotene in green leafy vegetables, green and yellow vegetables and fruits; vitamin E in vegetable oils, nuts and vegetables; bioflavonoids in most fruits, vegetables and grains; and indoles in citrus fruits and vegetables. Lentinan appears to be the active principle of the shiitake mushroom.

It is of interest that free oxygen radicals appear to play major roles in cancer and that many of the substances found in foods known to be protective against cancer are antioxidants. Most of the body's antioxidants are derived from dietary vitamins and minerals.

The Formula

1) Diet. Decrease intake of fat, particularly of the saturated variety, ideally to 20 percent (and not higher than 30 percent) of total dietary calories. Increase intake of carbohydrates, mainly of the complex type, to about 65 percent of dietary calories. Keep intake of red meats to a minimum. The closer you can get to a vegetarian-type diet, the better. Increase the amount of fiber-rich foods, such as whole-grain cereals (bran, oatmeal, and wheat, except for those allergic to wheat), fruits, vegetables and beans. Eat more cruciferous vegetables such as cabbage, broccoli, kohlrabi, brussels sprouts and cauliflower. Increase the amounts of fruits and dark green leafy vegetables in your diet. Try out shiitake mushroom and some of the seaweeds. Avoid the use of foods preserved by salt-pickling, salt-curing, smoking, and nitrite-cured foods. Avoid charred, burned and, when possible, browned foods. Reduce intake of cooked, heated and reheated fats and oils. Restrict intake of coffee to no more than two to four cups a day—maximum. You should limit alcohol consumption to no more than three to five average-potency drinks per week.

2) If you smoke, stop.

3) Use sunscreens if you spend much time outdoors.

4) Vitamin/mineral supplement. Choose the appropriate vitamin/mineral supplement for your age/gender/circumstances. (Review the various formulas.) Particularly important are beta-carotene, vitamin C, vitamin E and selenium. Recommended intakes of these micronutrients for cancer protection are: beta-carotene, 15 mg daily; vitamin C, 500–1,000 mg daily; vitamin E, 200–400 IUs daily; selenium 50–200 mg daily. The upper numbers are particularly recommended for those

with risk factors (family history, environmental exposure) for developing cancer.

Formula for Weight Loss

Note: *Permanent* weight loss is not an easy thing to accomplish. But it *is* possible. Excess weight is accumulated as fat. The amount of fat that a person accumulates is directly proportional to the fat content of his/her diet. As we have seen, the fat content of the standard American diet is much too high. Cutting your fat intake to 20 percent of your caloric intake, increasing your carbohydrate intake to 65 percent (mainly complex carbohydrates), using only low-fat dairy products and increasing your dietary fiber intake to 45–60 grams daily are steps that are *obligatory* if one is to achieve *permanent* weight loss. This diet is not only the best possible diet for permanent weight loss but also helps protect against cardiovascular disease, cancer, high blood pressure and diabetes.

Many people still think that the sugar in sweets is the principal cause of weight gain. The real culprit in most sweets (such as ice cream, cake, cookies and chocolate), however, is *not* the sugar but the fat. A diet high in complex carbohydrates and fiber is the perfect substitute for these sweets and fats, not only because it is very healthy but also because it is quite *filling*. Soluble dietary fiber forms a gel in your stomach, which helps fill it up. Many people have found that a tablespoon of pectin or psyllium fiber in water or orange or tomato juice, taken about fifteen to thirty minutes before each meal, is very helpful in their weight reduction programs. Supplementary L-carnitine, L-arginine, L-lysine and L-ornithine have also been used as weight-reduction aids, though studies are lacking to evaluate their usefulness, if any.

Couple dietary change with exercise and you will be starting a program that will help you maintain good health and optimum weight *for life*. Walking is an excellent exercise choice. Walking just one mile will burn up about 100 calories. So if you walk thirty minutes daily at a fairly brisk pace you will easily burn up about 1,000 calories in a week. If you walk an hour at the same pace you can burn 2,000 calories. Burning about 3,500 calories is equivalent to the loss of one pound. You will definitely lose weight if you change your dietary habits, as outlined above, and if you exercise regularly. The weight *won't* come off as quickly as it typically does when you go on a very low calorie diet, but once it comes off it is much more likely to *stay* off—for good.

The Formula

1) Diet. Decrease intake of fat, particularly saturated fat, to no more than 20 percent of your total caloric intake. Increase carbohydrate intake (mainly of the complex kind) to about 65 percent of total caloric intake. Keep intake of red meats to a minimum. Stick to low-fat dairy products. Avoid sweets as much as possible. If you absolutely require some sweets, there are ice creams now available that are low-fat and low-calorie. There are also low fat and non-fat yogurts. Increase your fiber intake to 45 to 60 grams daily. Women should generally restrict total caloric intake from 1,000 to 1,200 calories daily and men from 1,200 to 1,400 calories daily while trying to lose weight. Weight loss is about one-half to one pound weekly on this type of diet and more if you exercise regularly. Do *not* further restrict calories as this will prove counterproductive in the long run.

2) Exercise. Try to do exercises that will burn 2,000 calories weekly. Walking briskly for thirty minutes daily expends 1,000 calories per week; sixty minutes of walking daily burns 2,000 calories. You also use calories in your normal activities of daily living, such as walking up and down stairs, gardening, house cleaning, fixing things at home, etc.

3) Vitamin/mineral supplement. Choose the appropriate vitamin/mineral supplement based on your age/gender and other considerations discussed in this section. (Review the various formulas.) Add iron (if it is not already in the basic formula you choose) for a total of 10 to 15 mg daily (see Basic Formula for Men for recommended forms). Also add 50 to 100 mcg of vitamin K if it is not already in your formula.

3) Supplementary fiber. A tablespoon of psyllium fiber blended in water or orange or tomato juice, taken fifteen to thirty minutes before meals, can be very beneficial in a weight-reduction program.

4) Other. Those interested in substances for which claims have been made with respect to weight reduction should review the sections of L-carnitine, L-arginine, L-ornithine and L-lysine.

Formula for Athletes

Note: Energy is defined as the ability to do work. Runners, other athletes and all persons performing exercise necessarily are doing more physical work than those who live more sedentary lives. The energy that is required for these activities is derived from the burning of the foodstuffs (carbohydrates, fats and proteins) to produce the carrier of biologic energy, the molecule known as adenosine triphosphate, or ATP. ATP is mainly produced by the process known as oxidative phosphorylation. This process produces a certain amount of free-radical activity which increases the more the process is used. Those who engage in regular exercise produce more of these harmful free radicals and thus need more antioxidant protection.

A recent study indicates that supplementary vitamin E (400 IU daily) improves physical endurance at high altitudes. Another study suggests that soldiers taking L-tyrosine supplements at 6 grams daily do better physically and mentally at high altitudes than those who do not. No adverse effects were noted. Both vitamin E and L-tyrosine appear to produce effects which could have enormous significance for endurance athletes, mountain climbers, skiers and other athletes performing at high altitudes. Women athletes have been found to require higher amounts of vitamin B_2 (riboflavin). Endurance athletes have to be especially careful to maintain adequate magnesium intake. Suboptimal magnesium intake can significantly impair performance. Long-distance runners have been known to become iron deficient because of several factors, including the continuous pounding of their feet. Athletes exercising in areas that are polluted (such as Los Angeles) have been reported to have increased incidences of colds, flus and respiratory problems. This is most likely due to increased toxic free radical oxygen production caused by such pollutants as ozone.

Athletes require fluid replacement and the best form of fluid replacement is plain, unadulterated water. Endurance athletes also require carbohydrate replenishment. This is best supplied as glucose polymers, also known as maltodextrin.

The Formula

1) Vitamin/mineral supplement. Choose the appropriate basic vitamin/mineral supplement for your age/gender/condition (review the various formulas). All supply antioxidant protection. Vitamin E recommendation for *all* endurance athletes and for mountain climbers, skiers and anyone performing at high altitudes is 400 IU daily. Long-distance runners should add 10–15 mg of iron daily to their supplement program if it is not already included. Adequate riboflavin

is present in the basic formulas (enough to cover any additional need of a female athlete). The basic formulas also include adequate magnesium for all athletes.

2) L-tyrosine. Many athletes, especially those subjected to hypoxic conditions, such as those at high altitude, may profit from supplementary L-tyrosine. Start with 500 milligrams three times daily about thirty minutes to one hour before meals or on an empty stomach. The dose can be increased to 2 grams three times a day on an empty stomach. Those with high blood pressure should not take L-tyrosine except with their physician's consent and supervision. Those taking anti-depressants of the MAO inhibitor type should not use L-tyrosine. Before taking this amount of tyrosine, discuss it with your doctor and have him/her review the relevant material in this book.

3) Fluid replacement. Water is the best fluid replacement. Period. For endurance athletes, the addition of glucose polymer (maltodextrin) to the water is a good source of carbohydrate (and thus of energy).

4) Other. Those interested in substances for which claims have been made with respect to increased stamina, muscle building, etc., should review the sections on such substances (see Index) as L-arginine, bee pollen, boron, branched chain amino acids, L-carnitine, coenzyme Q_{10}, cytochrome C, flower pollen, ginseng, glandulars, inosine, L-lysine, Mexican sarsaparilla, octacosanol, L-ornithine, pangamic acid, pantothenic acid, phosphorus and succinate.

Formula for Smokers, Non-smokers Exposed to Cigarette Smoke and Those Exposed to High Levels of Environmental Pollutants

Notes: Many of the toxic elements in cigarette smoke are oxidants, generators of toxic oxygen forms that can cause molecular, cellular and tissue damage. Cigarette smoke contains high amounts of nitrogen oxides, which are themselves free radicals. Nitrogen oxides can react with polyunsaturated fatty acids found in cellular membranes, causing rancidification, rigidification and death of cells. Vitamin E, in particular, protects against these reactions.

The cancer-causing potential of cigarette smoking is well established. Lung cancer associated with smoking accounts for more cancer deaths than any other form of malignancy. Again it is free-radical activity that is believed to be the basic carcinogenic factor in smoking. Smoking also causes emphysema and increases the risk of heart attacks, strokes and clots in the legs. And it makes peptic ulcers slower to heal.

Non-smokers can also be affected by the noxious agents in cigarette smoke. One study found that the non-smoking wives of husbands who smoked died of cancer at *twice* the rate of wives whose husbands didn't smoke. An enormous number of people are sensitive to cigarette smoke and have problems breathing in its presence.

We are being exposed not only to cigarette smoke but also to a greater number of air pollutants coming from automobile and factory exhausts. Air pollutants include nitrogen oxides, ozone and sulfur oxides. When inhaled, these substances generate toxic forms of oxygen that damage our bodies. Radon gas is another problem, one that causes at least 10,000 deaths from lung cancer every year. Radon is a gas which is a decay product of uranium. Those living in air-tight homes located over natural uranium deposits are at risk for radon poisoning. Radon damage to the lungs also occurs by a free oxygen radical mechanism.

Antioxidants, clearly, are the first line of defense for those exposed to air pollutants. Some protection is afforded by substances such as beta-carotene, vitamin C, vitamin E, zinc, selenium, copper, folic acid and vitamin B_{12}. A 1988 report in the medical literature indicated that precancerous lesions in the airways of smokers were *reversed* after the smoker received megadoses of folic acid and vitamin B_{12} daily for several months. The dose of folic acid used in the study was 10 mg and that of vitamin B_{12}, 500 mcg.

The Formula

1) Stop smoking. This is easier said than done, but try to.

2) Vitamin/mineral supplement. Choose the appropriate basic vitamin/mineral supplement for your age/gender/condition (review the various formulas). In addition, beta-carotene is recommended at 15 mg or 25,000 IUs, vitamin E at 400 IUs, selenium at 200 mcg, vitamin C at 500–1,000 mg, folic acid at 800 mcg, vitamin B_{12} at 500 mcg, zinc at 15–30 mg and copper at 1.5–3 mg.

3) Megadose folic acid and vitamin B_{12}. Folic acid at 10 mg daily and vitamin B_{12} at 500 mcg daily have been shown to reverse precancerous bronchiole (airway) lesions in smokers. *This regimen should only be used with your physician's consent and supervision.*

Formula for Those with Inhalant (Respiratory) and Food Allergies/ Sensitivities

Note: The field of allergy has been dominated by folklore, fantasy, fable, contradiction and some science. Fortunately, science is finally taking the lead. Allergies have to do with heightened reactions of the immune system to things that enter the body from the environment, such as dust and pollens. Sometimes the body is "allergic" even to itself. Allergic reactions produce inflammatory processes, such as itchy, runny eyes (conjunctivitis), itchy, congested, runny nose (rhinitis) or wheezing, cough and chest tightness (asthma). Inhalant allergies to such things as pollens, dust, molds, dander and mites can be tested for, and there are treatments for these allergies. These treatments include antihistamines, bronchodilators, atropine-like substances, cromolyn sodium, cortisone-type steroids and "shots" or immunotherapy.

While the field of respiratory allergies has become more rational in terms of both diagnosis and treatment, the field of food allergies has not fared as well, mainly because we do not have reliable tests for food allergies. In fact, it is unclear whether what is called food allergy really *is* an allergy. Allergies require mediation by the immune system, sensitivities do not. Currently available allergy tests are *not* appropriate, in most cases, for testing food sensitivities.

Probably the best way to discover what foods one is sensitive to is to use an elimination diet. Wheat and dairy products are the foods that usually cause the most problems. Exclude all wheat and dairy products from your diet for a few days and see how you do. If you become symptom free, then restore one by one those wheat and dairy products you excluded to determine *which* are the culprits. If you still have symptoms after eliminating wheat and dairy products, then you need to begin eliminating other suspect foods, such as shellfish, corn and eggs, to determine the source of your problems. Some really *are* allergic to certain foods, such as strawberries or shellfish. But these people usually react in a violent manner to these foods (with symptoms such as rash, swelling and difficulty in breathing).

Some nutrients have been found to be beneficial in the prevention and treatment of allergies and sensitivities. Vitamin C, at a dose of 1 gram daily, may help prevent some symptoms of allergic asthma. Vitamin B_6, in doses of 50 to 100 mg daily, can also help prevent and treat these asthmatic symptoms. Vitamin B_{12}, in doses of 500–1,000 mcg daily, may help with prevention and treatment of respiratory allergies in general.

There have been reports, mostly from Europe, that those with food sensitivities may experience relief by dissolving the contents of one to two capsules of cromolyn sodium in a tablespoon of warm water and taking this about fifteen minutes before meals. Cromolyn sodium is a prescription drug used in the treatment of allergic asthma. The capsules are normally used in a special inhaler, but no adverse effects have been reported from the oral use of this form of cromolyn sodium (except in some who are intolerant of lactose or milk sugar, which is used as a filler in the capsule). Cromolyn sodium, interestingly, is a flavonoid-like derivative of an herb used in Egyptian medicine. Other bioflavonoids have also shown anti-allergic effects.

The Formula

1) Diet. The two most common food sensitivities are to wheat and dairy products. Those who are sensitive to milk should also avoid fresh meat products, canned products and baked goods that contain dry milk solids. Check labels. Hydrolyzed protein can be made of wheat, corn, eggs or milk, so that, if you are sensitive to any of these, you should avoid hydrolyzed protein. Those who are sensitive to wheat should try, instead, oats, barley, buckwheat, millet, rice, rye, sorghum, corn and quinoa. Follow "elimination diet" instructions outlined in Note above.

2) Vitamin/mineral supplement. Choose the appropriate basic vitamin/mineral supplement for your age/gender/condition (review the various formulas). Vitamin B_{12} at 500 mcg daily is recommended for those with general respiratory allergies. Vitamin C is recommended at 500–1,000 mg daily for those with allergic asthmatic conditions. Vitamin B_6 is recommended at 50 mg daily for those with allergic asthma as a preventive measure and at 100 mg daily for those having an attack. Doses greater than 50 mg daily should not be taken for any prolonged periods of times because of the possibility of adverse neurologic symptoms.

3) Cromolyn sodium. *This requires supervision by your physician.* Those with food sensitivities may be helped by dissolving the ingredients of one to two capsules of cromolyn sodium in a tablespoon of warm water and taking this about fifteen minutes before meals. Cromolyn sodium is available as capsules for the Intal inhaler, used in the treatment of allergic asthma. Those sensitive to milk may be bothered by the lactose in the capsule.

4) Other. See sections on bioflavonoids. Review material on Estivin in that section.

Formula for Those with Arthritis, Headaches, Fibrositis and Other Painful Disorders

Note: For years, rheumatologists ridiculed the possibility that diet had anything to do with arthritis. Admittedly, many of the popular beliefs about the relationship between diet and arthritis were quite fanciful. However, there is now evidence that diet can indeed affect the symptoms of arthritis, and we are even beginning to understand why this should be the case.

First of all, let's clarify some points about arthritis. Arthritis means inflammation of joints. The inflammation process usually includes pain, swelling, a hot feeling in the affected area and redness. Substances known as prostaglandins are important contributors to the inflammatory process. These compounds are types of polyunsaturated fatty acids which are derived from dietary polyunsaturated fatty acids. There are so-called inflammatory prostaglandins, that is, those that promote inflammation, and anti-inflammatory prostaglandins, those which dampen the inflammatory response. The types of fatty acids that we eat can modulate the production of the various prostaglandins. Diets rich in fish that contain the omega-3 fatty acids (fish oils), for example, can reduce inflammation. The omega-3 fatty acids themselves, taken in supplementary form, can also be beneficial in the treatment of both osteoarthritis and rheumatoid arthritis.

Other nutrients and nutrient derivatives have also been found to be useful in the treatment of arthritis. There is some recent evidence that gamma-linolenic acid, or GLA, an omega-6 fatty acid found in evening primrose oil and blue-green algae, may be beneficial in the treatment of certain types of arthritis. An older study found that megadoses of the B vitamin pantothenic acid, 2 grams daily, relieved symptoms of rheumatoid arthritis. Some reports suggest that the herb feverfew may also be useful for rheumatoid arthritis. S-adenosylmethionine, or SAM, is a derivative of the amino acid L-methionine. It is presently being used in Europe as a drug for the treatment of arthritis and fibrositis. Results so far are encouraging, and its introduction into the U.S. drug marketplace is expected. Liniments and ointments containing the active principle of hot chili peppers, capsaicin, are often helpful as topical agents for the symptomatic treatment of such soft-tissue disorders as fibrositis. Examples of over-the-counter liniments containing 0.025 percent capsaicin are Heet and Sloan's liniment. Zostrix is a prescription ointment containing this same concentration of capsaicin.

Vitamin B_6, given at 200 mg daily, has been found useful in the treatment of carpal (wrist) and tarsal (ankle) tunnel syndromes. These are conditions in which bending the wrist backward or ankle forward is very painful.

The herb feverfew has been found to be beneficial for the preventive treatment of migraine headaches. Most of the studies have come out of England, where it has been demonstrated that the equivalent of two leaves of the feverfew plant in powder form, which comes to about 100 mg, when administered daily, has a significant effect in the prevention of recurrence of migraine headaches. The active ingredients are sesquiterpene lactones, principally parthenolide, and it appears that about 0.1 mg or 100 mcg of the active constituents are required for the preventive effect. The amount of the active principle varies in different feverfew plants, making herbal preparations frequently unreliable. Better quality control and standardization are badly needed in herbal marketing. Diet is also important in the management of migraine headaches. Chocolates and certain wines, for example, can provoke migraine attacks.

The Formula

1) Diet. A diet like the one proposed in the Formula for Cholesterol Control should be followed. Include in the diet fatty fish (such as tuna and salmon); get at least one serving three times weekly. Migraine sufferers should stay away from chocolates, red wines and any other food which causes exacerbations of their headaches. Keeping a daily food journal is often helpful in determining what those foods are.

2) Vitamin/mineral supplement. Choose the basic appropriate vitamin/mineral supplement (review the various formulas) for your age/gender/condition.

3) Omega-3 fatty acids. Two to three grams of eicosapentaenoic acid, or EPA, have been found to be beneficial for the treatment of arthritis (both osteoarthritis and rheumatoid arthritis). *Consult with your physician regarding this.* Also, check your fish oil supplement to determine how much EPA each capsule contains. Stay away from fish oil products containing vitamin A and D because of potential toxicity from megadoses of these vitamins.

4) Gamma-linolenic acid (GLA). One to two grams of GLA daily may be helpful for the symptoms of rheumatoid arthritis. *Check with your physician about this.*

5) Pantothenic acid. One to two grams daily may be beneficial to those with rheumatoid arthritis. No adverse effects have been reported at these doses, *but check with your physician before starting it.*

6) Vitamin B_6 (pyridoxine). Vitamin B_6 at 200 mg daily may help

with the symptoms of carpal and tarsal tunnel syndromes. *Take this only with your physician's consent and supervision.* Don't take B_6 supplements in amounts greater than 50 mg daily for prolonged periods of time unless advised to do so by your physician (who should then carefully monitor you for any adverse neurologic side effects).

7) Feverfew. One hundred mg daily of feverfew containing 0.1 mg of the active principles, sesquiterpene lactones, may help in preventing recurrences of migraines. It is important to note that commercial preparations of feverfew vary greatly in their active constituents.

8) Capsaicin. Liniments containing 0.025 percent capsaicin, such as Heet and Sloan's liniment, are frequently helpful in relieving symptoms of fibrositis, muscle tenderness and other soft-tissue afflictions when used topically.

9) Other. See sections on S-adenosylmethionine (SAM), DMSO and DL-phenylalanine.

Formula for Hospitalized Patients (Surgical and Medical) and Those Scheduled for Surgery

Note: During the past fifteen years, several studies have shown that a surprisingly high percentage of hospitalized patients suffer from malnutrition (protein-calorie deficiencies, as well as vitamin and mineral deficiencies), and this appears to worsen the longer these patients remain in the hospital. This is obviously very detrimental to the patients' progress; if anyone needs optimal nutrition it is the typical hospitalized individual. Fortunately, awareness of this situation is growing; the patient's nutritional status is being given more and better attention in many hospitals. This is particularly true of *macro*nutrition, that is, protein, carbohydrate, fat content of the diet and total calories in the diet. Only recently has attention been given to *micro*nutrient content of the diet (vitamins and minerals).

It is certainly prudent of those who are hospitalized for surgical or medical reasons, for those scheduled for surgery and for those planning hospitalization for any reason to be taking a good vitamin/mineral supplement for nutritional insurance *before, during, and following hospitalization.* Consult with your physician regarding any vitamin/mineral supplement you may be using. He/she may have specific suggestions. There are a number of vitamins, minerals and other nutritional substances that may help speed healing of injuries, surgical wounds and so on. Zinc, for example, has been found to be useful in patients who tend to heal slowly, especially when given in relatively high doses (about 150 milligrams daily). *These higher doses, however, should be taken only under a physician's supervision.*

The Formula

1) Vitamin/mineral supplement. Choose the appropriate basic vitamin and mineral supplement for your age/gender/condition after reviewing the various formulas in this section. Increase daily intake of zinc to 30 milligrams and copper to 3 milligrams.

2) Other. Review sections on L-arginine, L-ornithine, vitamin A, aloe vera and alginates.

Formula for Those with Chronic Fatigue Syndrome

Chronic fatigue is a very common (and growing) problem. It may be due to iron deficiency, iron deficiency anemia, other types of anemia, an underactive or overactive thyroid, an autoimmune disease such as rheumatoid arthritis or systemic lupus erythematosus, infectious diseases such as Lyme disease or viral syndromes, allergic disorders or malignancy. Chronic fatigue is one thing, chronic fatigue syndrome (CFS) another. CFS is a highly controversial entity in medicine. Some doubt that it's real, and nobody is sure what causes it. It is usually characterized by myriad symptoms including malaise, recurrent sore throats, swelling of lymph nodes in the neck and groin areas, intermittent mild fevers, headaches, memory disturbances, chronic aches and pains all over the body, irritability, sleep problems, and depression, just to name the most common symptoms. It often occurs in young adults (though it can strike at any age), affects women more often than men, usually starts with a flu-like illness and often afflicts those who were previously very physically active. Many of those with CFS do *not* have any detectable abnormal laboratory values. But there is a subset of CFS patients whose symptoms can apparently be explained by recurrence of viral infections, usually cytomegalovirus (CMV) and, less commonly, Epstein-Barr virus (EBV).

Things that are helpful in this syndrome include dietary modification, mild exercise, stress reduction and the use of nutritional supplements. The amino acid L-tyrosine, taken at 1.5 to 6 grams daily, has also been found to be useful. Some CFS sufferers say they are helped by some of the substances used in chronic viral syndromes (see next section). A drug available in Europe called S-adenosylmethionine (SAM), which is a derivate of the amino acid L-methionine, is showing promise in the treatment of some of the symptoms of CFS, especially the aches, pains and depression.

The Formula

1) Diet. I recommend the diet discussed in the Formula for Cholesterol Control section. Add edible seaweeds and shiitake mushrooms. Also, natural licorice could be beneficial (see discussion of licorice).

2) Exercise. Although many with CFS believe that they can't even drag themselves out of bed, mild exercise, such as walking at a leisurely pace twenty to thirty minutes at least three times weekly, is encouraged. Increase the pace slowly. Most of my CFS patients feel better once they start mild exercise. Slow warm-ups and cool-downs are strongly recommended.

3) Stress reduction. Include deep-breathing exercises, meditation and massage.

4) Vitamin/mineral supplement. Check out the various vitamin and mineral regimens and choose the one that seems most appropriate to your life situation. Add to it from the following:

5) L-tyrosine. If you want to use this amino acid, start with 500 milligrams about thirty minutes to an hour before each meal for a total of 1,500 milligrams daily. You can gradually increase the dose to a total of 6,000 milligrams (6 grams) daily divided into three doses. No adverse effects are expected at this dose. Do not use tyrosine if you have high blood pressure except with your physician's consent. Do not use tyrosine if you are taking an MAO inhibitor type of anti-depressant. If the L-tyrosine works, you should feel "brighter," more energetic and less depressed. *Use of tyrosine should be discussed and monitored by your physician.*

5) Other. See next formula. Also, see sections on S-adenosylmethionine and piracetam.

Formula for Chronic Viral Syndromes (HIV Infection, ARC, AIDS, Herpes, CMV, EBV)

Note: By now, virtually everyone has heard of AIDS (acquired immune deficiency syndrome). What many do not know is that AIDS does not *have* to be fatal. There are those with AIDS who have survived in relatively good health for several years now. An ever increasing number are surviving longer and longer. The secret is to pay attention to *details*. These include diet, exercise, stress-reduction, use of supplements, immune enhancers, anti-viral agents and taking steps to *prevent* the diseases associated with AIDS.

A study performed a few years ago indicated that a few AIDS patients who followed a macrobiotic diet fared better than those consuming a more typical American diet. Unfortunately, there have been no follow-up studies to confirm this. Nonetheless, it makes some sense. A macrobiotic diet is, among other things, a low-cholesterol, low-fat, high-complex-carbohydrate and high-dietary-fiber diet. The membrane of the HIV virus that plays a role in AIDS is rich in cholesterol. Decreasing the amount of cholesterol in the viral membrane disrupts it and can even inactivate it. In addition, there is evidence that cells of immunity may become more effective if the cholesterol contents of their membranes are lowered. Thus, a cholesterol-lowering diet may be useful in two vital ways. An *increase* in the amount of *polyunsaturated* fatty acids in immune cell membranes should make them more fluid and should likewise enhance their activity. An increase in these same substances in the HIV membranes should *reduce* viral activity. Macrobiotic diets are rich in polyunsaturated fatty acids.

Several substances, most not yet approved by the FDA or not approved specifically for use in AIDS, are, nonetheless, being tried out by AIDS, ARC and other HIV-infected individuals in an effort to enhance their immune systems and for their possible anti-viral activities. *AL 721* (see discussion elsewhere) appears to have some (but limited) immunostimulatory effects, and there are some reports of clinical improvement among those taking it. *Naltrexone* is also being used; it is a pure opiate antagonist which is used at higher doses to treat opiate addiction and at much lower doses appears to have some immunostimulatory effects. *Isoprinosine* is another, better studied immune stimulant. Other *possible immune stimulants* that are being used by HIV-infected individuals include *disulfiram, shiitake mushrooms, flower pollen, DHEA* (*dehydroepiandrosterone*) and some of the minerals, especially zinc, selenium and germanium. Substances that are being used as *possible anti-viral agents* include *dextran sulfate*, an *aloe vera* drink rich in the polysaccharide *Carrisyn* and the herb *licorice*.

Some individuals with various of the herpes viruses, including recurrent cytomegalovirus (CMV) and Epstein-Barr virus (CBV), are also trying out some unapproved substances in pursuit of relief from their symptoms. (See discussion under Formula for Those with Chronic Fatigue Syndrome.) About 15 to 20 percent of those with chronic fatigue syndrome may, in fact, be suffering from recurrences of CMV or EBV infections. Isoprinosine, a drug that has been approved in many countries but not yet in the U.S., is said by some sufferers of chronic fatigue to hasten recovery. It has been shown to be effective, in a number of studies, against herpes simplex.

Note that in the formula below, several of the substances listed are either not FDA approved (or are not approved for use in this context) or are not presently available in the United States. The names and dosages of some of the more promising substances are provided in order to indicate what is being used by HIV-infected individuals and by some others with chronic viral syndromes. *Anyone wishing to use these substances should do so only under a knowledgeable physician's supervision and with informed consent.*

The Formula

1) Diet. I recommend the diet outlined in the Formula for Cholesterol Control. Add edible seaweeds and shiitake mushrooms.

2) Exercise. Develop a mild aerobic exercise program, such as walking thirty to sixty minutes at least three times a week.

3) Stress-reduction. Include deep (diaphragmatic) breathing exercises, meditation, message, visualization and other relaxation techniques.

4) Vitamin/mineral supplement. Review the various vitamin and mineral regimens in this section and select the one that appears most appropriate to your circumstances. Take zinc at 30 mg daily, copper at 3 mg daily and selenium at 200 micrograms daily.

5) Isoprinosine. Those who use this substance for chronic viral syndromes due to CMV, EBV and some other herpes infections typically take 2 to 3 grams daily in divided doses. It is not available in the United States but is in Mexico and many countries of Europe. It can cause elevation of uric acid levels and may aggravate gout in those predisposed to these problems.

6) Other substances being used by HIV-infected individuals: AL 721 at 10 to 20 grams daily; naltrexone at 1.75 mg six days a week; disulfiram (Antabuse), 750 mg one day each week (cannot drink alcohol

at the same time); dextran sulfate, 1,200–2,400 mg daily; aloe vera drink rich in Carrisyn, yielding 1,000 mg of Carrisyn daily. Review sections in the book on all of the above substances.

7) Still other substances for which beneficial claims have been made: Review sections on ampligen, BHT, carrageenan, DHEA, flower pollen, germanium, ginseng, chlorella, imuthiol, lentinan, licorice, monolaurin, ozone, Saint John's wort, thymosin, transfer factor, Wobe Mugos enzymes. Refer to index in order to find the appropriate sections.

Formula for Colds

Good news. Contrary to popular belief, there *are* things we can do to treat colds, decrease their duration and cut down on the number of them. Antihistamines and decongestants can treat some of the symptoms. Vitamin C, at one to two grams daily during the course of a cold, can, in many cases, reduce the number of days a cold lasts. Taking an aspirin or two right at the *very beginning* of cold symptoms may help abort the cold; aspirin has immune-boosting activity and inhibits bradykinin, a substance that helps sustain colds. You might also try 50 mg of zinc picolinate or zinc gluconate lozenges at the first hint of a cold and then take 25 mg of zinc every two hours until the symptoms abate. Take the zinc only during your normal waking hours—not after you go to bed—and discontinue after five days if you haven't been helped; discontinue sooner if symptoms go away.

FIFTEEN

Consumer Concerns:

Questions and

Answers

Q—What are the most important things to look for on a product label?

A—First you'll want to look to see what's in the product. Note quantities and the balance of nutrients. Compare these with the regimens I recommend. You'll also want to pay attention to the source of each nutrient, which is usually shown in parentheses right after the name of the nutrient. Again, compare with the information provided earlier. Pay attention to what *isn't* in the product, too. Are there some things that should be there that are entirely missing? Check out the list of additives. Use common sense here; if you can find a similar product with far fewer additives, buy that one. And when it comes to comparing cost, don't just look at price. You must look at price in terms of number of tablets or capsules in the container *and* in terms of the amount of nutrient in each tablet or capsule. Bottles of the same product put out by different manufacturers may be about the same size and still contain significantly different amounts of nutrients. If there are very large differences in price, check the labels again. One may be much more expensive because it is chelated or in timed-release form. (See information on these below.) Check seals to make sure that the product is tightly capped for freshness. Do not be swayed by "brand name." Just because you've seen a product heavily advertised does not mean that it is any better than a less advertised product. Look for an expiration date and don't buy beyond that date. The lack of an expiration date, however, should not be any cause for rejecting the product. Most products sell well before their potency is compromised by having been on the shelf too long.

Q—How can I be sure the vitamins, minerals and other supplements I buy are fresh and have full potency?

A—Unfortunately, you cannot be absolutely certain of this. If you look carefully at the labels on some products you will find an "expiration date" beyond which you should not buy the product. There are a few companies that stress the "freshness" and "potency" of their products and "guarantee" same through certain dates. Whether these guarantees really have any practical value is doubtful. Most products will, in fact, sell well before their potency is seriously compromised. The products that boast of full potency and freshness in expensive full-color ads tend, not surprisingly, to be higher priced than a lot of other products, and there is no evidence they really are any fresher. Look for expiration dates on labels but don't be alarmed if you don't find any. (Inclusion of expiration dates is not required.) Instead, look for a good outer and inner seal on product bottles and be cautious about buying from the bargain bin; products therein may very likely have been on the shelf too long.

Q—Once I've opened a bottle of vitamins or minerals should I store the container in the refrigerator?

A—No, unless product label instructs otherwise, keep supplements in a dry, dark place away from sunlight and heat, but don't put them in the refrigerator, where dampness may damage them. Keep lids tightened when not in use; buy products that are packaged in opaque containers that will not permit easy penetration by sunlight. If you buy a large container, you might consider putting a supply good for a couple of weeks or a month in a smaller opaque container so that you are not constantly exposing your main supply to fresh air each time you open the bottle or jar. Some supplements, for example, oil-based ones, will age more quickly than others. It's best to buy these supplements in smaller quantities so that you use them up before they rancidify. And if you buy large quantities of vitamin C, yeasts or other supplements in powder, granular, or loose form, be sure to follow the instructions above regarding use of large quantities of supplements.

Q—Are "natural" vitamins really better than "synthetic" ones? And if the label doesn't say "natural" should I assume the product is synthetic?

A—This is one of the most confusing issues facing the consumer. And many supplement manufacturers have done everything they can to take advantage of that confusion. Consumers all over the world are being persuaded to pay far more than natural food-supplement products than for synthetic ones. The advertising claims imply that only the natural products provide full potency and that the synthetic products are somehow "bad" or deficient. Many of the natural vitamin C products, for example, actually contain only a small amount of ascorbic acid derived from natural sources. A "rose hip" vitamin C is generally 90 percent or more synthetic. Moreover, the so-called natural products go through most of the same "unnatural" processing procedures that the synthetic ones do. *The fact is, in any event, that natural and synthetic versions of the same substance are necessarily chemically identical.* There is absolutely no reason, therefore, to expect that the action of the two versions will be different in any respect. The situation is most confusing with respect to vitamin E. Vitamin E is a mixture of several substances, the most active of which is d-alpha-tocopherol. Natural and synthetic d-alpha-tocopherol have identical vitamin E activity. Synthetic mixtures, such as d-alpha-tocopherol, however, may differ in activity when compared to natural mixtures of vitamin E.

Q—Are products that claim to be free of artificial preservatives, dyes, etc., better than others?

A—It depends upon what others you are comparing them to; if everything else is equal I would certainly prefer a product that was not loaded down with preservatives and artificial colors. Examine labels carefully and avoid those products that seem to have a long list of additives, such as coloring agents, preservatives, binders, fillers. There is some speculation that additives may cause serious health problems in people who take megadose quantities of supplements containing these extraneous substances. They may not cause problems in small amounts, but when you ingest enough of them, a variety of adverse reactions, including a number of allergies, may arise.

Q—Is it really necessary to worry about quality control in supplements? Doesn't the FDA monitor all that for us?

A—The Food and Drug Administration requires that supplement manufacturers list all of the active ingredients that go into their products. Manufacturers who fail to do this or who do not deliver what they say they are delivering on their labels can get into legal difficulty if detected. In fact, however, monitoring is sporadic and compliance uneven. But it is my impression, based on some chemical analyses, that most manufacturers deliver what they say they do, in terms of nutrient content.

Q—I've heard that mineral supplements do no good unless they are chelated. Is this true and what does it mean?

A—A number of supplement products are advertised as "chelated." These products usually cost more than non-chelated products. Chelation is a process that is supposed to make minerals more readily absorbable by altering their electrical charge, and in some cases this is true. The bioavailability of most non-chelated minerals, however, is sufficient when taken in the sort of combinations/regimens recommended earlier in this book.

Q—What is the best form in which to take supplements—pills, capsules, powders, liquids?

A—This may depend upon the individual supplement and the individual consumer. There are some people, for example, who cannot swallow pills without choking or panicking. Obviously those people need another way of taking supplements. Pills and tablets are best for most people. Nutrients can be tightly bound together in this form and protected against oxidation and rancidification. Fat-soluble vitamins such as vitamins A, E and D, on the other hand, are often conveniently packaged in gelatin capsules, and these are fine, too. The capsules, in fact, often obviate the need for additional preservatives because they provide such a good seal by themselves. Powders, crystals and granules are often the forms in which vitamin C is sold in larger quantities. Generally these forms will have no additives at all, which is certainly an advantage. Cost is usually lower, too. Some manufacturers are now producing "insurance" formulas made up of all the needed vitamins and minerals in powder form that can be mixed with juices and the like. And drops are also available for those who can't tolerate pills or capsules.

Q—Are "timed-release" capsules or tablets worth spending extra money on?

A—No. The idea of getting continuous antioxidant protection is an important one, but you can generally achieve satisfactory results by taking your supplements in divided doses, ideally three times a day, once with each meal. Time-released forms of iron are not reliably absorbed.

Q—There seem to be all kinds of different forms of various vitamins; how do I know which is best?

A—I have provided the form I believe is best for each vitamin and mineral. Special confusion prevails with respect to vitamin C. Labels may indicate that vitamin C is "derived from" everything from palm to corn to rose hips. What you want to be aware of is *how much* of the vitamin you are getting. This is more important than where it is coming from, unless you are allergic to one of the sources. Vitamin E is another nutrient that comes in many different forms. Stick to those products that get vitamin E from d-alpha-tocopherol. "Mixed tocopherols," another source of vitamin E, include forms for which there is no evidence of nutritional benefit.

Q—Are hair-analysis tests a good way of determining which supplements a person needs?

A—Claims are made that analysis of hair will yield information on mineral stores in the body. Unfortunately, hair analysis is a highly unreliable means of determining any mineral deficiency. Apart from the fact that mineral content of hair does not necessarily reflect mineral content in bodily tissue, there are all sorts of variables that can bias the results of these tests. In general, unless there is reason to suspect a particular vitamin/mineral deficiency, you can best determine your micronutrient needs by reading the analyses of the various nutrients discussed in this book.

Q—Are there other tests to determine nutritional deficiencies?

A—Yes. There are some good tests to determine vitamin deficiencies, fewer for mineral deficiencies. These are blood tests. There are also blood and urine tests to determine amino acid deficiencies. Consult your physician for further information.

Q—Should people with candidiasis avoid supplements containing yeast?

A—Candidiasis is a yeast infection, but the yeast involved is entirely different from nutritional yeasts. There is no evidence that these nutritional yeasts in any way aggravate this infection. There are, however, yeast-free nutritional supplements for those who are sensitive or allergic to yeasts.

Q—Is it better to take nutrients individually or in combinations?

A—As a general rule it is not practical or desirable to take your nutrients individually, except for therapeutic indications. Generally it is best to take a one-a-day or insurance formula and, then, to "amplify" this with additional or other nutrients, as needed. Proper balance is needed in most cases in order for nutrients to work optimally.

Q—What is the difference between one-a-day and insurance formulas?

A—A one-a-day is, as the name suggests, a vitamin-mineral supplement you take once a day. It typically contains the U.S. RDAs for the vitamins and variable amounts of minerals. In one-a-days, mineral doses are often much below the U.S. RDAs, especially for magnesium and calcium. In many cases, essential minerals, such as selenium, chromium, boron and molybdenum, are not even included in one-a-days. It is virtually impossible to pack the U.S. RDAs of all the essential vitamins and minerals into a single pill of a size that can comfortably be swallowed.

The answer to this problem is the so-called insurance formula which *does* contain all the essential vitamins and minerals in U.S. RDA or greater amounts. With an insurance formula, you typically take three to six tablets daily, usually with meals.

Q—Are "stress formulas" really helpful?

A—Unfortunately, most of those preparations labeled "stress formulas" really do little to help us cope with stress. On the other hand, there are nutrients which appear promising in this context but, alas, are seldom, if ever, included in these formulas. These include such substances as tyrosine, magnesium and vitamin E.

SIXTEEN

Drug/Vitamin/Mineral

Interactions

There are some combinations of drugs/vitamins/minerals that can be potentially dangerous or that can negate the effect of either the drugs or the nutrients. For further information, see individual nutrient analyses.

Alcohol—Diminishes the stores or interferes with the body's absorption of thiamin, riboflavin, niacinamide, pyridoxine, folic acid, calcium, iron, zinc, magnesium, selenium, vitamins B_{12}, C, A and D.

Antacids—Over-the-counter aluminum-containing antacids may, if used regularly, interfere with the calcium status in bone.

Anti-Convulsants—Phenytoin (Dilantin), phenobarbitol and primodone (mysoline) may interfere with folic acid (folacin) and vitamins D and K.

Aspirin (and Other Non-steroidal Anti-inflammatory Agents)
—May interfere with the absorption and activity of vitamin C, folic acid and iron.

Cholesterol-Lowering Drugs—Questran may interfere with the status of vitamins A, B_{12}, D, E, K and with folic acid and calcium. Clofibrate (Atromid-S) may interfere with vitamin B_{12} and iron status and colestipol (colestid) with vitamins A, D, E, K, and with folic acid and calcium.

Diuretics (Such as Hydrochlorothiazide and Furosemide)—May interfere with potassium, magnesium and zinc and result in deficiencies in all.

Fiber—Fiber products such as Metamucil are used as bulk laxatives to lower cholesterol, to improve blood sugar control in diabetics and for weight reduction. Long-term use of these products can negatively affect zinc, iron, manganese, copper, beta-carotene and vitamin B_2 (riboflavin).

Laxatives—Long-term use of the stool-softeners Colace and Surfac can adversely affect vitamins A and D. Long-term use of mineral oil can lead to deficiencies in vitamins A, D, E and K. Also see Fiber above.

Oral Contraceptives—May interfere, in particular, with pyridoxine (vitamin B_6) and folic acid.

Steroids—Chronic use of cortisone-type steroids can cause breakdown of protein in bone and produce osteoporosis-like disorders. Supplemental calcium is desirable.

Sunscreens—Sunscreens of SPF (sun protective factor) 8 or above also block formation of vitamin D in the skin. As more of us use sunscreens (a good idea), increase in dietary and supplementary vitamin D becomes more important.

Bibliography

CONTENTS

ABBREVIATIONS

Acta Dermatovener. (Acta Dermato-Venereologica)

Acta Neuro. Scand. (Acta Neurologica Scandinavica)

Acta Pathol. Microbiol. Scand. B. (Acta Pathologica et Microbiologica Scandinavica Section B)

Am. Heart J. (American Heart Journal)

Am. J. Cardiol. (American Journal of Cardiology)

Am. J. Clin. Nutr. (American Journal of Clinical Nutrition)

Am. J. Epidemiol. (American Journal of Epidemiology)

Am. J. Med. (American Journal of Medicine)

Am. J. Psychiatry (American Journal of Psychiatry)

Am. J. Surg. (American Journal of Surgery)

Am. J. Vet. Res. (American Journal of Veterinary Research)

Ann. Clin. Res. (Annals of Clinical Research)

Ann. Intern. Med. (Annals of Internal Medicine)

Ann. N.Y. Acad. Sci. (Annals of the New York Academy of Sciences)

Ann. Rev. Nutr. (Annual Review of Nutrition)

Ann. Surg. (Annals of Surgery)

Anticancer Res. (Anticancer Research)

Arch. Orthop. Trauma Surg. (Archives of Orthopedic and Traumatic Surgery)

Bioinorg. Chem. (Bioinorganic Chemistry)

Biol. Trace Elem. Res. (Biological Trace Element Research)

Br. J. Ca. (British Journal of Cancer)

Br. J. Derm. (British Journal of Dermatology)

Br. Med. J. (British Medical Journal)

Ca. Res. (Cancer Research)

Can. Med. Assoc. J. (Canadian Medical Association Journal)

Clin. Physiol. (Clinical Physiology)

Compr. Ther. (Comprehensive Therapeutics)

Conn. St. Med. J. (Connecticut State Medical Journal)

Curr. Ther. Res. (Current Therapeutic Research)

Fed. Proc. (Federation Proceedings)

Infect. Immun. (*Infection and Immunity*)

Int. J. Vit. Nutr. Res. (*International Journal for Vitamin and Nutrition Research*)

J. Am. Acad. Derm. (*Journal of the American Academy of Dermatology*)

J. Am. Coll. Nutr. (*Journal of the American College of Nutrition*)

J. Am. Med. Assoc. (*Journal of the American Medical Association*)

J. Am. Pod. Assoc. (*Journal of the American Podiatry Association*)

J. Chron. Dis. (*Journal of Chronic Diseases*)

J.N.C.I. (*Journal of the National Cancer Institute*)

J. Nutr. (*Journal of Nutrition*)

J. Nutr. Sci. Vitaminol. (*Journal of Nutrition Science and Vitaminology*)

J. Par. Ent. Nutr. (*Journal of Parenteral and Enteral Nutrition*)

J. Reprod. Med. (*Journal of Reproductive Medicine*)

J. Sch. Health (*Journal of the School of Health*)

J. Surg. Oncol. (*Journal of Surgical Oncology*)

J. Urol. (*Journal of Urology*)

J. Vitaminol. (*Journal of Vitaminology*)

Med. J. Aust. (*Medical Journal of Australia*)

M.M.W.R. (*Morbidity and Mortality Weekly Reports*)

N. Eng. J. Med. (*New England Journal of Medicine*)

Neurobiol. Aging (*Neurobiology of Aging*)

Nutr. Cancer (*Nutrition and Cancer*)

Nutr. Rev. (*Nutrition Reviews*)

Proc. Nat. Acad. Sci. (*Proceedings of the National Academy of Science*)

Res. Com. Chem. Path. Pharm. (*Research Communications in Chemical Pathology and Pharmacology*)

Rev. Can. Biol. (*Revue Canadienne de Biologie*)

Scand. J. Rheumatol. (*Scandinavian Journal of Rheumatology*)

Soc. Neurosc. (*Society of Neurosciences*)

Surg. Gynec. Obstet. (*Surgery Gynecology and Obstetrics*)

Toxicol. Path. (*Toxicology and Pathology*)

Trans. Am. Neurol. Assoc. (*Transactions of the American Neurological Association*)

VITAMINS

Vitamin A/Beta-Carotene

Alexander M, Neumark H and Miller RG. Oral beta-carotene can increase the number of OKT4 + cells in human blood. *Immunology Letters.* 9:221–224, 1985.

Bendich A. Carotenoids and the immune response. *J. Nutr.* 119:112–115, 1989.

Bendich A. The safety of beta-carotene. *Nutr. Cancer.* 11:207–214, 1988.

Bendich A and Langseth L. Safety of vitamin A. *Am. J. Clin. Nutr.* 49:358–371, 1989.

Bendich A and Olson JA. Biological action of carotenoids. *FASEB J.* 3:1927–1932, 1989.

Boyd AS. An overview of the retinoids. *Am. J. Med.* 86:568–574, 1989.

Burton GW and Ingold KU. Beta-carotene: An unusual type of lipid antioxidant. *Science.* 224:569–573, 1984.

Ellis CN and Voorhees JJ. Etetinate therapy. *J. Am. Acad. Derm.* 16:267–291, 1987.

Gerber LE and Erdman JW Jr. Effect of dietary retinyl acetate, beta-carotene and retinoic acid on wound healing in rats. *J. Nutr.* 112:1555, 1982.

Goldfarb MT et al. Topical tretinoin therapy: Its use in photoaged skin. *J. Am. Acad. Derm.* 21:645–650, 1989.

Hong WK et al. 13-cis-retinoic acid in the treatment of oral leukoplakia. *N. Eng. J. Med.* 315:1501–1505, 1986.

Krinsky NI. Carotenoids and cancer in animal models. *J. Nutr.* 119:123–126, 1989.

Kune GA et al. Serum levels of beta-carotene, vitamin A and zinc in male lung cancer cases and controls. *Nutr. Cancer.* 12:169–176, 1989.

Levenson SM et al. Supplemental vitamin A prevents the acute radiation-induced defect in wound healing. *Ann. Surg.* 200:494–512, 1984.

Lowe NJ, Lazarus V and Matt L. Systemic retinoid therapy for psoriasis. *J. Am. Acad. Derm.* 19:186–191, 1988.

Mallkovsky M et al. Enhancement of specific immunity in mice fed a diet enriched in vitamin A acetate. *Proc. Nat. Acad. Sci.* 80:6322, 1983.

Matthews-Roth MM. Antitumor activity of beta-carotene, canthaxanthin and phytoene. *Oncology.* 39:33–37, 1982.

Menkes MS et al. Serum beta-carotene, vitamins A and E, selenium and the risk of lung cancer. *N. Eng. J. Med.* 315:1250–1254, 1986.

Micksche M et al. Stimulation of immune response in lung cancer patients by vitamin A therapy. *Oncology.* 34:234–238, 1977.

Moon RC. Comparative aspects of carotenoids and retinoids as chemopreventive agents for cancer. *J. Nutr.* 119:127–134, 1989.

Murakoshi M et al. Inhibitory effects of alpha-carotene on proliferation of the human neuroblastoma cell line GOTO. *J.N.C.I.* 81:1649–1652, 1989.

Oishi K et al. A case study of prostatic cancer with reference to dietary habits. *Prostate.* 12:179–190, 1988.

Palgi A. Vitamin A and lung cancer: A perspective. *Nutr. Cancer.* 6:105–120, 1984.

Patty I et al. Controlled trial of vitamin A therapy in gastric ulcer. *Lancet.* 2:876, 1982.

Peto R et al. Can dietary beta-carotene materially reduce human cancer rates? *Nature.* 290:201–208, 1981.

Salonen JT et al. Risk of cancer in relation to serum concentrations of selenium and vitamins A and E: Matched case-control analysis of prospective data. *Br. Med. J.* 290:417–420, 1985.

Seifter E et al. Impaired wound healing in streptozotocin diabetes: Prevention by supplemental vitamin A. *Ann. Surg.* 194:42, 1981.

Seifter E et al. Moloney murine sarcoma virus tumors in CBA/J mice: Chemopreventive and chemotherapeutic actions of supplemental beta-carotene. *J.N.C.I.* 68:835–840, 1982.

Seifter E et al. Morbidity and mortality reduction by supplemental vitamin A or beta-carotene in mice given total body gamma radiation. *J.N.C.I.* 73:1167–1177, 1984.

Seifter E. et al. Regression of C3HBA mouse tumor due to X-ray therapy combined with supplemental beta-carotene or vitamin A. *J.N.C.I.* 71:409–417, 1983.

Shekelle RB et al. Dietary vitamin A and risk of cancer in the Western Electric study. *Lancet.* 2:1185, 1981.

Sklan D. Vitamin A in human nutrition. *Progress in Food and Nutrition Science.* 11:39–55, 1987.

Som S, Chatterjee M and Banerjee MR. Beta-carotene inhibition of 7,12–dimethylbenz[a]anthracene-induced transformation of murine mammary cells in vitro. *Carcinogenesis.* 5:937–940, 1984.

Sommer A et al. Impact of vitamin A supplementation on childhood mortality. *Lancet.* 1:1169–1173, 1986.

Stich HF, Rosin MP and Vallerjera MO. Reduction with vitamin A and beta-carotene administration of proportion of micronucleated buccal mucosal cells in Asian betel nut and tobacco chewers. *Lancet.* 1:1204, 1984.

Tomita Y et al. Augmentation of tumor immunity against syngeneic tumors in mice by beta-carotene. *J.N.C.I.* 78:679, 1987.

Watson RR and Moriguchi S. Cancer prevention by retinoids: role of immunological modification. *Nutrition Research.* 5:663–675, 1985.

Weiss JS et al. Topical tretinoin improves photoaged skin: A double-blind, vehicle-controlled study. *J. Am. Med. Assoc.* 259:527–532, 1988.

Willett WC et al. Vitamins A, E and carotene: Effects of supplementation on their plasma levels. *Am. J. Clin. Nutr.* 38:559–566, 1983.

Ziegler RG. A review of epidemiologic evidence that carotenoids reduce the risk of cancer. *J. Nutr.* 119:116–122, 1989.

Vitamin B$_1$ (Thiamine)

Anderson SH, Vickery CA and Nicol AD. Adult thiamine requirement and the continuing need to fortify processed cereals. *Lancet.* 2:85–89, 1986.

Anonymous. Beriberi can complicate TPN. *Nutr. Rev.* 45(8):239–243, 1987.

Anonymous, Deaths associated with thiamine-deficient total parenteral nutrition. *M.M.W.R.* 38(3):43–46, 1989.

Blass JP et al. Thiamine and Alzheimer's disease: A pilot study. *Archives of Neurology.* 45:833–835, 1988.

Campbell CH. The severe lacticacidosis of thiamine deficiency: Acute pernicious or fulminating beriberi. *Lancet.* 2:446–449, 1984.

Centerwall BS and Criqui MH. Prevention of the Wernicke-Korsakoff syndrome. *N. Eng. J. Med.* 299:285–289, 1978.

Larrieu AJ et al. Beneficial effects of cocarboxylase in the treatment of experimental myocardial infarctions in dogs. *American Surgeon.* 53:721–725, 1987.

Mandel H et al. Thiamine-dependent beriberi in the "thiamine-responsive anemia syndrome." *N. Eng. J. Med.* 311:836–838, 1984.

Skelton WP and Skelton NK. Thiamine deficiency neuropathy: It's still common today. *Postgraduate Medicine.* 85(8):301–306, 1989.

Vitamin B$_2$ (Riboflavin)

Belko AZ et al. Effects of exercise on riboflavin requirements of young women. *A. J. Clin. Nutr.* 37:509–517, 1983.

Munoz N. et al. Effect of riboflavin, retinol, and zinc on micronuclei of buccal mucosa and of esophagus: A randomized double-blind intervention study in China. *J.N.C.I.* 79:687–691, 1987.

Powers HJ, Wright AJA and Fairweather-Tait JJ. The effect of riboflavin deficiency in rats on the absorption and distribution of iron. *British Journal of Nutrition.* 59:381–387, 1988.

Roe DA, Kelkwarf H and Stevens J. Effect of fiber supplements on the apparent absorption of pharmacologal doses of riboflavin. *Journal of the American Dietetic Association.* 88:211–213, 1988.

Vitamin B$_3$ (Niacin)

Canner PL et al. Fifteen year mortality in coronary drug project patients: Long term benefit with niacin. *Journal of the American College of Cardiology.* 8:1245–1255, 1986.

Carlson LA, Hamsten A and Asplund A. Pronounced lowering of serum levels of lipoprotein Lp(a) in hyperlipidemic subjects treated with nicotinic acid. *Journal of Internal Medicine.* 226:271–276, 1989.

Hawkins D. Orthomolecular psychiatry: Treatment of schizophrenia. In: Hawkins D and Pauling L (eds.). *Orthomolecular Psychiatry.* San Francisco: WH Freeman and Company, pp. 667–668, 1973.

Henderson LM. Niacin. *Ann. Rev. Nutr.* 3:289–307, 1983.

Hoffer A. Treatment of arthritis by nicotinic acid and nicotinamide. *Can. Med. Assoc. J.* 81:235, 1959.

Kaufman W. Niacinamide therapy for joint mobility: Therapeutic reversal of a common clinical manifestation of the "normal" aging process. *Conn. St. Med. J.* 17:584, 1953.

Knopp RH et al. Contrasting effects of unmodified and time release forms of niacin on lipoproteins in hyperlipidemic subjects: Clue to mechanism of action of niacin. *Metabolism.* 34:442, 1985.

Lawson T. Nicotinamide stimulates the repair of carcinogen-induced DNA damage in the hamster pancreas in vivo. *Anticancer Res.* 3:207, 1983.

Luria MH. Effect of low-dose niacin on high density lipoprotein cholesterol and total cholesterol/high density lipoprotein cholesterol ratio. *Archives of Internal Medicine.* 148:2493–2495, 1988.

Vogue P et al. Nicotinamide may extend remission phase in insulin-dependent diabetes. *Lancet.* 1:619, 1987.

Yamada K et al. Preventive and therapeutic effects of large-dose nicotinamide injections on diabetes associated with insulinitis. *Diabetes.* 31:749, 1982.

Yovos JG et al. Effects of nicotinic acid therapy on plasma lipoproteins and very low density lipoprotein apoprotein C subspecies in hyperlipoproteinerria. *Journal of Clinical Endocrinology and Metabolism.* 54:1210–1215, 1982.

Vitamin B$_6$

Abraham GE and Hargrove J. Effect of vitamin B$_6$ on premenstrual symptomatology in women with premenstrual tension syndromes: A double-blind cross-over study. *Infertility.* 3:155–165, 1980.

Adams PW et al. Influence of oral contraceptives, pyridoxine (vitamin B$_6$) and tryptophan on carbohydrate metabolism. *Lancet.* 1:759, 1976.

Amadio PC. Pyridoxine as an adjunct in the treatment of carpal tunnel syndrome. *Journal of Hand Surgery.* 10:237–241, 1985.

Anonymous. Can B$_6$ add to asthma therapy? *Medical World News.* P. 63, August 11, 1986.

Baumblat MJ and Winston F. Pyridoxine and the pill. *Lancet.* 1:832, 1970.

Collipp PJ et al. Pyridoxine treatment of childhood bronchial asthma. *Annals of Allergy.* 35:93–97, 1975.

DiSorbo DM and Litwack G. Vitamin B$_6$ kills hepatoma cells in culture. *Nutr. Cancer.* 3(4):216–222, 1982.

DiSorbo DM and Nathanson L. High dose pyridoxal supplemented culture medium inhibits the growth of a human malignant melanoma cell line. *Nutr. Cancer.* 5(1):10–15, 1983.

DiSorbo DM, Wagner R Jr. and Nathanson L. In vivo and in vitro inhibition of B$_{16}$ melanoma growth by B$_6$. *Nutr. Cancer.* 7:43, 1985.

Duvoisin RC, Yahr MD and Cote LD. Pyridoxine reversal of L-dopa effects in Parkinsonism. *Trans. Am. Neurol. Assoc.* 95:81, 1969.

Ellis JM. Treatment of carpal tunnel syndrome with vitamin B$_6$. *Southern Medical Journal.* 80:882–884, 1987.

Folkers K et al. Biochemical evidence for a deficiency of vitamin B$_6$ in the carpal tunnel syndrome based on a cross-over clinical study. *Proc. Nat. Acad. Sci.* 75:3410, 1978.

Goutieres F and Aicardi J. Atypical presentations of pyridoxine dependent seizures: a treatable cause of intractable epilepsy in infants. *Annals of Neurology.* 17:117–120, 1985.

Gridley DS et al. In vivo and in vitro stimulation of cell mediated immunity by vitamin B$_6$. *Nutrition Research.* 8:201–207, 1988.

Kasdan ML and James CJ. Carpal tunnel syndrome and vitamin B$_6$. *Plastic and Reconstructive Surgery.* 80:882–884, 1987.

Molimard R et al. Impairment of memorization by high doses of pyridoxine in man. *Biomedicine.* 32:88, 1982.

Parry GJ and Bresdesen DE. Sensory neuropathy with low-dose pyridoxine. *Neurology.* 35:1466, 1985.

Reynolds RD and Natta CL. Depressed plasma and erythrocyte pyridoxal phosphate in asthmatics. *Fed. Proc.* 43:470, 1984.

Rimland B, Calloway and Dreyfus P. The effect of high doses of vitamin B$_6$ on autistic children: A double-blind cross-over study. *Am. J. Psychiatry.* 135:472, 1978.

Schaumberg H et al. Sensory neuropathy from pyridoxine abuse. *N. Eng. J. Med.* 309:445–448, 1983.

Talbott MC, Miller LT and Kerkvliet NI. Pyridoxine supplementation: Effect on lymphocyte responses in elderly persons. *Am. J. Clin. Nutr.* 46:659, 1987.

Wason S, Lacouture PG and Lovejoy FH, Jr. Single high-dose pyridoxine treatment for isoniazid overdose. *J. Am. Med. Assoc.* 246:1102–1104, 1981.

Vitamin B₁₂

Anonymous. Vitamin B₁₂ confirmed as effective sulfite allergy blocker. *Allergy Observer.* 4(2):1, March–April 1987.

Beck WS. Cobalamin and the nervous system (editorial). *N. Eng. J. Med.* 318:1752–1754, 1988.

Bruce G. The myth of vegetarian B₁₂. *East West.* Pp. 44–55, May 1988.

Burkes RS et al. Low serum cobalamin levels occur frequently in the acquired immune deficiency syndrome and related disorders. *European Journal of Haematology.* 38:141–147, 1988.

Harriman GR et al. Vitamin B₁₂ malabsorption in patients with acquired immunodeficiency syndrome. *Archives of Internal Medicine.* 149:2039–2041, 1989.

Heimburger et al. Improvement in bronchial squamous metaplasia in smokers treated with folate and vitamin B₁₂. *Am. J. Clin. Nutr.* 45:866, 1987.

Herbert V. B₁₂ deficiency in AIDS (Letter). *J. Am. Med. Assoc.* 260:2837, 1988.

Jacobsen DW, Simon RA and Singh M. Sulfite oxidase deficiency and cobalamin protection in sulfite sensitive asthmatics (SSA) (Abstract). *Journal of Allergy and Clinical Immunology* (Supplement). 73:135, 1984.

Lindenbaum J et al. Neuropsychiatric disorders caused by cobalamin deficiency in the absence of anemia or macrocytosis. *N. Eng. J. Med.* 318:1720–1727, 1988.

Biotin

Bonjour JP. Biotin in human nutrition. *Ann. N.Y. Acad. Sci.* 447:97–104, 1985.

Marshall MW. The importance of biotin—an update. *Nutrition Today.* Pp. 26–30, November–December, 1987.

Shelley WB and Shelley ED. Uncombable hair syndrome: Observations on response to biotin and occurrence in siblings with ectodermal dysplasia. *J. Am. Acad. Derm.* 13:97–102, 1985.

Sydenstricker VP et al. Observations on the "egg white injury" in man and its cure with biotin concentrate. *J. Am. Med. Assoc.* 118:1199–1200, 1942.

Folic Acid

Biale Y and Lewenthal H. Effect of folic acid supplementation on congenital malformations due to anticonvulsive drugs. *European Journal of Obstetrics, Gynecology and Reproductive Biology.* 18:211–216, 1984.

Brown WT et al. High dose folic acid treatment of fragile (X) males. *American Journal of Medical Genetics.* 23:263–271, 1986.

Butterworth CE et al. Improvement in cervical cysplasia associated with folic acid therapy in users of oral contraceptives. *Am. J. Clin. Nutr.* 35:73, 1982.

Froster-Iskenius U et al. Folic acid treatment in males and females with fragile -(X)- syndrome. *American Journal of Medical Genetics.* 23:272–289, 1986.

Hagerman RJ et al. Oral folic acid versus placebo in the treatment of males with the fragile -(X)- syndrome. *American Journal of Medical Genetics.* 23:241–262, 1986.

Heimburger DC et al. Improvement in bronchial squamous metaplasia in smokers treated with folate and vitamin B₁₂. *J. Am. Med. Assoc.* 259:1525–1530, 1988.

Hillman RS and Steinberg SE. The effects of alcohol on folate metabolism. *Annual Review of Medicine.* 33:345–354, 1982.

Kopjas TL. Effect of folic acid on collateral circulation in diffuse chronic arteriosclerosis. *Journal of the American Geriatrics Society.* 14:1187–1192, 1966.

Lashner BA et al. Effect of folate supplementation on the incidence of dysplasia and cancer in chronic ulcerative colitis: A case controlled study. *Gastroenterology.* 97:255–259, 1989.

Mills JL et al. The absence of a relation between the periconceptional use of vitamins and neural-tube defects. *N. Eng. J. Med.* 321:430–435, 1989.

Milunsky A et al. Multivitamin/folic acid supplementation in early pregnancy reduces the prevalence of neural tube defects. *J. Am. Med. Assoc.* 262:2847–2852, 1989.

Pantothenic Acid and Pantethine

Aprahamian M et al. Effects of supplemental pantothenic acid on wound healing: Experimental study in rabbit. *Am. J. Clin. Nutr.* 41:578–589, 1985.

Arsenio L et al. Effectiveness of long-term treatment with pantethine in patients with dyslipidemia. *Clinical Therapeutics.* 8:537–541, 1986.

Avogaro P., Bittolo Bon G and Fusello M. Effect of pantethine on lipids, lipoproteins and apolipoproteins in man. *Curr. Ther. Res.* 33:488, 1983.

Barton-Wright EC and Elliott WA. The pantothenic acid metabolism of rheumatoid arthritis. *Lancet.* 2:862–863, 1963.

Bertolini S et al. Lipoprotein changes induced by pantethine in hyperlipoproteinemic patients: Adults and children. *International Journal of Clinical Pharmacology Therapy and Toxicology.* 24:630–637, 1986.

Bon GB et al. In vitro effect of pantethine on platelet aggregation. *Curr. Ther. Res.* 40:464, 1986.

Carrara P et al. Pantethine reduces plasma cholesterol and the severity of arterial lesions in experimental hypercholesterolemic rabbits. *Atherosclerosis.* 53:255–264, 1984.

Gaddi A et al. Controlled evaluation of pantethine: A natural hypolipidemic compound, in patients with different forms of hyperlipoproteinemia. *Atherosclerosis.* 50:73–83, 1984.

General Practitioner Research Group. Calcium pantothenate in arthritic conditions. *Practitioner.* 224:208–211, 1980.

Gensini GF et al. Changes in fatty acid composition of the single platelet phospholipids induced by pantethine treatment. *International Journal of Clinical Pharmacology Research.* 5:309–318, 1985.

Hoffman B et al. Effect of pantethine on platelet functions in vitro. *Curr. Ther. Res.* 41:791–801, 1987.

Litoff D, Scherzer H and Harrison J. Effects of pantothenic acid supplementation on human exercise. *Medicine and Science in Sports and Exercise.* 17:287 (Abstract 17), 1985.

Maggi GC, Donati and Criscuoli G. Pantethine: A physiological lipomodulating agent in the treatment of hyperlipidemia. *Curr. Ther. Res.* 32:380–386, 1982.

Nice C et al. The effects of pantothenic acid on human exercise capacity. *Journal of Sports Medicine.* 24:26–29, 1984.

Watanabe A et al. Lowering of blood acetaldehyde but not ethanol concentrations by pantethine following alcohol ingestion: Different effects in flushing and nonflushing subjects. *Alcoholism: Clinical and Experimental Research.* 9(3):272–276, 1985.

Vitamin C

Anderson R et al. Ascorbic acid neutralizes reactive oxidants released by hyperactive phagocytes from cigarette smokers. *Lung.* 166:149–159, 1988.

Anderson R et al. The effects of increasing weekly doses of ascorbate on certain cellular and humoral immune functions in normal volunteers. *Am. J. Clin. Nutr.* 33:71, 1980.

Banic S and Kosak M. Prevention of post-transfusion hepatitis by vitamin C. *Int. J. Vit. Nutr. Res. Suppl.* 19:41, 1979.

Bordia AK. The effect of vitamin C on blood lipids, fibrinolytic activity and platelet adhesiveness in patients with coronary artery disease. *Atherosclerosis.* 35:181–187, 1980.

Bright-See E. Vitamin C and cancer prevention. *Seminars in Oncology.* 10(3):294–298, 1983.

Cameron E and Pauling L. Supplemental ascorbate in the supportive treatment of cancer: Prolongation of survival times in terminal human cancer. *Proc. Nat. Acad. Sci.* 73:3685, 1976.

Connor HJ et al. Effect of increased intake of vitamin C on the mutagenic activity of gastric juice and intragastric concentrations of ascorbic acid. *Carcinogenesis.* 6:1675–1676, 1985.

Cordova C et al. Influence of ascorbic acid on platelet aggregation in vitro and in vivo. *Atherosclerosis.* 41:15–19, 1982.

Creagan ET et al. Failure of high-dose vitamin C (ascorbic acid) therapy to benefit patients with advanced cancer. *N. Eng. J. Med.* 301:687, 1979.

Dahl H and Degre M. The effect of ascorbic acid on production of human interferon and the antiviral activity in vitro. *Acta Pathol. Microbiol. Scand. B.* 84:280, 1976.

Finley EB and Cerlewski FL. Influence of ascorbic acid supplementation on copper status in young adult men. *Am. J. Clin. Nutr.* 37:553–556, 1983.

Fraser RC et al. The effect of variations in vitamin C intake on the cellular immune response of guinea pigs. *Am. J. Clin. Nutr.* 33:839, 1980.

Frei B, England L and Ames BN. Ascorbate is an outstanding antioxidant in human blood plasma. *Proc. Nat. Acad. Sci.* 86:6377–6381, 1989.

Gonzales ER. Sperm swim singly after vitamin C therapy (Report). *J. Am. Med. Assoc.* 249:2747–2751, 1983.

Henderson H. Vitamin C Rx with haloperidol? *Medical Tribune.* 26(25):51, September 4, 1985.

Karlowski TR et al. Ascorbic acid for the common cold: A prophylactic and therapeutic trial. *J. Am. Med. Assoc.* 231:1038, 1975.

Krivit W et al. Prevention of cyclophosphamide (CYT) induced hemorrhagic cystitis (HC) by use of ascorbic acid (AA) to reduce urinary PH (Abstract). *American Society of Clinical Oncology.* 2:27, 1983.

Kuodell RG et al. Vitamin C prophylaxis for post transfusion hepatitis lack of effect in a controlled trial. *Am. J. Clin. Nutr.* 34:20, 1981.

Kyrtopoulos SA. Ascorbic acid and the formation of N-nitroso compounds: Possible role of ascorbic acid in cancer prevention. *Am. J. Clin. Nutr.* 45:1344–1350, 1987.

Leibovitz B and Siegel BV. Ascorbic acid, neutrophil function and the immune response. *Int. J. Vit. Nutr. Res.* 48:159, 1978.

Migliozzi JA. Effect of ascorbic acid on tumor growth. *Br. J. Ca.* 35:448, 1977.

Mirvish SS. Effects of vitamins C and E on N-nitroso compound formation, carcinogenesis and cancer. *Cancer 58* (Suppl.):1842–1850, 1986.

Moertel CG et al. High-dose vitamin C versus placebo in the treatment of patients with advanced cancer who have had no prior chemotherapy. *N. Eng. J. Med.* 312:137–141, 1985.

Mohsenin V, Dubois AB and Douglas JS. Effect of ascorbic acid on response to methacholine challenge in asthmatic subjects. *American Review of Respiratory Disease.* 127:143–147, 1983.

O'Connor HJ et al. Effect of increased intake of vitamin C on the mutagenic activity of gastric juice and intragastric concentrations of ascorbic acid. *Carcinogenesis.* 6:1675, 1985.

Pauling L. Evolution and the need for ascorbic acid. *Proc. Nat. Acad. Sci.* 67:1643–1648, 1970.

Pauling L. The significance of the evidence about ascorbic acid and the common cold. *Proc. Nat. Acad. Sci.* 68:2678–2681, 1971.

Rebec GV et al. Ascorbic acid and the behavioral response to haloperidol: Implications for the action of antipsychotic drugs. *Science.* 227:438–440, 1985.

Romney SL et al. Plasma vitamin C and uterine cervical dysplasia. *American Journal of Obstetrics and Gynecology.* 151:976–980, 1985.

Sarji E et al. Decreased platelet vitamin C in diabetes mellitus: Possible role in hyperaggregation. *Thrombosis Research.* 15:639, 1979.

Shilotri PG and Bhat KS. Effect of megadoses of vitamin C on bactericidal activity of leukocytes. *Am. J. Clin. Nutr.* 30:1077, 1977.

Siegel BV. Enhanced interferon response to murine leukemia virus by ascorbic acid. *Infect. Immun.* 10:409, 1974.

Siegel BV and Morton JI. Vitamin C and immunity: Influence of ascorbate on prostaglandin E_2 synthesis and implications for natural killer cell activity. *Int. J. Vit. Nutr. Res.* 54:339, 1984.

Sobala GM et al. Ascorbic acid in the human stomach. *Gastroenterology.* 97:357–363, 1989.

Spanhake EW and Menkes HA. Vitamin C—new tricks for an old dog (Editorial). *American Review of Respiratory Disease.* 127:139–140, 1983.

Tannenbaum SR and Mergena W. Reaction of nitrite with vitamins C and E. *Ann. N.Y. Acad. Sci.* 355:267–277, 1980.

Taylor TV et al. Ascorbic acid supplementation in the treatment of pressure sores. *Lancet.* 2:544, 1974.

Vanderjagt DJ and Garry PJ. Significance of vitamin C in the elderly. *Geriatric Medicine Today.* 8(10):85–100, 1989.

Wassertheil-Smoller et al. Dietary vitamin C and uterine cervical dysplasia. *Am. J. Epidemiol.* 114:714, 1981.

Vitamin D

Anonymous. Vitamin D: New perspectives (Editorial). *Lancet.* 1:1122–1123, 1987.

Crowle AJ, Ross EJ and May MH. Inhibition by $1,25(OH)_2$—vitamin D_3 of the multiplication of virulent tubercle bacilli in cultured human macrophages. *Infect. Immun.* 55:2945–2950, 1987.

DeLuca HF. The vitamin D story: A collaborative effort of basic science and clinical medicine. *FASEB J.* 2:224–236, 1988.

Garland C et al. Dietary vitamin D and calcium and risk of colorectal cancer: A 19-year prospective study in men. *Lancet.* 1:307–309, 1985.

Garland CF and Garland FC. Do sunlight and vitamin D reduce the likelihood of colon cancer? *International Journal of Epidemiology.* 9:227–231, 1980.

Harju E et al. High incidence of low serum vitamin D concentration in patients with hip fracture. *Arch. Orthop. Trauma Surg.* 103:408, 1985.

Matsuoka LY et al. Sunscreens suppress cutaneous vitamin D_3 synthesis. *Journal of Clinical Endocrinology and Metabolism.* 64:1165–1168, 1987.

Parfitt AM et al. Vitamin D and bone health in the elderly. *Am. J. Clin. Nutr.* 36:1014, 1982.

Sowers MR, et al. The association of intakes of vitamin D and calcium with blood pressure among women. *Am. J. Clin. Nutr.* 42:135, 1985.

Vitamin E

Bjorneboe GA et al. Diminished serum concentration of vitamin E in alcoholics. *Annals of Nutrition and Metabolism.* 32:56–61, 1988.

Blumberg JB. Vitamin E requirements during aging. In: Hayaishi O and Mino M (eds.), *Clinical and Nutritional Aspects of Vitamin E*. Elsevier Science Publishers, pp. 53–61, 1987.

Calabrese E et al. Influence of dietary vitamin E on susceptibility to ozone exposure. *Bulletin of Environmental Contamination and Toxicology.* 34:417–422, 1985.

Corwin M, Gordon RK and Shloss J. Studies of the mode of action of vitamin E in stimulating T-cell mitogenesis. *Scandinavian Journal of Immunology.* 14:565–571, 1981.

Ernster VL et al. Vitamin E and benign breast "disease": A double-blind randomized clinical trial. *Surgery.* 97:490, 1985.

Finer NN et al. Effect of intramuscular vitamin E on frequency and severity of rentrolental fibroplasia: A controlled trial. *Lancet.* 1:1087, 1982.

FitzGerald GA and Bush AR. Endogenous prostacyclin and thromboxane biosynthesis during chronic vitamin E therapy in man. *Ann. N.Y. Acad. Sci.* 393:209, 1982.

Gillilan RE, et al. Quantitative evaluation of vitamin E in the treatment of angina pectoris. *Am. Heart J.* 93:444, 1977.

Haegar K. Long-term treatment of intermittent claudication with vitamin E. *Am. J. Clin. Nutr.* 27:1179, 1974.

Horvath PM and Ip C. Synergistic effect of vitamin E and selenium in the chemo-prevention of mammary carcinogenesis in rats. *Ca. Res.* 43:5335, 1983.

Jandak J, Steiner M and Richardson PD. Alpha tocopherol, an effective inhibitor of platelet adhesion. *Blood.* 73:141–149, 1989.

Kamimura M. Anti-inflammatory activity of vitamin E. *J. Vitaminol.* 18:204, 1972.

Kanofsky JD and Kanofsky PB. Prevention of thromboembolic disease by vitamin E. *N. Eng. J. Med* 305:173, 1981.

Livingstone PD and Jones C. Treatment of intermittent claudication with vitamin E. *Lancet.* 2:602, 1958.

Locitzer K. Long-term vitamin E may avert cataracts (Report). *Medical Tribune.* Pp. 9–11, July 20, 1989.

Lohr JB et al. Alpha-tocopherol in tardive dyskinesia. *Lancet.* 1:913–914, 1987.

London RF et al. The effect of vitamin E on mammary dysplasia: A double-blind study. *Obstetrics and Gynecology.* 65:104–106, 1985.

London RS. Efficacy of alpha-tocopherol in the treatment of the premenstrual syndrome. *J. Reprod. Med.* 32:400, 1987.

Nockels CF. Protective effects of supplemental vitamin E against infection. *Fed. Proc.* 38:2134, 1979.

Pacht ER et al. Deficiency of vitamin E in the alveolar fluid of cigarette smokers. *Journal of Clinical Investigation.* 77:789–796, 1986.

Oski FA. Vitamin E—a radical defense (Editorial). *N. Eng. J. Med.* 303:454–455, 1980.

Pinsky MJ. Treatment of intermittent claudication with alpha-tocopherol. *J. Am. Pod. Assoc.* 70:454, 1980.

Prasad JS. Effect of vitamin E supplementation on leukocyte function. *Am. J. Clin. Nutr.* 33:606, 1980.

Sharif R et al. Vitamin E supplementation in smokers. *Am. J. Clin. Nutr.* 47:758 (abstract), 1988.

Simon-Schnass I and Pabst H. Influence of vitamin E on physical performance. *Int. J. Vit. Nutr. Res.* 58:49–54, 1988.

Sitrin MD et al. Vitamin E deficiency and neurological disease in adults with cystic fibrosis. *Ann. Intern. Med.* 107:51–54, 1987.

Sokol RJ. Vitamin E and neurologic function in man. *Free Radical Biology & Medicine.* 6:189–207, 1989.

Stryker WS. The relation of diet, cigarette smoking and alcohol consumption to plasma beta-carotene and alpha-tocopherol levels. *Am. J. Epidemiol.* 127:283–296, 1988.

Sundaram GS et al. Alpha-tocopherol and serum lipoproteins. *Lipids.* 16:223–227, 1981.

Tanaka J. Vitamin E and immune response. *Immunology.* 38:727–734, 1979.

Trickler D and Shkler G. Prevention by vitamin E of experimental oral carcinogenesis. *J.N.C.I.* 78:165–169, 1987.

Williams HTG, Fenna D and MacBeth RA. Alpha tocopherol in the treatment of intermittent claudication. *Surg. Gynec. Obstet.* 132:662, 1971.

Vitamin K

Chelbowski RT, Akman SA and Block JB. Vitamin K in the treatment of cancer. *Cancer Treatment Reviews.* 12:49–63, 1985.

Hart JP et al. Circulating vitamin K_1 levels in fractured neck of femur. *Lancet.* 2:283, 1984.

Houschka PV, Liam JB and Gallop PM. Vitamin K and mineralization. *Trends in Biochemical Sciences.* 3:75–78, 1978.

Tomita A. Postmenopausal osteoporosis ^{47}Ca study with vitamin K_2. *Clinical Endocrinology.* 19:731–736, 1971.

MINERALS

Boron

Nielsen FH. Boron—an overlooked element of potential nutritional importance. *Nutrition Today*. Pp. 4–7, January–February 1988.

Nielsen FH et al. Effect of dietary boron on mineral, estrogen, and testosterone metabolism in postmenopausal women. *FASEB J*. 1:394–397, 1987.

Calcium

Ackley S, Barrett-Conner E and Suarez L. Dairy products, calcium and blood pressure. *Am. J. Clin. Nutr*. 38:457, 1983.

Albanese AA et al. Calcium nutrition and skeletal and alveolar bone loss. *Nutrition Reports International*. 31:741–755, 1985.

Amschler DH. Calcium intake: A lifelong proposition. *J. Sch. Health*. 55:360, 1985.

Appleton GVN et al. Inhibition of intestinal carcinogenesis by dietary supplementation with calcium. *British Journal of Surgery*. 74:523, 1987.

Belizan J and Villar J. The relationship between calcium intake and edema-, proteinuria- and hypertension-gestosis: An hypothesis. *Am. J. Clin. Nutr*. 33:2202, 1980.

Belizan JM et al. Preliminary evidence of the effect of calcium supplementation on blood pressure in normal pregnant women. *American Journal of Obstetrics and Gynecology*. 146:175, 1983.

Belizan JM et al. Reduction of blood pressure with calcium supplementation in young adults. *J. Am. Med. Assoc*. 249:1161, 1983.

Bierenbaum ML, Fleischman AL and Raichelson RI. Long term human studies on the lipid effects of oral calcium. *Lipids*. 7:202, 1972.

Carlson LA et al. Effect of oral calcium upon serum cholesterol and triglycerides in patients with hyperlipidemia. *Atherosclerosis*. 14:391, 1971.

Ellis FR, Holesch S and Ellis JW. Incidence of osteoporosis in vegetarians and omnivores. *Am. J. Clin. Nutr*. 25:555, 1972.

Garland C et al. Dietary vitamin D and calcium and risk of colorectal cancer: A 19-year prospective study in men. *Lancet*. 1:307–309, 1985.

Goei GS, Galston JL and Abraham GE. Dietary patterns of patients with premenstrual tension. *Journal of Applied Nutrition*. 34:69, 1982.

Harvey JA, Zobita MM and Pak CYC. Calcium citrate: Reduced propensity for the crystallization of calcium oxalate in urine resulting from induced hypercalciuria of calcium supplementation. *Journal of Clinical Endocrinology*. 61:391–393, 1985.

Heilbrun LK et al. Colon cancer and dietary fat, phosphorus and calcium in Hawaiian-Japanese men. *Am. J. Clin. Nutr*. 43:306, 1986.

Holbrook TL, Barrett-Connor E and Winegard DL. Dietary calcium and risk of hip fracture: 14-year prospective population study. *Lancet*. 2:1046–1049, 1988.

Horowitz M et al. The effect of calcium supplements on plasma alkaline phosphatase and urinary hydroxyproline in postmenopausal women. *Hormone and Metabolic Research*. 17:311, 1985.

Lee CJ, Lawler GS and Johnson GH. Effect of supplementation of the diets with calcium and calcium-rich foods on bone density of elderly females with osteoporosis. *Am. J. Clin. Nutr*. 34:819–823, 1981.

Lipkin M and Newmark A. Effect of added dietary calcium on colonic epithelial-cell proliferation in subjects at high risk for familial colonic cancer. *N. Eng. J. Med*. 313:1381–1384, 1985.

Lyle RM et al. Blood pressure and metabolic effects of calcium supplementation in normotensive white and black men. *J. Am. Med. Assoc*. 257:1772–1776, 1987.

McCarron DA. Calcium: Confirming an inverse relationship. *Hospital Practice*. Pp. 229–244, February 15, 1989.

McCarron DA, Morris CD and Cole C. Dietary calcium in human hypertension. *Science*. 217:267, 1982.

McCarron DA et al. Blood pressure and nutrient intake in the United States. *Science*. 224:1392–1398, 1984.

Nepper Holm C and Hessov I. Effects of calcium treatment on urinary stone index after intestinal bypass for obesity. *Digestion*. 22:255, 1981.

Nicar MJ and Pak CYC. Calcium bioavailability from calcium carbonate and calcium citrate. *Journal of Clinical Endocrinology*. 61:391–393, 1985.

Parrot-Garcia M and McCarron DA. Calcium and hypertension. *Nutr. Rev*. 42:205, 1984.

Pence BC and Buddingh F. Inhibition of dietary fat promotion of colon carcinogenesis by supplemental calcium or vitamin D. *Proceedings of the American Association of Cancer Research*. 28:154, 1987.

Recker RR. Calcium absorption and achlorhydria. *N. Eng. J. Med*. 313:70–73, 1985.

Recker RR, Saville PD and Heaney RP. Effect of estrogens and calcium carbonate on bone loss in postmenopausal women. *Annals of Internal Medicine*. 87:649, 1977.

Resnick LM, Nicholson JP and Laragh JH. Outpatient

therapy of essential hypertension with dietary calcium supplementation. *Journal of the American College of Cardiology.* 3:616, 1984.

Riggs BL et al. Effect of the fluoride/calcium regimen on vertebral fracture occurrence in postmenopausal osteoporosis. *N. Eng. J. Med.* 306:446, 1982.

Riis B, Thomsen K and Christiansen C. Does calcium supplementation prevent postmenopausal bone loss? *N. Eng. J. Med.* 316:173–177, 1987.

Rozen P et al. Oral calcium suppresses increased rectal epithelial proliferation of persons at risk of colorectal cancer. *Gut.* 30:650–655, 1989.

Sandler RB et al. Postmenopausal bone density and milk consumption in childhood and adolescence. *Am. J. Clin. Nutr.* 42:270, 1985.

Wargovich MJ et al. Calcium ameliorates the toxic effect of deoxycholic acid on colonic epithelium. *Carcinogenesis.* 4:1205, 1983.

Yacowitz H, Fleischman AL and Bierenbaum ML. Effect of oral calcium upon serum lipids in man. *Br. Med. J.* 1:1352–1354, 1965.

Chromium

Abraham AS et al. The effect of chromium on established atherosclerotic plaques in rabbits. *Am. J. Clin. Nutr.* 33:2294–2298, 1980.

Anderson RA. Chromium metabolism and its role in disease processes in men. *Clinical Physiology and Biochemistry.* 4:31–41, 1986.

Anderson RA and Kozlovsky AS. Chromium intake, absorption and excretion of subjects consuming self-selected diets. *Am. J. Clin. Nutr.* 4:1177–1183, 1985.

Anderson RA et al. Chromium supplementation of humans with hypoglycemia. *Fed. Proc.* 43:471, 1984.

Anderson RA et al. Effect of chromium supplementation on urinary Cr excretion of human subjects and correlation of Cr excretion with selected clinical parameters. *J. Nutr.* 113:276–281, 1983.

Anderson RA et al. Effects of supplemental chromium on patients with symptoms of reactive hypoglycemia. *Metabolism.* 35:351–355, 1987.

Bunker W et al. The uptake and excretion of chromium by the elderly. *Am. J. Clin. Nutr.* 39:799–802, 1984.

Canfield W. Chromium, glucose tolerance and serum cholesterol in adults. In: Shapcott D and Hubert J (eds.), *Chromium in Nutrition and Metabolism.* Amsterdam: Elsevier, 1979, p. 145.

Check WA. And if you add chromium, that's even better. *J. Am. Med. Assoc.* 247:3046, 1982.

Elias AN, Grossman MK and Valenta LJ. Use of the artificial beta cell (ABC) in the assessment of peripheral insulin sensitivity: Effect of chromium supplementation in diabetes. *General Pharmacology.* 15:535–539, 1984.

Elwood JC, Nash DT and Streeten DHP. Effect of high chromium brewer's yeast on human serum lipids. *J. Amer. Coll. Nutr.* 1:263, 1982.

Freiberg JM et al. Effects of brewer's yeast on glucose tolerance. *Diabetes.* 24:433, 1975.

Freund H, Atamian S and Fischer JE. Chromium deficiency during total parenteral nutrition. *J. Am. Med. Assoc.* 241:496–498, 1979.

Glinsmann WH and Mertz W. Effect of trivalent chromium on glucose tolerance. *Metabolism.* 15:510–520, 1966.

Jeejeebhoy KN et al. Chromium deficiency, glucose intolerance and neuropathy reversed by chromium supplementation in a patient receiving long-term total parenteral nutrition. *Am. J. Clin. Nutr.* 3:531–538, 1977.

Kozlovsky AS et al. Effects of diets high in simple sugars on urinary chromium losses. *Metabolism.* 35:515–518, 1986.

Liu VJK et al. Effects of high-chromium yeast-extract supplementation on serum lipids, serum insulin and glucose tolerance in older women. *Fed. Proc.* 36:1123, 1977.

Martinez OB. Dietary chromium and effect of chromium supplementation on glucose tolerance of elderly Canadian women. *Nutrition Research.* 5:609–620, 1985.

Mertz W. Chromium—an overview. In: Shapcott D and Huber J (eds.), *Chromium in Nutrition and Metabolism.* Amsterdam: Elsevier, 1979, pp. 1–14.

Mertz W. Effects and metabolism of glucose tolerance factor. *Nutr. Rev.* 33:129, 1975.

Mossop RT. Effects of chromium III on fasting blood glucose, cholesterol and cholesterol HDL levels in diabetics. *Central African Journal of Medicine.* 29:80–82, 1983.

Newman HAI et al. Serum chromium and angiographically determined coronary artery disease. *Clinical Chemistry.* 24:541–544, 1978.

Offenbacher EG and Pi-Sunyer FX. Beneficial effects of chromium-rich yeast on glucose tolerance and blood lipids in elderly subjects. *Diabetes.* 29:919–925, 1980.

Offenbacher EG and Pi-Sunyer FX. Chromium in human nutrition. *Ann. Rev. Nutr.* 8:543–563, 1988.

Potter JF et al. Glucose metabolism in glucose-intolerant older people during chromium supplementation. *Metabolism.* 34:199–204, 1985.

Press RI, Geller J and Evans GW. The effect of chromium picolinate on serum cholesterol and apolipoprotein fractions in human subjects. *Western Journal of Medicine* 152:41–45, 1990.

Riales R and Albrink MJ. Effects of chromium chloride supplementation on glucose tolerance and serum lipids including high-density lipoprotein of adult men. *Am. J. Clin. Nutr.* 34:2670–2678, 1981.

Saner G. *Chromium in Nutrition and Disease.* New York: Alan R. Liss, Inc., 1980, p. 129.

Schroeder HA. Chromium deficiency in rats: A syndrome stimulating diabetes mellitus with retarded growth. *J. Nutr.* 88:439, 1966.

Schroeder HA, Nason AP and Tipton IH. Chromium deficiency as a factor in atherosclerosis. *J. Chron. Dis.* 23:123–142, 1970.

Simonoff M et al. Low plasma chromium in patients with coronary artery and heart disease. *Biol. Trace Elem. Res.* 6:431, 1984.

Uusitupa MI et al. Effect of inorganic chromium supplementation on glucose tolerance, insulin response, and serum lipids in noninsulin-dependent diabetics. *Am. J. Clin. Nutr.* 38:404–410, 1983.

Copper

Anonymous. Copper deficiency and hypercholesterolemia. *Nutr. Rev.* 45(4):116–117, 1987.

Askari A, Long CL and Blakemore WS. Zinc, copper and parenteral nutrition in cancer: A review. *J. Par. Ent. Nutr.* 4:561–571, 1980.

Klevay LM. Coronary heart disease: The zinc/copper hypothesis. *Am. J. Clin. Nutr.* 28:764–774, 1975.

Klevay LM. The ratio of zinc to copper of diets in the United States. *Nutrition Reports International.* 11:237–242, 1975.

Klevay LM et al. Effects of a diet low in copper on a healthy man. *Clinical Research.* 28:758, 1980.

Klevay LM et al. Evidence of dietary copper and zinc deficiencies. *J. Am. Med. Assoc.* 241:1916–1918, 1979.

Pfeiffer CC and Iliev. A study of zinc deficiency and copper excess in schizophrenics. *International Review of Neurobiology. 1* (Supplement):141–165, 1972.

Reiser S et al. Effect of copper intake on blood cholesterol and its lipoprotein distribution in men. *Nutrition Reports International.* 36:641–649, 1987.

Shore D et al. CSF copper concentrations in chronic schizophrenia. *Am. J. Psychiatry.* 140:754–757, 1983.

Sorenson JRJ. Copper complexes: A physiologic approach to treatment of chronic diseases. *Compr. Ther.* 11(4):49, 1985.

Sorenson JRJ. Copper complexes: A unique class of anti-arthritic drugs. *Progress in Medicinal Chemistry.* 15:211–260, 1978.

Soskel NT et al. A copper-deficient zinc-supplemented diet produces emphysema in pigs. *American Review of Respiratory Disease.* 126:316, 1982.

Tilson MD. Decreased hepatic copper levels: A possible chemical marker for the pathogenesis of aortic aneurysms in man. *Archives of Surgery.* 117:1212–1213, 1982.

Walker WR and Keats DM. An investigation of the therapeutic value of the "copper bracelet"-dermal assimilation of copper in arthritic rheumatoid conditions. *Agents and Actions.* 6:454–459, 1976.

Williams DM. Copper deficiency in humans. *Seminars in Hematology.* 20:118–128, 1983.

Fluorine

Bernstein DS et al. Prevalence of osteoporosis in high-and-low fluoride areas in North Dakota. *J. Am. Med. Assoc.* 198:85–90, 1966.

Bikle DD, Fluoride treatment of osteoporosis: A new look at an old drug. *Ann. Intern. Med.* 98:1013, 1983.

Clements NC Jr. and Mooradian AD. Sodium fluoride in the treatment of osteoporosis. *Drug Therapy.* Pp. 69–80, May 1989.

Glenn FB, Glenn WD III and Duncan RC. Fluoride tablet supplementation during pregnancy for caries immunity: A study of the offspring produced. *American Journal of Obstetrics and Gynecology.* 143:560, 1982.

Heaney RP et al. Fluoride therapy for the vertebral crush fracture syndrome: A status report. *Ann. Intern. Med.* 111:678–680, 1989.

Leone NC et al. A roentgenologic study of a human population exposed to high-fluoride domestic water: A 10-year study. *American Journal of Roentgenology.* 74:874, 1955.

Mamelle N et al. Risk-benefit ratio of sodium fluoride treatment in primary vertebral osteoporosis. *Lancet.* 2:361–365, 1988.

Oestreicher A. Fluorides' fracture aid disputed (Report). *Medical World News.* October 23, 1989.

Pak CYC et al. Safe and effective treatment of osteoporosis with intermittent slow release sodium fluoride: Augmentation of vertebral bone mass and inhibition of fractures. *Journal of Clinical Endocrinology and Metabolism.* 68:150–159, 1989.

Richmond VL. Thirty years of fluoridation: A review. *Am. J. Clin. Nutr.* 41:129–138, 1985.

Schamshula RG and Barmes DE. Fluoride and health: Dental caries, osteoporosis and cardiovascular disease. *Ann. Rev. Nutr.* 1:427, 1981.

Simonen O and Laitinen O. Does fluoridation of

drinking-water prevent bone fragility and osteoporosis? *Lancet.* 2:432–433, 1985.

Germanium

Asai K. *Miracle Cure: Organic germanium.* Tokyo: Japan Publications, Inc., 1980.

Aso H et al. Antiviral activity of carboxyethylgermanium sesquioxide (Ge-132) in mice infected with influenza virus. *Journal of Biological Response Modifiers.* 8:180–189, 1989.

Matsusaka T et al. Germanium-induced nephropathy: Report of two cases and review of the literature. *Clinical Nephrology.* 30:341–345, 1988.

Sato I et al. Inhibition of tumor growth and metastasis in association with modification of immune response by novel organic germanium compounds. *Journal of Biological Response Modifiers.* 4:159–168, 1985.

Suzuki F, Brutkiewicz RR and Pollard RB. Cooperation of lymphokine(s) and macrophages in expression of antitumor activity of carboxyethylgermanium sesquioxide (Ge-132). *Anticancer Res.* 6:177–182, 1986.

Suzuki F. Brutkiewicz RB and Pollard RB. Ability of sera from mice treated with Ge-132, an organic germanium compound, to inhibit experimental murine ascites tumours. *Br. J. Ca.* 52:757–763, 1985.

Suzuki F, Brutkiewicz RB and Pollard RB. Importance of T-cells and macrophages in the antitumor activity of carboxyethylgermanium sesquioxide (Ge-132). *Anticancer Res.* 5:479–484, 1985.

Iodine

Anonymous. Iodine relieves pain of fibrocystic breasts (Report). *Medical World News.* P. 25, January 11, 1988.

Becker DV et al. The use of iodine as a thyroidal blocking agent in the event of a reactor accident. *J. Am. Med. Assoc.* 252:659–661, 1984.

Iron

Anonymous. Iron deficiency and mental development. *Nutr. Rev.* 41(8):235–237, 1983.

Bates CJ, Powers HJ and Thurnham DI. Vitamins, iron and physical work. *Lancet.* 2:313–314, 1989.

Beard J and Myfanwy B. Iron deficiency and thermoregulation. *Nutrition Today.* 23(5):41–45, September–October, 1988.

Beutler E, Larsh SE and Gurney CW. Iron therapy in chronically fatigued nonanemic women: A double-blind study. *Ann. Intern. Med.* 52:378–394, 1960.

Blake DK et al. The importance of iron in rheumatoid disease. *Lancet.* 2:1142, 1981.

Dallman PR. Iron deficiency and the immune response. *Am. J. Clin. Nutr.* 46:329–334, 1987.

Dhur A, Galan P and Hercberg S. Iron status, immune capacity and resistance to infections. *Comparative Biochemistry and Physiology.* 94A:11–19, 1989.

Edgerton VR et al. Iron-deficiency anaemia and its effect on worker productivity and activity patterns. *Br. Med. J.* 2:1546–1549, 1979.

Hershko C, Peto TEA and Weatherall DJ. Iron and infection. *Br. Med. J.* 296:660–664, 1988.

Hunding A, Jordahl R and Pauley PE. Runners anemia and iron deficiency. *Acta Medica Scandinavica.* 209:315–318, 1981.

Kuvibidila S. Iron deficiency, cell-mediated immunity and resistance against infections: Present knowledge and controversies. *Nutrition Research.* 7:989–1003, 1987.

Lampe JW, Slavin JL and Apple FS. Poor iron status of women runners training for a marathon. *International Journal of Sports Medicine.* 7:111–114, 1986.

Lozoff B et al. Developmental deficits in iron-deficient infants: Effects of age and severity of iron lack. *Journal of Pediatrics.* 10:948–952, 1982.

Ohira Y et al. Work capacity, heart rate and blood lactate response to iron treatment. *British Journal of Haematology.* 41:365–372, 1979.

Sacks P and Houchin DN. Comparative bioavailability of elemental iron powders for repair of iron deficiency anemia in rats: Studies of efficacy and toxicity of carboxyl iron. *Am. J. Clin. Nutr.* 31:566–573, 1978.

Scrimshaw NS. Functional consequences of iron deficiency in human populations. *J. Nutr. Sci. Vitaminol.* 30:47–63, 1984.

Stevens RG et al. Body iron stores and the risk of cancer. *N. Eng. J. Med.* 319:1047–1052, 1988.

Walter T, Kovalskys J and Stekel AL. Effect of mild iron deficiency on infant mental development scores. *Journal of Pediatrics.* 102:519–522, 1983.

Magnesium

Abraham G. Nutritional factors in the etiology of the premenstrual tension syndromes. *J. Reprod. Med.* 28:446–464, 1983.

Altura BM et al. Magnesium deficiency and hypertension: Correlation between magnesium-deficient diets and microcirculatory changes in situ. *Science.* 223:1315, 1984.

Anderson TW et al. Ischemic heart disease, water

hardness and myocardial magnesium. *Can. Med. Assoc. J.* 113:199, 1975.

Anonymous. Hypomagnesemia found in 25% of eating disorders (Report). *Internal Medicine News.* 21(3):47, July 1–14, 1988.

Buckley JE. Hypomagnesemia after cisplatin combination chemotherapy. *Archives of Internal Medicine.* 144:2347–2348, 1984.

Chipperfield B and Chipperfield JR. Heart-muscle magnesium, potassium and zinc concentrations after sudden death from heart-disease. *Lancet.* 2:293, 1973.

Chipperfield B and Chipperfield JR. Magnesium and the heart. *Am. Heart J.* 93:679, 1977.

Cohen L and Kitzes R. Magnesium sulfate and digitalis-toxic arrhythmias. *J. Am. Med. Assoc.* 249: 2808–2810, 1983.

Crawford T and Crawford MD. Prevalence and pathological changes of ischemic heart disease in a hard-water and in a soft-water area. *Lancet.* 1:229, 1967.

Dubey A and Solomon R. Magnesium, myocardial ischaemia and arrhythmias: The role of magnesium in myocardial infarction. *Drugs.* 37:1–7, 1989.

Dyckner T and Wester PO. Effect of magnesium on blood pressure. *Br. Med. J.* 286:1847, 1983.

Dyckner T and Wester PO. Intracellular potassium after magnesium infusion. *Br. Med. J.* 1:882, 1978.

Embry CK and Lippmann S. Use of magnesium sulfate in alcohol withdrawal. *American Family Physician.* 35:167–170, 1987.

Franz KB. Physiologic changes during a marathon, with special reference to magnesium. *J. Am. Coll. Nutr.* 4:187–194, 1985.

Henderson DG, Schierup J and Schodt T. Effect of magnesium supplementation on blood pressure and electrolyte concentrations in hypertensive patients receiving long term diuretic treatment. *Br. Med. J.* 293:664, 1986.

Hueston WJ. Prevention and treatment of preterm labor. *American Family Physician.* 40(5):139–146, 1989.

Iseri LT, Chung P and Tobis J. Magnesium therapy for intractable ventricular tachyarrhythmias in normomagnesemic patients. *Western Journal of Medicine.* 138:823–828, 1983.

Johnasson G et al. Effects of magnesium hydroxide in renal stone disease. *J. Am. Coll. Nutr.* 1:179, 1982.

Johnson CJ, Peterson DP and Smith EK. Myocardial tissue concentrations of magnesium and potassium in men dying suddenly from ischemic heart disease. *Am. J. Clin. Nutr.* 32:967, 1979.

Liu L, Borowski G and Rose LI. Hypomagnesemia in a tennis player. *The Physician and SportsMedicine.* 11(5):79–80, 1983.

Malkiel-Shapiro B and Bersohn I. Magnesium sulphate in coronary thrombosis. *Br. Med. J.* 1:292, 1960.

Marier JR. Cardioprotective contribution of hard waters to magnesium intake. *Rev. Can. Biol.* 37:115, 1978.

Melnick I et al. Magnesium therapy of recurrent calcium oxalate urinary calculi. *J. Urol.* 105:119, 1971.

Molloy DW. Hypomagnesemia and respiratory-muscle weakness in the elderly. *Geriatric Medicine Today.* 6(2):53–61, 1987.

Nielsen FH. Dietary magnesium, manganese and boron affect the response of rats to high dietary aluminum. *Magnesium.* 7:133–147, 1988.

Okayama H et al. Bronchadilating effect of intravenous magnesium sulfate in bronchial asthma. *J. Am. Med. Assoc.* 257:1076–1078, 1987.

Paolisso G et al. Improved insulin response and action by chronic magnesium administration in aged NIDDM subjects. *Diabetes Care.* 12:265–269, 1989.

Peterson DR, Thompson DJ and Nam J-M. Water hardness, arteriosclerotic heart disease, and sudden death. *Am. J. Epidemiol.* 92:90, 1970.

Raloff J. New misgivings about low magnesium (Report). *Science News.* 133:356, 1988.

Rasmussen HS et al. Influence of magnesium substitution therapy on blood lipid composition in patients with ischemic heart disease. *Archives of Internal Medicine.* 149:1050–1053, 1989.

Rasmussen HS et al. Intravenous magnesium in acute myocardial infarction. *Lancet.* 1:234–235, 1986.

Resnick LM, Gupta RK and Laragh JH. Intracellular free magnesium in erythrocytes of essential hypertension: Relation to blood pressure and serum divalent cations. *Proc. Nat. Acad. Sci.* 81:6511, 1984.

Rolla G et al. Reduction of histamine-induced bronchoconstriction by magnesium in asthmatic subjects. *Allergy.* 42:186–188, 1987.

Ruddell H et al. Effect of magnesium supplementation in patients with labile hypertension. *J. Am. Coll. Nutr.* 6:445, 1987.

Seelig M and Heggtveit A. Magnesium interrelationships in ischemic heart disease: A review. *Am. J. Clin. Nutr.* 27:59–79, 1974.

Sjogren A, Edvinsson L and Fallgren B. Magnesium deficiency in coronary artery disease and cardiac arrhythmias. *Journal of Internal Medicine.* 226:213–222, 1989.

Skobeloff EM et al. Intravenous magnesium sulfate for the treatment of acute asthma in the emergency department. *J. Am. Med. Assoc.* 262:1210–1213, 1989.

Specter MJ, Schweizer E and Goldman RH. Studies on magnesium's mechanism of action in digitalis-induced arrhythmias. *Circulation.* 52:1001, 1975.

Stendig-Lindberg G et al. Changes in serum magnesium concentration after strenuous exercise. *J. Am. Coll. Nutr.* 6(1):35–40, 1987.

Whang R and Aikawa JK. Magnesium deficiency and refractoriness to potassium repletion. *J. Chron. Dis.* 30:65, 1977.

Manganese

Doisy EA Jr. Effects of deficiency in manganese upon plasma levels of clotting proteins and cholesterol in man. In: Hoekstra JW et al. (eds.), *Trace Element Metabolism in Animals*, 2nd ed. Baltimore: University Park Press, 1974, pp. 668–670.

Donaldson J, McGregor D and LaBella F. Manganese toxicity: A model for free radical mediated neuro-degeneration? *Canadian Journal of Physiology and Pharmacology.* 60:1398–1405, 1982.

Frank BS, *Nucleic Acid and Antioxidant Therapy of Aging and Degeneration.* New York: Rainstone Publishing, 1977, pp. 158, 163.

Freeland-Graves JH. Manganese: An essential nutrient for humans. *Nutrition Today.* Pp. 13–19, November–December 1988.

Friedman BJ et al. Manganese balance and clinical observations in young men fed a manganese-deficient diet. *J. Nutr.* 117:133–143, 1987.

Mena I. Manganese poisoning. In: Vinken PJ and Bruyh GW (eds.), *Handbook of Clinical Neurology,* Vol. 36. Amsterdam: North Holland, 1979, pp. 217–237.

Pfeiffer CC, *Zinc and Other Micro-Nutrients.* New Canaan, Conn.: Keats Publishing, 1978, pp. 66–73.

Molybdenum

Anonymous. Molybdenum deficiency in TPN. *Nutr. Rev.* 45(11):337–341, 1987.

Coordinating Group for Research on Etiology of Esophageal Cancer in North China. The epidemiology and etiology of esophageal cancer in north China: A preliminary report. *Chinese Medical Journal.* 1(3):167–183, 1975.

Luo XM et al. Molybdenum and esophageal cancer in China. *Federation Proceedings.* Federation of the American Society for Experimental Biology. 46:928, 1981.

Rajagopalan KV. Molybdenum: An essential trace element. *Nutr. Rev.* 45(11):321–328, 1987.

Rajagopalan KV. Molybdenum: An essential trace element in human nutrition. *Ann. Rev. Nutr.* 8:401–427, 1988.

Yang CS. Research on esophageal cancer in China: A review. *Ca. Res.* 40:2633–2644, 1980.

Phosphorus

Berner YN and Shike M. Consequences of phosphate imbalance. *Ann. Rev. Nutr.* 8:121–148, 1988.

Dale G et al. Fitness, unfitness and phosphate. *Br. Med. J.* 294:939, 1987.

Dale G et al. Profound hypophosphatemia in patients collapsing after a "fun run." *Br. Med. J.* 292:447–448, 1986.

Knochel JP. Hypophosphatemia. *Western Journal of Medicine.* 134:15–26, 1981.

Potassium

Khaw K-T and Barrett-Connor E. Dietary potassium and stroke-associated mortality: A 12-year prospective population study. *N. Eng. J. Med.* 316:235–240, 1987.

Khaw K-T and Thom S. Randomized double-blind cross-over trial of potassium on blood pressure in normal subjects. *Lancet.* 2:1127–1129, 1982.

Krishna GG, Miller E and Kapoor S. Increased blood pressure during potassium depletion in normotensive men. *N. Eng. J. Med.* 320:1177–1182, 1989.

Kurtz TW et al. "Salt-sensitive" essential hypertension in men: Is the sodium ion alone important? *N. Eng. J. Med.* 317:1043–1048, 1987.

Langford HG. Dietary potassium and hypertension: Epidemiologic data. *Ann. Intern. Med.* 98(Part 2):770–772, 1983.

MacGregor GA et al. Moderate potassium supplementation in essential hypertension. *Lancet.* 2:567–570, 1982.

Meneely GR and Battarbee HD. High sodium–low potassium environment and hypertension. *Am. J. Cardiol.* 38:768–785, 1976.

Ophir O et al. Low blood pressure in vegetarians: The possible role of potassium. *Am. J. Clin. Nutr.* 37:755–762, 1983.

Skrabal F, Aubock J and Hortnagl H. Low sodium/high potassium diet for prevention of hypertension: Probable mechanism of action. *Lancet.* 2:895, 1981.

Selenium

Broghamer WL, McConnell KO and Blotcky AL. Relationship between serum selenium levels and patients with carcinoma. *Cancer.* 37:1384, 1976.

Burney PGJ, Comstock GW and Morris JS. Serologic precursors of cancer: Serum micronutrients and the subsequent risk of pancreatic cancer. *Am. J. Clin. Nutr.* 49:895–900, 1989.

Clark L. The epidemiology of selenium and cancer. *Fed. Proc.* 44:2584–2589, 1985.

Dworkin BM et al. Selenium deficiency in the acquired immunodeficiency syndrome. *J. Par. Ent. Nutr.* 10:405–407, 1986.

Ip C. Interaction of vitamin C and selenium supplementation in the modification of mammary carcinogenesis in rats. *J.N.C.I.* 77:299, 1986.

Ip C. Selenium inhibition of chemical carcinogenesis. *Fed. Proc.* 44: 2573–2578, 1985.

Kiremidjian-Schumacher L and Stotzky G. Selenium and immune responses. *Environmental Research.* 42:277–303, 1987.

Kok FJ et al. Decreased selenium levels in acute myocardial infarction. *J. Am. Med. Assoc.* 261:1161–1164, 1989.

Kok FJ et al. Selenium status and chronic disease mortality: Dutch epidemiological findings. *International Journal of Epidemiology.* 16:329–331, 1987.

Korpella H et al. Decreased serum selenium in alcoholics as related to liver structure and function. *Am. J. Clin. Nutr.* 42:147–151, 1985.

McConnell KP et al. The relationship of dietary selenium and breast cancer. *J. Surg. Oncol.* 8:67, 1980.

Menkes MS et al. Serum beta-carotene, vitamins A and E, selenium and risk of lung cancer. *N. Eng. J. Med.* 315:1250–1254, 1986.

Moore JA, Noive R and Wells IC. Selenium concentrations in plasma of patients with arteriographically defined coronary atherosclerosis. *Clinical Chemistry.* 30:1171–1173, 1984.

Oster O et al. The serum selenium concentration of patients with acute myocardial infarction. *Ann. Clin. Res.* 18:36, 1986.

Perry HM Jr and Erlanger MW. Prevention of cadmium-induced hypertension by selenium. *Fed. Proc.* 33:357, 1974.

Salonen JT. Association between serum selenium and the risk of cancer. *Am. J. Epidemiol.* 120:342–349, 1984.

Salonen JT et al. Association between cardiovascular death and myocardial infarction and serum selenium in a matched-pair longitudinal study. *Lancet.* 2:175, 1982.

Salonen JT et al. Risk of cancer in relation to serum concentrations of selenium and vitamins A and E: Matched case control analysis of prospective data. *Br. Med. J.* 290:417–420, 1985.

Schrauzer GN. Selenium and cancer: A review. *Bioinorg. Chem.* 5:275, 1976.

Schrauzer GN, White DA and Schneider CJ. Cancer mortality correlation studies III: Statistical associations with dietary selenium intakes. *Bioinorg. Chem.* 7:23–34, 1977.

Shamberger RJ et al. Antioxidants and cancer: I. Selenium in the blood of normals and cancer patients. *J.N.C.I.* 50:863, 1973.

Stead RJ et al. Selenium deficiency and possible increased risk of carcinoma in adults with cystic fibrosis. *Lancet.* 2:862–863, 1985.

Tolonen M, Halme and Sarna S. Vitamin E and selenium supplementation in geriatric patients. *Biol. Trace Elem. Res.* 7:161, 1985.

Van Vleet JF et al. Effect of selenium-vitamin E on adriamycin-induced cardiomyopathy in rabbits. *Am. J. Vet. Res.* 39:997, 1978.

Whanger PD. Selenium and heavy metal toxicity. In: Spallholz JE, Martin JL and Ganther HE (eds.), *Selenium in Biology and Medicine.* Westport: AVI Publishing, 1981, p. 230.

Willett WC et al. Prediagnostic serum selenium and risk of cancer. *Lancet.* 2:130–133, 1983.

Yang G et al. Endemic selenium intoxication of humans in China. *Am. J. Clin. Nutr.* 37:872–881, 1983.

Yu S-Y et al. Regional variation of cancer mortality incidence and its relation to selenium levels in China. *Biol. Trace Elem. Res.* 7:21–29, 1985.

Silicon

Carlisle EM. The nutritional essentiality of silicon. *Nutr. Rev.* 40:193–198, 1982.

Schwarz K. A bound form of silicon in glycosaminoglycans and polyuronides. *Proc. Nat. Acad. Sci.* 70:1608–1612, 1973.

Schwarz K. Silicon, fibre and atherosclerosis. *Lancet.* 1:454–456, 1977.

Vanadium

Anonymous. Vanadium, vitamin C and depression. *Nutr. Rev.* 40:293–295, 1982.

Heyliger CE, Tahiliani AG and McNeill JH. Effect of vanadate on elevated blood glucose and depressed cardiac performance of diabetic rats. *Science.* 227:1474, 1985.

Naylor GJ. Vanadium and manic-depressive psychosis. *Nutrition and Health.* 3:79, 1984.

Naylor GJ and Smith AHW. Vanadium: A possible aetiological factor in manic-depressive illness. *Psychological Medicine.* 11:249–256, 1981.

Zinc

Brewer GJ et al. Oral zinc therapy for Wilson's disease. *Ann. Intern. Med.* 99:314–320, 1983.

Brody I. Topical treatment of recurrent herpes simplex and post-herpetic erythema multiforme with low concentrations of zinc sulfate solution. *Br. J. Derm.* 104:191–194, 1981.

Bulbena EG. Zinc compounds, a new treatment in peptic ulcer. *Drugs Under Experimental and Clinical Research.* 15(2):83–89, 1989.

Carruthers R. Oral zinc in cutaneous healing. *Drugs.* 6:164, 1973.

Chandra RK. Excessive intake of zinc impairs immune responses. *J. Am. Med. Assoc.* 252:1443–1446, 1984.

Cohen C. Zinc sulphate and bed sores. *Br. Med. J.* 2:561, 1968.

Crouse SF et al. Zinc ingestion and lipoprotein values in sedentary and endurance-trained men. *J. Am. Med. Assoc.* 252:785, 1984.

DeWys W and Pories W. Inhibition of a spectrum of animal tumors by dietary zinc deficiency. *J.N.C.I.* 48:375–381, 1972.

Duchateau J et al. Beneficial effects of oral zinc supplementation on the immune response of old people. *Am. J. Med.* 70:1001–1004, 1981.

Eby GA, Davis DA and Halcomb WW. Reduction in duration of common colds by zinc gluconate lozenges in a double-blind study. *Antimicrobial Agents and Chemotherapy.* 25:20, 1984.

Fabris N et al. AIDS, zinc deficiency, and thymic hormone failure. *J. Am. Med. Assoc.* (Letter). 259:839–840, 1988.

Falutz J, Tsoukas C and Gold P. Zinc as a cofactor in human immunodeficiency virus-induced immunosuppression. *J. Am. Med. Assoc.* 259:2850–2851, 1988.

Fong LYY et al. Zinc deficiency and the development of esophageal and forestomach tumors in Sprague-Dawley rats fed precursors of N-nitroso-N-benzylmethylamine. *J.N.C.I.* 72:419–425, 1984.

Fraker PJ et al. Interrelationships between zinc and immune function. *Fed. Proc.* 45:1479, 1986.

Freeland-Graves JH et al. Effect of zinc supplementation on plasma high-density lipoprotein cholesterol and zinc. *Am. J. Clin. Nutr.* 35:988, 1982.

Frommer DJ. The healing of gastric ulcers by zinc sulphate. *Med. J. Aust.* 2:793, 1975.

Greaves MW and Ive FA. Double-blind trial of zinc sulphate in the treatment of chronic venous leg ulceration. *Br. J. Derm.* 87:632, 1972.

Habib FK. Zinc and the steroid endocrinology of the human prostate. *Journal of Steroid Biochemistry.* 9:403–407, 1978.

Hansen MA, Fernandes G and Good RA. Nutrition and immunity: The influence of diet on autoimmunity and the role of zinc in the immune response. *Ann. Rev. Nutr.* 2:151–177, 1982.

Hooper PL et al. Zinc lowers high-density lipoprotein cholesterol levels. *J. Am. Med. Assoc.* 244:1960–1961, 1980.

Kinlaw WB et al. Abnormal zinc metabolism in type II diabetes mellitus. *Am. J. Med.* 75:273–277, 1983.

Lally EV and Crowley JP. An element of uncertainty: The clinical significance of zinc deficiency in rheumatoid arthritis. *Internal Medicine.* 8(1):98–107, 1987.

Leissner KH, Fjelkegard B and Tisell LS. Concentration and content of zinc in the human prostate. *Investigative Urology.* 18:32–35, 1980.

McClain CJ and Su L. Zinc deficiency in the alcoholic: A review. *Alcoholism.* 7:5–10, 1983.

Michaelsson G. Oral zinc in acne. *Acta Dermatovener (Supplement).* 89:87, 1980.

Myers MB and Cherry G. Zinc and the healing of chronic leg ulcers. *Am. J. Surg.* 120:77, 1970.

Newsome DA et al. Oral zinc in macular degeneration. *Archives of Ophthalmology.* 106:192–198, 1988.

Pories WJ et al. Acceleration of wound healing in man with zinc sulphate given by mouth. *Lancet.* 1:1069, 1969.

Rasker JJ and Kardaun SH. Lack of beneficial effect of zinc sulphate in rheumatoid arthritis. *Scand. J. Rheumatol.* 11:168, 1982.

Rosoff B. Studies of zinc in hormal and neoplastic prostatic tissues. In: *The Prostatic Cell: Structure and Function.* New York: Alan R. Liss, 1981, pp. 447–457.

Russell RM et al. Zinc and the special senses. *Ann. Intern. Med.* 99:227–239, 1983.

Schachner L. The treatment of acne: A contemporary review. *Pediatric Clinics of North America.* 30:501–510, 1983.

Sergeant GR, Galloway RE and Gueri MC. Oral zinc sulphate in sickle cell ulcers. *Lancet.* 2:891, 1970.

Simkin PA. Treatment of rheumatoid arthritis with oral zinc sulphate. *Agents Action Suppl.* 8:587–596, 1981.

Verm KC, Saini AS and Dhamija SK. Oral zinc sulfate therapy in acne vulgaris: A double-blind trial. *Acta Dermatovener.* 60:337–340, 1980.

AMINO ACIDS

L-Arginine (and Ornithine)

Albina JE et al. Arginine metabolism in wounds. *American Journal of Physiology.* 254:E459–E467, 1988.

Barbul A. Arginine: Biochemistry, physiology and therapeutic implications. *J. Par. Ent. Nutr.* 10:227–238, 1986.

Barbul A et al. Arginine stimulates lymphocyte immune response in healthy human beings. *Surgery.* 90:244–251, 1981.

Barbul A et al. Immunostimulatory effects of arginine in normal and injured rats. *Journal of Surgical Research.* 29:228–235, 1980.

Barbul A et al. Arginine: Supplemental arginine, wound healing, and thymus: Arginine-pituitary interaction. *Surgical Forum.* 29:93, 1978.

Barbul A et al. Thymic stimulatory actions of arginine. *J. Par. Ent. Nutr.* 4:446–449, 1980.

Barbul A et al. Thymotropic and wound-healing promoting agent. *Surgical Forum.* 28:101–103, 1977.

Isidori A, Lo Monaco A and Cappa M. A study of growth hormone release in man after oral administration of amino acids. *Current Medical Research and Opinion.* 7:475–481, 1981.

Milner JA and Stepanovich LV. Inhibitory effect of dietary arginine on growth of Ehrlich ascites tumor cells in mice. *J. Nutr.* 109:489–494, 1979.

Moncada S, Palmer RMJ and Higgs EA. Biosynthesis of nitric oxide from L-arginine. *Biochemical Pharmacology.* 38:1709–1715, 1989.

Moriguchi S et al. Functional changes in human lymphocytes and monocytes after in vitro incubation with arginine. *Nutrition Research.* 7:719–729, 1987.

Pryme IF. The effects of orally administered L-arginine HCL on the development of myeloma tumours in Balb/c mice following the injection of single cell suspensions, cell aggregates or tumor fragments; and on the growth of two ascites tumour cell lines. *Cancer Letters.* 5:19, 1978.

Rettura G et al. Supplemental arginine increases thymic cellularity in normal and murine sarcoma virus-inoculated mice and increases the resistance to murine sarcoma virus tumor. *J. Par. Ent. Nutr.* 3:409–416, 1979.

Schachter A et al. Treatment of oligospermia with the amino acid arginine. *J. Urol.* 110:311–313, 1973.

Seifter E et al. Arginine: An essential amino acid for injured rats. *Surgery.* 84:224–230, 1978.

Seifter E et al. Supplemental arginine increases survival in mice undergoing local tumor excision. *J. Par. Ent. Nutr.* 5:589, 1980.

Takeda Y et al. Inhibitory effect on L-arginine on growth of rat mammary tumors induced by 7,12-dimethylbenz(a)anthracene. *Ca. Res.* 35:2390–2393, 1975.

L-Aspartic Acid

Ahlborg B, Ekelund LG and Nilsson CG. Effect of potassium-magnesium-aspartate on the capacity for prolonged exercise in man. *Acta Physiologica Scandinavia.* 74:238–245, 1968.

Hagan RD et al. Absence of effect of potassium-magnesium aspartate on physiologic responses to prolonged work in aerobically trained men. *International Journal of Sports Medicine.* 3:177–181, 1982.

Hicks JT. Treatment of fatigue in general practice: A double-blind study. *Clinical Medicine.* 71:85–90, 1964.

Nieper HA and Blumberger K. Electrolyte transport therapy of cardiovascular diseases. In: Bajusz E (ed.), *Electrolytes and Cardiovascular Diseases,* Volume 2. Basel/New York: S. Karger, 1966, pp. 141–173.

Sener AI et al. Comparison of the suppressive effects of L-aspartic acid and chlorpromazine and diazepam treatments on opiate abstinence syndrome signs in man. *Arzneimittel-Forschung.* 36:1684–1686, 1986.

Branched-Chain Amino Acids

Anonymous. Branched-chain amino acids reverse hepatic encephalopathy. *Internal Medicine News.* 18(18):5, 1985.

Anonymous. Parkinson's researchers try amino acid therapy. *Medical World News.* P. 26, November 8, 1982.

Baker AL. Amino acids in liver disease: A cause of hepatic encephalopathy? (Editorial). *J. Am. Med. Assoc.* 242:355–356, 1979.

Bower RH, Kern KA and Fischer JE. Use of a branched-chain amino acid enriched solution in patients under metabolic stress. *Am. J. Surg.* 149:266–270, 1985.

Cerra FB et al. Branched chains support postoperative protein synthesis. *Surgery.* 92:192–199, 1982.

Freund H et al. The role of the branched-chain amino acids in decreasing muscle catabolism in vivo. *Surgery.* 83:611–618, 1978.

Okada A et al. Branched-chain amino acids metabolic support in surgical patients: A randomized, controlled trial in patients with subtotal or total gastrectomy in sixteen (16) Japanese institutions. *J. Par. Ent. Nutr.* 12:332–337, 1987.

Plaitakas A et al. Pilot trial of branched-chain amino acids in amyotrophic lateral sclerosis. *Lancet.* 1:1015–1018, 1988.

L-Cysteine (and Glutathione)

Anderson R, Theron AJ and Ras GJ. Regulation by the antioxidants ascorbate, cysteine and dapsone of the increased extracellular and intracellular generation of reactive oxidants by activated phagocytes from cigarette smokers. *American Review of Respiratory Diseases.* 135:1027–1032, 1987.

Campbell NR, Reade PG and Radden BG. Effect of cysteine on the survival of mice with transplanted malignant thymoma. *Nature.* 251:158–159, 1974.

Forman HJ, Rotman EI and Fisher AB. Role of selenium and sulfur-containing amino acids in protection against oxygen toxicity. *Laboratory Investigation.* 49:148–153, 1983.

Lieber CS. The influence of alcohol on nutritional status. *Nutr. Rev.* 46:241–254, 1988.

Meister A. New aspects of glutathione biochemistry and transport: Selective alteration of glutathionine metabolism. *Nutr. Rev.* 42:397–410, 1984.

Meister A. Selective modification of glutathione metabolism. *Science.* 220:472–477, 1983.

Oeriu S and Vochitu E. The effect of the administration of compounds which contain sulfhydryl groups on the survival rates of mice, rats and guinea pigs. *Journal of Gerontology.* 20:417, 1965.

Springe et al. Protectants against acetaldehyde toxicity: Sulfhydryl compounds and ascorbic acid. *Fed. Proc.* Federation of the American Society for Experimental Biology, Abstract No. 172. P. 233, March 1974.

L-Glutamine/L-Glutamic Acid

Astin AW and Ross S. Glutamic acid and intelligence. *Psychological Bulletin.* 57:429–443, 1960.

Bulus N et al. Physiological importance of glutamine. *Metabolism.* 38(8): Supplement 1, pp. 1–5, 1989.

Fincle LP. The effect of L-glutamine on psychiatric hospitalized alcoholic patients. *Bedford Research.* Bedford, Massachusetts. Veteran's Administration Hospital. 7(1):2, January 2, 1961.

Fincle LP. Experiments in treating alcoholics with glutamic acid and glutamine. *Biochemical and Nutritional Aspects of Alcoholism.* Proceedings of symposium sponsored by The Christopher D. Smithers Foundation and The Clayton Foundation Biochemical Institute. The University of Texas, Austin, 1964, pp. 26–37.

Flot, Carry and Rosier. Some clinical results in the treatment of alcoholism with L-glutamic acid monoamide. *Le Journal de Medecine de Lyon.* 45:1067–1080, 1964.

Jackson DV et al. Amelioration of vincristine neurotoxicity by glutamic acid. *Am. J. Med.* 84:1016–1022, 1988.

Mebane AH. L-glutamine and mania (Letter). *Am. J. Psychiatry.* 141:1302–1303, 1984.

Ravel JM et al. Reversal of alcohol toxicity by glutamine. *Journal of Biological Chemistry.* 214:497, 1955.

Rogers LL and Pelton RB. Glutamine in the treatment of alcoholism. *Quarterly Journal of Studies on Alcohol.* 18:581, 1957.

Rogers LL, Pelton RB and Williams RJ. Voluntary alcohol consumption by rats following administration of glutamine. *Journal of Biological Chemistry.* 214:503–506, 1955.

Shive W. Glutamine as a metabolic agent protecting against alcohol poisoning. *Biochemical and Nutritional Aspects of Alcoholism.* Proceedings of symposium sponsored by The Christopher D. Smithers Foundation and The Clayton Foundation Biochemical Institute. The University of Texas, Austin, 1964, pp. 17–25.

Glycine

Barbeau A. Preliminary study of glycine administration in patients with spasticity. *Neurology.* 24:392, 1974.

Davidoff RA. Antispasticity drugs: Mechanism of action. *Annals of Neurology.* 17:107–116, 1985.

Stern P and Bakonjic R. Glycine therapy in seven (7) cases of spasticity: A pilot study. *Pharmacology.* 12:117–119, 1974.

Histidine

Gerber DA. Treatment of rheumatoid arthritis with histidine. *Clinical Research.* 17:351, 1969.

McCarty M. Supplementary histidine may promote suppressor T cell activity. *Medical Hypothesis.* (In press.)

Pinals RS et al. Treatment of rheumatoid arthritis with L-histidine: A randomized, placebo-controlled, double-blind trial. *Journal of Rheumatology.* 4:414, 1977.

L-Lysine

DiGiovanna JJ and Blank H. Failure of lysine in frequently recurrent herpes simplex infection: Treatment and prophylaxis. *Archives of Dermatology.* 120:48–51, 1984.

Griffith RS et al. Success of L-lysine therapy in frequently recurrent herpes simplex infection. *Dermatologica.* 175:183–190, 1987.

Griffith RS, Norins AL and Kagan C. A multicentered study of lysine therapy in herpes simplex infection. *Dermatologica.* 156:257–267, 1978.

Isidori A, LaMonaco A and Cappa M. A study of growth hormone release in man after oral administration of amino acids. *Current Medical Research and Opinion.* 7:475–481, 1981.

Kagan C. Lysine therapy for herpes simplex. *Lancet.* 1:137, 1974.

McCune MA et al. Treatment of recurrent herpes simplex infections with L-lysine monohydrochloride. *Cutis.* 34:366–373, 1984.

Simon CA, VanMelle GD and Ramelet AA. Failure of lysine in the therapy of herpes simplex. *Journal of Antimicrobial Chemotherapy.* 12:489–496, 1983.

L-Methionine and Taurine

Azuma J et al. Therapeutic effect of taurine in congestive heart failure: A double-blind crossover trial. *Clinical Cardiology.* 8:276, 1985.

Barbeau A. Zinc, taurine and epilepsy. *Archives of Neurology.* 30:52, 1974.

Barbeau A et al. The neuropharmacology of taurine. *Life Sciences.* 17:669–678, 1975.

Belli DC et al. Taurine improves the absorption of a fat meal in patients with cystic fibrosis. *Pediatrics.* 80:517–523, 1987.

Chesney RW. Taurine: Its biological role and clinical implications. *Advances in Pediatrics.* 22:1–42, 1985.

Geggel HS et al. Nutritional requirements for taurine in patients receiving long-term parenteral nutrition. *N. Eng. J. Med.* 312:142–146, 1985.

Hayes KC. Taurine requirements in primates. *Nutr. Rev.* 43(3):65–70, 1985.

Hayes KC, Carey RE and Schmidt SY. Retinal degeneration associated with taurine deficiency in the cat. *Science.* 188:949–951, 1975.

Hayes KC and Sturman JA. Taurine in metabolism. *Ann. Rev. Nutr.* 1:401–425, 1981.

Kulkowski EC and Maturo J. Hypoglycemic properties of taurine: Not mediated by enhanced insulin release. *Biochemical Pharmacology.* 33:2835–2838, 1984.

Lampson WG, Kramer JH and Schaefer SW. Potenti-ation of the actions of insulin by taurine. *Canadian Journal of Physiology and Pharmacology.* 61:457–463, 1983.

Pion PD. Myocardial failure in cats associated with low plasma taurine: A reversible cardiomyopathy. *Science.* 237:764–768, 1987.

Takahashi R and Nakane Y. Clinical trial of taurine in epilepsy. In: Barbeau A and Huxtable RJ (eds.), *Taurine and Neurological Disorders.* New York: Raven Press, 1978, p. 375.

Takihara K et al. Beneficial effect of taurine in rabbits with chronic congestive heart failure. *Am. Heart J.* 112:1278, 1986.

L-Phenylalanine, D-Phenylalanine, DL-Phenylalanine

Balagot RC and Ehrenpreis S. Continuing studies of D-phenylalanine induced analgesia in mice and humans. *Anesthesiology.* 51:S231, 1979.

Beckman H et al. DL-Phenylalanine versus imipramine: A double-blind controlled study. *Archiv für Psychiatrie und Nervenkrankheiten.* 227:49, 1979.

Beckman VH and Ludolph E. DL-phenylalanine as antidepressant. *Arzneimittel-Forschung.* 28:1283–1284, 1978.

Blum K et al. Enkephalinase inhibition: Regulation of ethanol intake in genetically predisposed mice. *Alcohol.* 4:449–456, 1987.

Budd K. Use of D-phenylalanine, an enkephalinase inhibitor, in the treatment of intractable pain. *Advances in Pain Research and Therapy.* 5:305, 1983.

Cheng RS and Pomeranz B. A combined treatment with D-amino acids and electroacupuncture produces a greater analgesia than either treatment alone; naloxone reverses these effects. *Pain.* 8:231–236, 1980.

Ehrenpreis S. D-phenylalanine and other enkephalinase inhibitors as pharmacological agents: Implications for some important therapeutic application. *Substance and Alcohol Actions/Misuse.* 3:231–239, 1982.

Ehrenpreis S et al. Further studies on the analgesic activity of D-phenylalanine (DPA) in mice and humans. In: Way EL (ed.), *Endogenous and Exogenous Opiate Agonists and Antagonists.* New York: Pergamon Press, 1980, pp. 379–381.

Ehrenpreis S et al. Naloxone reversible analgesia in mice produced by D-phenylalanine and hydrocinnamic acid, inhibitors of carboxypeptidase A. *Advances in Pain Research and Therapy.* 3:479–487, 1979.

Hyodo M, Kitada T and Hosoka E. Study on the enhanced analgesic effect induced by phenylalanine during acupuncture analgesia in humans. *Advances in Pain Research and Therapy.* 5:577, 1983.

Kravitz HM, Sabelli HC and Fawcett J. Dietary supplements of phenylalanine and other amino acid precursors of brain neuroamines in the treatment of depressive disorders. *Journal of the American Osteopathic Association.* 84:119, 1984.

Seltzer S, Marcus and Stoch R. Perspectives in the control of Chronic Pain by Nutritional Manipulation. *Pain.* 11:141–148, 1981.

Spatz H, Heller B, Nachon M and Fischer E. Effects of D-phenylalanine on clinical picture and phenylethylaminuria in depression. *Biological Psychiatry.* 10:235, 1975.

Walsh NE et al. Analgesic effectiveness of D-phenylalanine in chronic pain patients. *Archives of Physical Medicine and Rehabilitation.* 67:436, 1986.

L-Tryptophan

Anonymous. L-tryptophan interval therapy is effective in chronic insomnia. *Internal Medicine News.* 17(18):11, 1984.

Anonymous. Tryptophan aids adjustment to jet lag, shift work. *Internal Medicine News.* 20(4):53, 1987.

Brewerton TD and Reus VI. Lithium carbonate and L-tryptophan in the treatment of bipolar and schizophrenic disorders. *Am. J. Psychiatry.* 140:757–760, 1983.

Hartmann E. L-tryptophan: A rational hypnotic with clinical potential. *Am. J. Psychiatry.* 134:366, 1977.

Hartmann E, Chung R and Chien C-O. L-tryptophan and sleep. *Psychopharmacologia* (Berlin). 19:114–127, 1971.

Hartmann E and Spinweber CL. Sleep induced by L-tryptophan: Effect of dosages within the normal dietary intake. *Journal of Nervous and Mental Disease.* 167:497–499, 1979.

Hrboticky N et al. Effects of L-tryptophan on short term food intake in lean men. *Nutrition Research.* 5:595–607, 1985.

King RB. Pain and tryptophan. *Journal of Neurosurgery.* 53:44, 1980.

Leiter LA et al. Failure of L-tryptophan to improve weight loss in obese dieters. *Proceedings from the Fourth International Congress on Obesity.* 68A(Abstract), 1983.

Lyness WH. Effect of L-tryptophan pretreatment on d-amphetamine self administration. *Substance and Alcohol Actions/Misuse.* 4:305–312, 1983.

Rosecrans JS. The treatment of cocaine abuse with imipramine, L-tyrosine and L-tryptophan. Reported before the VII World Congress of Psychiatry, Vienna, Austria, 1983.

Seltzer S et al. The effects of dietary tryptophan on chronic maxillofacial pain and experimental pain tolerance. *Journal of Psychiatric Research.* 17:181, 1982.

Shpeen SE, Morse DR and Furst ML. The effect of tryptophan on postoperative endodontic pain. *Oral Surgery, Oral Medicine and Oral Pathology.* 58:446, 1984.

Wyatt RJ et al. Effects of L-tryptophan (a natural sedative) on human sleep. *Lancet.* 2:842, 1970.

Yoshida O et al. Relation between tryptophan metabolism and heterotropic recurrences of human urinary bladder tumors. *Cancer.* 25:773–780, 1970.

L-Tyrosine

Elwes RDC et al. Treatment of narcolepsy with L-tyrosine: Double-blind placebo-controlled trial. *Lancet.* 2:1067–1068, 1989.

Gelenberg AJ et al. Tyrosine for the treatment of depression. *Am. J. Psychiatry.* 137:622–623, 1980.

Gold MS et al. Cocaine withdrawal: Efficacy of tyrosine (Abstract). *Soc. Neurosc.* 9:157, 1983.

Goldberg IK. L-tyrosine in depression. *Lancet.* 2:364, 1980.

Goleman D. Food and brain: Psychiatrists explore use of nutrients in treating disorders (Report). *New York Times.* Pp. 15–18, March 1, 1988.

Laborit H and Valette N. The action of L-tyrosine and arachidonic acid on the experimental hypertension in rats: Physiopathogenic deductions. *Res. Com. Chem. Path. Pharm.* 8:489, 1974.

Mouret J et al. Treatment of narcolepsy with L-tyrosine. *Lancet.* 2:1458–1459, 1989.

Reimherr RW et al. An open trial of L-tyrosine in the treatment of attention deficit disorders, residual type. *Am. J. Psychiatry.* 144:1071–1073, 1987.

Reinstein DK, Lehnert H and Wurtman RJ. Dietary tyrosine suppresses the rise in plasma corticosterone following acute stress in rats. *Life Sciences.* 37:2157–2163, 1985.

Sved AF, Fernstrom JD and Wurtman RJ. Tyrosine administration reduces blood pressure and enhances brain norepinephrine release in spontaneously hypertensive rats. *Proc. Nat. Acad. Sci.* 76:3511–3514, 1979.

Tennant F. Stepwise detoxification from cocaine. *Postgraduate Medicine.* 84:225–235, 1988.

LIPIDS AND DERIVATIVES

AL 721

Grieco MH et al. Open study of AL 721 treatment of HIV-infected subjects with generalized lymphadenopathy syndrome: An eight week open trial and follow-up. *Antiviral Research.* 9:177–190, 1988.

Heron DS, Shinitzky M and Samuel D. Alleviation of drug withdrawal symptoms by treatment with a potent mixture of natural lipids. *European Journal of Pharmacology.* 83:253–261, 1982.

Lyte M and Shinitzky M. A special lipid mixture for membrane fluidization. *Biochimica et Biophysica Acta.* 812:133–138, 1985.

Rabinowich H et al. Augmentation of mitogen responsiveness in the aged by a special lipid diet AL 721. *Mechanisms of Ageing and Development.* 40:131–138, 1987.

Sarin PS et al. Effects of a novel compound (AL 721) on HTLV-III infectivity in vitro. *N. Eng. J. Med.* 313:1289–1290, 1985.

Shinitzky M and Haimovitz R. Dissemination and activity of AL 721 after oral administration. In: Hanin I and Ansell GB (eds.), *Lecithin: Technological, Biological and Therapeutic Aspects.* New York: Plenum Press, 1987, pp. 155–166.

Fish Oils/EPA and DHA

Allen BR et al. The effects on psoriasis of dietary supplementation with eicosapentaenoic acid. *Br. J. Derm.* 113:777, 1986.

Anderson GJ and Connor WE. On the demonstration of omega-3 essential-fatty-acid deficiency in humans (Editorial). *Am. J. Clin. Nutr.* 49:585–587, 1989.

Bang HO and Dyerberg J. Plasma lipids and lipoproteins in Greenlandic West Coast Eskimos. *Acta Medica Scandinavica.* 192:85–94, 1972.

Berlin E, Matusik EJ and Young C Jr. Effect of dietary fat on the fluidity of platelet membrane. *Lipids.* 15:604–608, 1980.

Bjorneboe A et al. Effect of dietary supplementation with eicosapentaenoic acid in the treatment of atopic dermatitis. *Br. J. Derm.* 117:463–469, 1987.

Catherine E et al. Topical eicosapentaenoic acid (EPA) in the treatment of psoriasis. *Br. J. Derm.* 120:581–584, 1989.

Chandra RK. There is more to fish than fish oils. *Nutrition Research.* 8:1–2, 1988.

Culp BR et al. The effect of dietary supplementation of fish oil on experimental myocardial infarction. *Prostaglandins.* 20:1021, 1980.

Davidson MH and Liebson PR. Marine lipids and atherosclerosis: A review. *Cardiovascular Reviews and Reports.* 7:461–468, 1986.

Dehmer GJ et al. Reduction in the rate of early restenosis after coronary angioplasty by a diet supplemented with n-3 fatty acids. *N. Eng. J. Med.* 319:733–740, 1988.

DiGiacomo RA, Kremer JL and Shah DM. Fish-oil dietary supplementation in patients with Raynaud's phenomenon: A double-blind, controlled, prospective study. *Am. J. Med.* 86:158–164, 1989.

Dougherty RM et al. Lipid and phospholipid fatty acid composition of plasma, red blood cells and platelets and how they are affected by dietary lipids: A study of normal subjects from Italy, Finland and the USA. *Am. J. Clin. Nutr.* 45:443–455, 1987.

Driss F et al. Inhibition of platelet aggregation and thromboxane synthesis after intake of small amount of eicosapentaenoic acid. *Thrombosis Research.* 36:389–396, 1984.

Fox PL and DiCorleto PE. Fish oils inhibit endothelial cell production of platelet-derived growth factor like protein. *Science.* 241:453–456, 1988.

Friday KE et al. The effect of omega-3 fatty acid supplementation on glucose homeostasis and plasma lipoproteins in type II diabetic subjects. *Am. J. Clin. Nutr.* 45:871, 1987.

Glauber H et al. Adverse effect of omega-3 fatty acids in non-insulin dependent diabetes mellitus. *Ann. Intern. Med.* 108:663–668, 1988.

Goodnight SH Jr., Harris WS and Connor WE. The effects of dietary omega-3 fatty acids on platelet composition and function in man: A prospective, controlled study. *Blood.* 58:880–885, 1981.

Gorlin R. The biological actions and potential clinical significance of dietary omega-3 fatty acids. *Archives of Internal Medicine.* 148:2043–2048, 1988.

Harris WS. Effect of a low saturated fat, low cholesterol fish oil supplement in hypertriglyceridemic patients: A placebo-controlled trial. *Ann. Intern. Med.* 109:465–470, 1988.

Hay CRM, Durber AP and Saynor R. Effect of fish oil on platelet kinetics in patients with ischaemic heart disease. *Lancet.* 1:1269, 1982.

Kamada T et al. Dietary sardine oil increases erythrocyte membrane fluidity in diabetic patients. *Diabetes.* 35:604–611, 1986.

Kamido H, Matsuzawa Y and Tarui S. Lipid composition of platelets from patients with atherosclerosis: Effect of purified eicosapentaenoic acid ethyl ester administration. *Lipids.* 23:917–923, 1988.

Kettler AH et al. The effect of dietary fish oil supplementation on psoriasis. *J. Am. Acad. Derm.* 18:1267–1273, 1988.

Knapp HR and Fitzgerald GA. The antihypertensive effects of fish oil: A controlled study of polyunsaturated fatty acid supplements in essential hypertension. *N. Eng. J. Med.* 320:1037–1043, 1989.

Kremer JM et al. Effects of manipulation of dietary fatty acids on clinical manifestations of rheumatoid arthritis. *Lancet.* 1:184–187, 1985.

Kremer JM et al. Fish oil fatty acid supplementation in active rheumatoid arthritis. *Ann. Intern. Med.* 106:497–506, 1987.

Kromhout D, Bosschieter EB and Coulander D de L. The inverse relation between fish consumption and 20-year mortality from coronary heart disease. *N. Eng. J. Med.* 312:1205–1209, 1985.

Leaf A and Weber PC. Cardiovascular effects of n-3 fatty acids. *N. Eng. J. Med.* 318:549–557, 1988.

Lee TH et al. Effect of dietary enrichment with eicosapentaenoic and docosahexaenoic acids on in vitro neutrophil and monocyte leukotriene generation and neutrophil function. *N. Eng. J. Med.* 312:1217, 1985.

Levine PH et al. Dietary supplementation with omega-3 fatty acids prolongs platelet survival in hyperlipidemic patients with atherosclerosis. *Archives of Internal Medicine.* 149:1113–1116, 1989.

Lorenz R et al. Platelet function, thromboxane formation and blood pressure control during supplementation of the western diet with cod liver oil. *Circulation.* 67:504, 1983.

McCarren T et al. Amelioration of severe migraine by fish oil (omega-3) fatty acids. *Am. J. Clin. Nutr.* 41:874, 1985.

Mori TA et al. New findings in the fatty acid composition of individual platelet phospholipids in man after dietary fish oil supplementation. *Lipids.* 22:744–750, 1987.

Norris P, Jones CJH and Weston MJ. Effect of dietary supplementation with fish oil on systolic blood pressure in mild essential hypertension. *Br. Med. J.* 293:105, 1986.

Phillipson BE et al. Reduction of plasma lipids, lipoproteins and apoproteins by dietary fish oils in patients with hypertriglyceridemia. *N. Eng. J. Med.* 312:1210, 1985.

Raloff J. No-fault fat: More praise for fish oil. *Science News.* 134:228, 1988.

Reich R, Royce L and Martin GR. Eicosapentaenoic acid reduces the invasive and metastatic activities of malignant tumor cells. *Biochemical and Biophysical Research Communications.* 160:559–564, 1989.

Sanders TAB. Fish and coronary artery disease (Editorial). *British Heart Journal.* 57:214–219, 1987.

Saynor R and Verel D. Eicosapentaenoic acid, bleeding time and serum lipids. *Lancet.* 2:272, 1982.

Saynor R, Verel D and Gillot T. The long term effect of dietary supplementation with fish lipid concentrate on serum lipids, bleeding time, platelets and angina. *Atherosclerosis.* 50:3–10, 1984.

Simons LA, Hickie JB and Balasubramaniam S. On the effects of dietary n-3 fatty acids (Maxepa) on plasma lipids and lipoproteins in patients with hyperlipidemia. *Atherosclerosis.* 54:75, 1985.

Von Schacky C. Prophylaxis of atherosclerosis with marine omega-3 fatty acids. *Ann. Intern. Med.* 107:890–899, 1987.

Weiner BH et al. Inhibition of atherosclerosis by cod-liver oil in a hyperlipidemic swine model. *N. Eng. J. Med.* 315:841–846, 1986.

Woodcock BE et al. Beneficial effect of fish oil on blood viscosity in peripheral vascular disease. *Br. Med. J.* 288:592, 1984.

Yetiv JZ. Clinical applications of fish oils. *J. Am. Med. Assoc.* 260:665–669, 1982.

Gamma-Linolenic Acid and Oil of Evening Primrose

Bamford JT, Gibson RW and Renier CM. Atopic eczema unresponsive to evening primrose oil (linoleic and gamma-linolenic acids). *J. Am. Acad. Derm.* 13:959–965, 1985.

Belch JJF et al. Effects of altering dietary essential fatty acids on requirements for non-steroidal anti-inflammatory drugs in patients with rheumatoid arthritis: A double-blind placebo controlled study. *Annals of the Rheumatic Diseases.* 47:96–104, 1988.

Belch JJF et al. Evening primrose oil (Efamol) in the treatment of Reynaud's phenomenon: A double-blind study. *Thrombosis and Haemostasis.* 54:490–494, 1985.

Darlington LG. Do diets rich in polyunsaturated fatty acids affect disease activity in rheumatoid arthritis? *Annals of the Rheumatic Diseases.* 47:169–172, 1982.

Hanifin JM. Diet, nutrition and allergy in atopic dermatitis. *J. Am. Acad. Derm.* 8:729–731, 1983.

Jantti JT et al. Evening primrose oil in rheumatoid arthritis: Changes in serum lipids and fatty acids. *Annals of the Rheumatic Diseases.* 48:124–127, 1989.

Kendler BS. Gamma-linolenic acid: Physiological effects and potential medical applications. *Journal of Applied Nutrition.* 39:79–93, 1987.

Melnik BC and Plewig G. Is the origin of atopy linked to deficient conversion of omega-6-fatty acids to prostaglandin E1? *J. Am. Acad. Derm.* 21:557–563, 1989.

Skogh M. Atopic eczema unresponsive to evening primrose oil (linoleic and gamma-linolenic acids). *J. Am. Acad. Derm.* 15:114–115, 1986.

Wright S and Burton JL. Oral evening primrose seed oil improves atopic eczema. *Lancet.* 2:1120–1122, 1982.

Inositol (Myo-Inositol) and Phosphatidylinositol

Clements RS Jr. Review of myo-inositol and sorbinil studies. *Clin. Physiol.* 5(Suppl. 5):90, 1985.

Clements RS Jr. and Darnell B. Myo-inositol content of common foods: Development of a high-myo-inositol diet. *Am. J. Clin. Nutr.* 33:1954–1967, 1980.

Clements RS Jr. et al. Dietary myo-inositol intake and peripheral nerve function in diabetic neuropathy. *Metabolism.* 28:477, 1979.

Gregersen G et al. Oral supplementation of myo-inositol: Effects on peripheral nerve function in human diabetics and concentration in plasma, erythrocytes, urine and muscle tissue in human diabetics and normals. *Acta Neuro. Scand.* 67:164, 1983.

Salway JG et al. Effect of myo-inositol on peripheral-nerve function in diabetics. *Lancet.* 2:1282–1284, 1978.

Lecithin/Phosphatidycholine/Choline

Atoba MA, Ayoola EA and Ogunseyinde O. Effect of essential phospholipid choline on the course of acute hepatitis-B infection. *Tropical Gastroenterology.* 6(2):96–99, 1985.

Bartus RT et al. Age related changes in passive avoidance retention: Modulation with dietary choline. *Science.* 209:302–303, 1980.

Bartus RT et al. Profound effects of combining choline and piracetam on memory enhancement and cholinergic function in aged rats. *Neurobiol. Aging.* 2:105, 1981.

Bertoni-Freddari C et al. Chronic dietary choline modulates synaptic plasticity in the cerebellar glomeruli of aging mice. *Mechanisms of Ageing and Development.* 30:1, 1985.

Cohen BM, Lipinski JF and Altesman RI. Lecithin in the treatment of mania: Double-blind, placebo-controlled trials. *Am. J. Psychiatry.* 139:1162–1164, 1982.

Editorial. Dietary choline and synaptic morphology in mice. *Nutr. Rev.* 45:25, 1987.

Gelenberg AJ, Doller-Wojcik JC and Growdon JH. Choline and lecithin in the treatment of tardive dyskinesia: Preliminary results from a pilot study. *Am. J. Psychiatry.* 136:772–776, 1979.

Growdon JH. Use of phosphatidylcholine in brain diseases: An overview. In: Hanin I and Ansell GB (eds.), *Lecithin: Technological, Biological and Therapeutic Aspects.* New York: Plenum Press, 1987, pp. 121–136.

Growdon JH, Wheeler MA and Graham HN. Plasma choline responses to lecithin-enriched soup. *Psychopharmacology.* 20:603–606, 1984.

Growdon JH et al. Lecithin can suppress tardive dyskinesia. *N. Eng. J. Med.* 298:1029–1030, 1978.

Growdon JH et al. Oral choline administration to patients with tardive dyskinesia. *N. Eng. J. Med.* 297:524–527, 1977.

Hanin I and Ansell GB (eds.). *Lecithin: Technological, Biological and Therapeutic Aspects.* New York: Plenum Press, 1987.

Jackson IV et al. Treatment of tardive dyskinesia with lecithin. *Am. J. Psychiatry.* 136:1458–1460, 1979.

Jenkins PJ et al. Use of polyunsaturated phosphatidyl choline in HBsAg negative chronic active hepatitis: Results of prospective double-blind controlled trial. *Liver.* 2:77–81, 1982.

Kosina F et al. Essential cholinephospholipids in the treatment of virus hepatitis (translated from Czech). *Casopis Lekaru Ceskych.* 120:957–960, August 13, 1981.

Little A et al. A double-blind, placebo controlled trial of high-dose lecithin in Alzheimer's disease. *Journal of Neurology, Neurosurgery and Psychiatry.* 48:736–742, 1985.

Ma W-C. A cytopathological study of acute and chronic morphinism in the albino rat. *Chinese Journal of Physiology.* 5:251–278, 1931.

Mohs RC et al. Choline chloride effects on memory in the elderly. *Neurobiol. Aging.* 1:21, 1980.

Rosenberg GS and Davis KL. The use of cholinergic precursors in neuropsychiatric diseases. *Am. J. Clin. Nutr.* 36:709, 1982.

Shelly ED and Shelley WD. The fish odor syndrome: Trimethylaminuria. *J. Am. Med. Assoc.* 251:253–255, 1984.

Visco G. Polyunsaturated phosphatidylcholine in association with vitamin B complex in the treatment of acute viral hepatitis B (translated from Italian). *Clinica Terapeutica.* 114:183–188, 1985.

Wood JL and Allison RG. Effects of consumption of choline and lecithin on neurological and cardiovascular systems. *Fed. Proc.* 41:3015–3021, 1982.

Wurtman RJ, Hefti F and Melamed E. Precursor control of neurotransmitter synthesis. *Pharmacological Reviews*. 32:315–335, 1981.

Wurtman RJ, Hirsch MJ and Growdon JH. Lecithin consumption raises serum-free-choline levels. *Lancet*. 2:68–69, 1977.

Zeisel SH. Dietary choline: Biochemistry, physiology and pharmacology. *Ann. Rev. Nutr.* 1:95–121, 1981.

Liposomes

Ostro MJ. Liposomes. *Scientific American*. 256(1):102–111, 1987.

Zoler ML. Liposomes safely, quickly shrink cholesterol plaques (Report). *Medical World News*. Pp. 94–95, April 25, 1988.

Lipotropes/Activated Lipotropes

Bell KM et al. S-adenosylmethionine treatment of depression: A controlled clinical trial. *Am. J. Psychiatry*. 145:1110–1114, 1988.

Carney MWP, Toone BK and Reynolds EH. S-adenosylmethionine and effective behavior. *Am. J. Med.* 83 (Supplement 5A):104–106, 1987.

DeLeo D. S-adenosylmethionine as an antidepressant. *Curr. Ther. Res.* 41:865–870, 1987.

Kakihana M et al. Effects of CDP-choline on neurologic deficits and cerebral glucose metabolism in a rat model of cerebral ischemia. *Stroke*. 19:217–222, 1988.

Newberne PM, Nauss KM and deCamargo JLV. Lipotropes, immunocompetence, and cancer. *Ca. Res.* (Supplement). 43:2426s–2434s, 1983.

Proceedings of a Symposium. Osteoarthritis: The clinical picture, pathogenesis, and management

with studies on a new therapeutic agent, S-adenosylmethionine. *Am. J. Med.* 83(Supplement 5A), 1987.

Salvadorini F et al. Clinical evaluation of CDP-choline (Nicholin) efficacy as antidepressant treatment. *Curr. Ther. Res.* 18:513–520, 1975.

Tavoni A et al. Evaluation of S-adenosylmethionine in primary fibromyalgia. *Am. J. Med.* 83(Supplement 5A):107–110, 1987.

Monolaurin and Caprylic Acid

Hierholzer JC and Kabara JJ. In vitro effects of monolaurin compounds on enveloped RNA and DNA viruses. *Journal of Food Safety*. 4:1–12, 1982.

Kabara JJ. Lipids as host-resistance factors of human milk. *Nutr. Rev.* 38(2):65–73, 1980.

Kabara N et al. Fatty acids and derivatives as antimicrobial agents. *Antimicrobial Agents and Chemotherapy*. 2:23–28, 1972.

Sands J, Auperin D and Snipes W. Extreme sensitivity of enveloped viruses, including herpes simplex, to long-chain unsaturated monoglycerides and alcohols. *Antimicrobial Agents and Chemotherapy*. 15:67–73, 1979.

Phosphatidylserine and Phosphatidylethanolamine

Toffano G. The therapeutic value of phosphatidylserine effect in the aging brain. In: Hanin I and Ansell GB (eds.), *Lecithin: Technological, Biological and Therapeutic Aspects*. New York: Plenum Press, 1987, pp. 137–146.

NUCLEIC ACIDS

DNA and RNA

Aarons S et al. Immune RNA therapy as an effective adjuvant immunotherapy after surgery: An animal model. *J. Surg. Onc.* 23:21, 1983.

Brodsky I and Strayer DR. Therapeutic potential of Ampligen. *American Family Physician*. 36(4):253–256, 1987.

Cameron DE et al. Effects of ribonucleic acid on memory defect in the aged. *Am J. Psychiatry*. 120:320–325, 1963.

Fanslow WC et al. Effect of nucleotide restriction and supplementation on resistance to experimental murine candidiasis. *J. Par. Ent. Nutr.* 12:49–52, 1988.

Frank BS. *Nucleic Acid and Antioxidant Therapy of Aging and Degeneration*. New York: Rainstone Publishing, 1977.

Johnson AG. Immunomodulating effects of synthetic polynucleotides. *Journal of Biological Response Modifiers*. 4:481–483, 1985.

Kulkarni AD et al. Effect of dietary nucleotides on response to bacterial infections. *J. Par. Ent. Nutr.* 10:169–171, 1986.

Lacour J et al. Adjuvant treatment with polyadenylic • polyuridylic acid (poly A • poly U) in operable breast cancer. *Lancet*. 2:161–164, 1980.

Michelson AM, Lacour F and Lacour J. Polyadenylic • polyuridylic acid in the cotreatment of cancer. *Proceedings of the Society for Experimental Biology and Medicine*. 179:1–8, 1985.

Montefiori DC, Robinson WE Jr. and Mitchell WM. Mismatched ds RNA (Ampligen) induces protection against genomic variants of the human immunodeficiency virus type I (HIV-1) in a multiplicity of target cells. *Antiviral Research.* 9:47–56, 1988.

Nodine JH et al. A double-blind study of the effect of ribonucleic acid in senile brain disease. *Am. J. Psychiatry.* 123:1257–1259, 1967.

Newman EA and Grossman MI. Effect of nucleic acid supplements in the diet on rate of regeneration of liver in rats. *American Journal of Physiology.* 164:251–253, 1951.

Odens M. Prolongation of the life span in rats. *Journal of the American Geriatrics Society.* 21:450–451, 1973.

Pilch YH. Immunotherapy of cancer with "immune" RNA. *Am. J. Surg.* 132;631–637, 1976.

Werner EG et al. Dual biological activity of apurinic acid on human lymphocytes: Induction of interferon-gamma and protection from human immunodeficiency virus in vitro. *Antiviral Research.* 9:191–204, 1988.

Wiltrout RH et al. Immunomodulation of natural killer activity by polyribonucleotides. *Journal of Biological Response Modifiers.* 4:512–517, 1985.

Adenosine

Anonymous. Adenosine revisited (Editorial). *Lancet.* 2:927–928, 1985.

Belhassen B and Pelleg A. Acute management of paroxysmal supraventricular tachycardia: Verapamil, adenosine triphosphate or adenosine? *Am. J. Cardiol.* 25:225, 1985.

Belhassen B et al. Comparative clinical and electrophysiologic effects of adenosine triphosphate and verapamil on paroxysmal reciprocating junctional tachycardia. *Circulation.* 77:795, 1988.

Clarke B et al. Rapid and safe termination of supraventricular tachycardia in children by adenosine. *Lancet.* 1:299, 1987.

Drury AN and Szent-Gyorgi A. The physiological activity of adenine compounds with especial reference to their action upon the mammalian heart. *Journal of Physiology* (London). 68:213–237, 1929.

Greco R et al. Treatment of paroxysmal supraventricular tachycardia in infancy with digitals, adenosine-5′-triphosphate and verapamil: A comparative study. *Circulation.* 66:504–508, 1982.

Pelleg A. Cardiac cellular electrophysiologic actions of adenosine and adenosine triphosphate. *Am. Heart J.* 110:688–693, 1985.

Sklars S et al. Herpes zoster: The treatment and prevention of neuralgia with adenosine monophosphate. *J. Am. Med. Assoc.* 253:1427–1430, 1985.

Somlo E. Adenosine triphosphate in paroxysmal tachycardia. *Lancet.* 268:1125, 1955.

Inosine and Isoprinosine

Campoli-Richards DM, Sorkin EM and Heel RC. Inosine pranobex. *Drugs.* 32:383–424, 1986.

Glasky A et al. Isoprinosine in progressive generalized lymphadenopathy-kinetics of action and clinical response. *International Journal of Immunopathology.* 7, 3(Abstracts):318, 1985.

Scandinavian Isoprinosine Study Group, Hidovre, Denmark. Isoprinosine reduced clinical progression in HIV infected patients in a double blind placebo controlled study (Abstract). *Fifth International Conference on AIDS.* P. 219, 1989.

Tsang KY et al. In vitro restoration of immune responses in aging humans by isoprinosine. *International Journal of Immunopharmacology.* 7:199–206, 1985.

Tsang PH et al. Modulation of T- and B- lymphocyte functions by isoprinosine in homosexual subjects with prodromata and in patients with Acquired Immune Deficiency Syndrome (AIDS). *Journal of Clinical Immunology.* 4:469–478, 1984.

Wiedermann D, Wiedermannova D and Lokaj J. Immunorestoration in children with recurrent respiratory infections treated with isoprinosine. *International Journal of Immunopharmacology.* 9:947–949, 1987.

Orotic Acid

Bailey LE. The effect of orotic acid on excitation-contraction coupling in dystrophic hamster hearts. In: Shibata and Bailey (eds.), *Recent Development in Cardiac Muscle Pharmacology.* Tokyo: Igaku-Shoin, 1982, pp. 1–12.

Donohoe JA et al. The action of orotic acid as a positive inotropic agent during the acute phase of myocardial hypertrophy. *Australian and New Zealand Journal of Medicine.* 4:542–548, 1974.

O'Sullivan WJ. Orotic acid. *Australian and New Zealand Journal of Medicine.* 3:417–422, 1973.

Pshennikova MG, Meerson FZ and Teraevo NG. The influence of folic acid and orotic acids and actinomycin on the contractile function of the myocardium in hyperfunction of the heart. *Kardiologia.* 6(4):54, 1966.

Robinson JL et al. Assessment in humans of hypolipidemia induced by orotic acid. *Am. J. Clin. Nutr.* 41:605–608, 1985.

Simonson E and Berman R. New approach in treatment of cardiac decompensation in U.S.S.R. *Am. Heart J.* 86:117–123, 1973.

HERBS

General

Beijing Medical College. *Dictionary of Traditional Chinese Medicine*. San Francisco: China Books and Periodicals, Inc., 1985.

Carper J. *The Food Pharmacy*. New York: Bantam Books, 1988.

Chang HM, Yeung HW, Tso W-W and Koo A. *Advances in Chinese Medicinal Materials Research*. Philadelphia: World Scientific, 1985.

Chang RS and Yeung HW. Inhibition of growth of human immunodeficiency virus in vitro by crude extracts of Chinese medicinal herbs. *Antiviral Research*. 9:163–176, 1988.

Duke JA. *Handbook of Medicinal Herbs*. Boca Raton, Fla.: CRC Press, Inc., 1985.

Duke JA and Ayensu ES. *Medicinal Plants of China*. Algonac, Mich.: Reference Publications, 1985.

Lust J. *The Herb Book*. New York: Bantam Books, 1980.

Murray M. *The 21st Century Herbal*. Bellevue, Wash.: Vita-Line, Inc., 1988.

Reynolds JEF (ed.). *Martindale: The Extra Pharmacopoeia*. London: The Pharmaceutical Press, 1989.

Tyler VE. *The New Honest Herbal*. Philadelphia: George F Stickley Co., 1987.

Weiss RF. *Herbal Medicine*. Beaconsfield, England: Beaconsfield Publishers Ltd, 1988.

Alfalfa

Bell D. The effect of canavanine on herpes simplex virus replication. *Journal of General Virology*. 22:319–330, 1974.

Berjis M and Green MH. Selective cytotoxicity of L-canavanine in tumorigenic Madin-Darby canine kidney T_1 cells. *Chemico-Biological Interactions*. 60:305–315, 1986.

Green MH et al. Antitumor activity of L-canavanine against L 1210 murine leukemia. *Ca. Res*. 40:535–537, 1980.

Malinow MR et al. Systemic lupus erythematosus-like syndrome in monkey fed alfalfa sprouts: Role of a nonprotein amino acid. *Science*. 216:415–417, 1982.

Roberts JL and Hayashi JA. Exacerbation of SLE associated with alfalfa ingestion (Letter). *N. Eng. J. Med*. 308:1361, 1983.

Rosenthal GA. The biological effects and mode of action of L-canavanine, a structural analogue of L-arginine. *Quarterly Review of Biology*. 52:155–178, 1977.

Aloe Vera and Derivatives

Grindlay D and Reynolds T. The aloe phenomenon: A review of the properties and modern uses of the leaf parenchyma gel. *Journal of Ethnopharmacology*. 16:117–151, 1986.

Klein AD and Penneys NS. Aloe vera. *J. Am. Acad. Derm*. 18:714–720, 1988.

Womble D and Helderman JH. Enhancement of alloresponsiveness of human lymphocytes by acemannan (Carrisyn). *International Journal of Immunopharmacology*. 10:967–974, 1988.

Angelica

Kimura Y et al. Effects of an active substance isolated from the roots of *Angelica shkiokana* on leukotriene and monohydroxyeicosatetreaenoic acid biosyntheses in human polymorphonuclear lymphocytes. *Planta Medica*. 53:521–525, 1988.

Shen SJ et al. Analysis and processing of Chinese herbal drugs, VI: The study of *Angelica radix*. *Planta Medica*. 53:377–378, 1987.

Astragalus

Hou YD et al. Effect of *Radix astragali seu hedysari* on the interferon system. *Chinese Medical Journal*. 94:35–40, 1981.

Sun Y et al. Immune restoration and/or augmentation of local graft versus host reaction by traditional Chinese medicinal herbs. *Cancer*. 52:70–73, 1983.

Capsicum/Hot Peppers

Bernstein JE. Capsaicin in postherpetic neuralgia. *Medical Times*. 117:113–115, 1989.

Bernstein JE et al. Treatment of chronic postherpetic neuralgia with topical capsaicin. *J. Am. Acad. Derm*. 17:93–96, 1987.

Fitzgerald M. Capsicum and sensory neurons. *Pain*. 15:109–130, 1983.

Graham DV, Smith JL and Opekun AR. Spicy food and the stomach: Evaluation by videoendoscopy. *J. Am. Med. Assoc*. 260:3473–3475, 1988.

Hawk RJ and Millikon LE. Treatment of oral postherpetic neuralgia with topical capsaicin. *International Journal of Dermatology*. 27:336, 1988.

Kumar N et al. Do chillies influence healing of duodenal ulcer? *Br. Med. J*. 288:1803–1804, 1984.

Ross DR and Varipapa RJ. Treatment of painful diabetic neuropathy with topical capsaicin (Letter). *N. Eng. J. Med.* 321:474–475, 1989.

Visudhiphan S et al. The relationship between high fibrinolytic activity and daily capsicum ingestion in Thais. *Am. J. Clin. Nutr.* 35:1452–1458, 1982.

Comfrey

Awang DVC. Comfrey. *Canadian Pharmacology Journal.* 120:101–104, 1987.

Mattocks AR. Toxic pyrrolizidine alkaloids in comfrey. *Lancet.* 2:1136–1137, 1980.

Ridker PM and McDermott. Comfrey tea and hepatic veno-occlusive disease. *Lancet.* 1:657–658, 1989.

Roitman JN. Comfrey and liver damage. *Lancet.* 1:944, 1981.

Cruciferous Vegetables

Lourau M and Lartigue O. Influence du regime alimentaire sur les effets biologiques produits par une irratiation unique de tout le corps (Rayons X). *Experientia.* 6:25, 1950.

Marchand LL et al: Vegetable consumption and lung cancer risks: A population based case-control study in Hawaii. *J.N.C.I.* 81:1158–1164, 1989.

Sparnins VL, Chuan J and Wattenberg LW. Enhancement of glutathione-S-transferase activity of the esophagus by phenols, lactones, and benzyl isothiocyanate. *Ca. Res.* 42:1205–1207, 1982.

Spector H and Calloway DH. Reduction of X-radiation mortality by cabbage and broccoli. *Proceedings of the Society for Experimental Biology and Medicine.* 100:405–407, 1957.

Temple NJ and Basu TK. Selenium and cabbage and colon carcinogenesis in mice. *J.N.C.I.* 79:1131–1134, 1987.

Wattenberg LW. Inhibition of carcinogenic hydrocarbons by benzyl isothiocyanate and related compounds. *J.N.C.I.* 58:395–398, 1977.

Wattenberg LW. Inhibition of carcinogen-induced neoplasia by sodium cyanate, tert-butyl isocyanate, and benzyl isothiocyanate administered subsequent to carcinogen exposure. *Ca. Res.* 41:2991–2994, 1981.

Wattenberg LW and Loub WD. Inhibition of polycyclic aromatic hydrocarbon-induced neoplasia by naturally occurring indoles. *Ca. Res.* 38:1410–1413, 1978.

Wattenberg LW et al. Dietary constituents altering the responses to chemical carcinogens. *Fed. Proc.* 35:1327–1331, 1976.

Echinacea

Bauer R et al. Immunological in vivo examinations of echinacea extracts. *Arzneimittel-Forschung/Drug Research.* 38:276–281, 1988.

Coeugniet EG and Elek E. Immunomodulation with *Viscum album* and *Echinacea purpurea* extracts. *Onkologie.* 10(3):27–33, 1987.

Stimpel M et al. Macrophage activation and induction of macrophage cytotoxicity by purified polysaccharide fractions from the plant *Echinacea purpurea.* *Infect. Immun.* 46:845–849, 1984.

Wacker A and Hilbig W. Virus inhibition by *Echinacea purpurea.* *Planta Medica.* 33:89, 1978.

Wagner VH et al. Immunostimulating polysaccharides (heteroglycans) of higher plants. *Arzneimittel-Forschung/Drug Research.* 35:1069–1075, 1985.

Feverfew

Heptinstall S et al. Extracts of feverfew inhibits granule secretion in blood platelets and polymorphonuclear leucocytes. *Lancet.* 1:1071–1073, 1985.

Johnson ES et al. Efficiency of feverfew as prophylactic treatment of migraine. *Br. Med. J.* 291:569–573, 1985.

Murphy JJ, Heptinstall S and Mitchell JRA. Randomized double-blind placebo-controlled trial of feverfew in migraine prevention. Lancet. 2:189–192, 1988.

Forskolin

Kreitmer W et al. Bronchodilator and antiallergy activity of forskolin. *European Journal of Pharmacology.* 111:1–8, 1985.

Garlic and Onions

Block E. The chemistry of garlic and onions. *Scientific American.* 252:114–119, March 1985.

Harris LJ. *The Book of Garlic.* Berkeley, Calif.: Aris Books/Harris Publishing Company, Inc., 1979.

Kendler BS. Garlic (*Allium sativum*) and onion (*Allium cepa*): A review of their relationship to cardiovascular disease. *Preventive Medicine.* 16:670–685, 1987.

Lau BHS, Adetumbi MA and Sanchez A. *Allium sativum* (garlic) and atherosclerosis: A review. *Nutrition Research.* 3:119–128, 1983.

Niukian K, Schwartz J and Shklar G. *In vitro* inhibitory effect of onion extract on hamster buccal pouch carcinogenesis. *Nutr. Cancer.* 10:137–144, 1987.

Srivastava KC. Onion exerts antaggregatory effects by altering arachidonic acid metabolism in platelets.

Prostaglandin Leukotrienes and Medicine. 24:43–50, 1986.

Weber N et al. Antiviral activity of *Allium sativum* (garlic). 88th Meeting American Society for Microbiology. Abstract A-126, p. 22, May 1988.

Wei-Cheng Y et al. Allium vegetables and reduced risk of stomach cancer. *J.N.C.I.* 81:162–164, 1989.

Ginger

Mowrey DB and Clayson DE. Motion sickness, ginger and psychophysics. *Lancet.* 1:655–657, 1982.

Ginkgo

Allard M. Treatment of old age disorders with *Ginkgo biloba* extract. *La Presse Medicale.* 15:1540–1545, 1986.

Bauer U. *Ginkgo biloba* extract in the treatment of lower limb arteritis. *La Presse Medicale.* 15:1546–1549, 1986.

Bauer U. 6-month double-blind randomised clinical trial of *Ginkgo biloba* extract versus placebo in two parallel groups in patients suffering from peripheral arterial insufficiency. *Arzneimittel-Forschung/Drug Research.* 34:716–720, 1984.

Gebner B, Voelp and Klasser M. Study of long-term action of a *Ginkgo biloba* extract on vigilance and mental performance as determined by means of quantitative pharmaco-EEG and psychometric measurements. *Arzneimittel-Forschung/Drug Research.* 35:1459–1465, 1985.

Haguenauer JP, Cantenot F, Koskas H and Pierart H. Treatment of disturbances of equilibrium with *Ginkgo biloba* extract. *La Presse Medicale.* 15:1569–1572, 1986.

Hindmarch I. Activity of *Ginkgo biloba* on short term memory. *La Presse Medicale.* 15:1592–1594, 1986.

Lebuisson DA, Leroy L and Rigal G. Treatment of senile macular degeneration with *Ginkgo biloba.* *La Presse Medicale.* 15:1556–1558, 1986.

Meyer B. A multicentre, randomized, double-blind drug versus placebo study of *Ginkgo biloba* extract in the treatment of tinnitus. *La Presse Medicale.* 15:1562–1564, 1986.

Pidoux B. Effects of *Ginkgo biloba* extract on functional activity of the brain. *La Presse Medicale.* 15:1588–1591, 1986.

Schaffler VK and Reeh PW. Double-blind study of the hypoxia-protective effects of a standardized *Ginkgo bilobae* preparation after repeated administration in healthy volunteers. *Arzneimittel-Forschung/Drug Research.* 35:1283–1286, 1985.

Taillandier J et al. *Ginkgo biloba* extract in the treatment of cerebral disorders due to ageing. *La Presse Medical.* 15:1583–1585, 1986.

Ginseng

Han BH et al. Chemical and biochemical studies on antioxidant components of ginseng. *Advances in Chinese Medicinal Materials Research.* Philadelphia: World Scientific Publishing Company, 1985, pp. 485–498.

Lee FC et al. Effects of *Panax ginseng* on blood alcohol clearance in man. *Clinical and Experimental Pharmacology & Physiology.* 14:543–546, 1987.

Takeda A, Yonezawa M and Katoh N. Restoration of radiation injury by ginseng, I: Responses of X-irradiated mice to ginseng extract. *Journal of Radiation Research.* 22:323–335, 1981.

Takeda A, Yonezawa M and Katoh N. Restoration of radiation injury by ginseng, II: Some properties of the radioprotective substances. *Journal of Radiation Research.* 22:336–343, 1981.

Zuin M et al. Effects of a preparation containing a standardized ginseng extract combined with trace elements and multivitamins against hepatotoxin-induced chronic liver disease in the elderly. *Journal of International Medical Research.* 15:276–281, 1987.

Kava Kava

Siegel RK. Herbal intoxication. *J. Am. Med. Assoc.* 236:473, 1976.

Licorice

Abe H et al. Effects of glycyrrhizin and glycyrrhetinic acid on growth and melanogenesis in cultured B_{16} melanoma cells. *European Journal of Cancer & Clinical Oncology.* 23:1549–1555, 1987.

Baba M and Shigeta S. Antiviral activity of glycyrrhizin against varicella-zoster virus in vitro. *Antiviral Research.* 7:99–107, 1987.

Ito M et al. Inhibitory effect of glycyrrhizin on the in vitro infectivity and cytopathic activity of the human immunodeficiency virus (HIV [HTLV-III/LAV]) *Antiviral Research.* 7:127–137, 1987.

Ito M et al. Mechanism of inhibitory effect of glycyrrhizin on replication of human immunodeficiency virus (HIV). *Antiviral Research.* 10:289–298, 1988.

Kiso Y et al. Mechanism of antihepatotoxic activity of glycyrrhizin, I: Effect on free radical generation and lipid peroxidation. *Planta Medica.* 50:298, 1984.

Nakashima H et al. A new anti-human immunodeficiency virus substance, glycyrrhizin sulfate: Endowment of glycyrrhizin with reverse transcriptase-inhibitory activity by chemical modification. *Japanese Journal of Cancer Research.* 78:767–771, 1987.

Parke DV. The biochemical pharmacology of carbenoxolone. *Acta Gastro Enterologica Belgica.* 46:437–447, 1983.

Pompei R et al. Glycyrrhizic acid inhibits virus growth, and inactivates virus particles. *Nature.* 281:689–690, 1979.

Stewart PM et al. Mineralocorticoid activity of liquorice: 11-beta hydrorxsteroid dehydrogenase deficiency comes of age. *Lancet.* 2:821–823, 1987.

Ligustrum

Sun Y et al. Immune restoration and/or augmentation of local graft versus host reaction by traditional Chinese medicinal herbs. *Cancer.* 52:70–73, 1983.

Milk Thistle

Floersheim GL et al. Effects of penicillin and silymarin on liver enzymes and blood clotting factors in dogs given a boiled preparation of *Amanita phalloides. Toxicology and Applied Pharmacology.* 46:455–462, 1978.

Valenzuela A, Guerra R and Garrido A. Silybin dihemisuccinate protects rat erythrocytes against phenylhydrazine-induced lipid peroxidation and hemolysis. *Planta Medica.* 53:402–405, 1987.

Valenzuela A, Guerra R and Videla LA. Antioxidant properties of the flavonoids silybin and (+)-cyanidanol-3: Comparison with butylated hydroxyanisole and butylated hydroxytoluene. *Planta Medica.* 52:438–440, 1986.

Valenzuela A, Lagos C and Schmidt K. Silymarin protection against hepatic lipid peroxidation induced by acute ethanol intoxication in the rat. *Biochemical Pharmacology.* 34:2209–2212, 1985.

Vengerovski AI et al. Liver protective action of silybinene in experimental CCL4 poisoning. *Farmakologiya I Toksikologiya.* 50:67–69, 1987.

Vogel G. A peculiarity among the flavonoids: Silymarin, a compound active on the liver. *Munich Proceedings of the International Bioflavonoid Symposium.* 461–480, 1981.

Wagner H. Antihepatotoxic flavonoids. *Progress in Clinical and Biology Research.* 213:319–331, 1986.

Wagner H et al. The chemistry of silymarin (silybim), the active principle of the fruits of *Silybum*

marianum (*L*) gaertn. (*Carduus marianus*) (L). *Arzneimittel-Forschung/Drug Research.* 18:688–696, 1968.

Mistletoe/Iscador

Bloksma N et al. Cellular and humoral adjuvant activity of a mistletoe extract. *Immunobiology.* 156:309–319, 1979.

Coeugniet EG and Elek E. Immunomodulation with *Viscum album* and *Echinacea purpurea* extracts. *Onkologie.* 10(3):27–33, 1987.

Kwaja T et al. Recent studies on the anti cancer activities of mistletoe and its alkaloids. *Oncology.* 43:42, 1986.

Rentea R, Lyon E and Hunter R. Biologic properties of Iscedor: A *Viscum album* preparation. *Laboratory Investigation.* 44:43–47, 1981.

Oats

Anand CL. Effect of *Avena sativa* on cigarette smoking. *Nature.* 233:496, 1971.

Connor J et al. The pharmacology of *Avena sativa. Journal of Pharmacy and Pharmacology.* 27:92–98, 1975.

Quinine

Fowler AW. Quinine for night cramps. *Br. Med. J.* 291:281, 1985.

Fowler AW. Relief of cramps. *Lancet.* 1:99, 1973.

Fung M-C and Holbrook JH. Placebo-controlled trial of quinine therapy for nocturnal leg cramps. *Western Journal of Medicine.* 151:42–44, 1989.

Henry J. Quinine for night cramps (Editorial). *Br. Med. J.* 291:3, 1985.

St. John's Wort (Hypericum)

Araya OS and Ford EJH. An investigation of the type of photosensitization caused by the ingestion of St. John's Wort (*Hypericum perforatum*) by calves. *Journal of Comparative Pathology.* 91:135–141, 1981.

Meruelo D, Lavie G and Lavie D. Therapeutic agents with dramatic antiretroviral activity and little toxicity at effective doses: Aromatic polycyclic diones hypericin and pseudohypericin. *Proc. Nat. Acad. Sci.* 85:5230–5234, 1988.

Muldner VH and Zoller M. Antidepressive effect of a *Hypericum* extract standardized to the active hypericine complex: Biochemistry and clinical studies. *Arzneimittel-Forschung/Drug Research.* 34:918–920, 1984.

Triphala

Inamdar MC and Rajarama Rao MR. Studies on the pharmacology of *Terminalia chebula* Retz. *Journal of Scientific and Industrial Research.* 21C:345–348, 1962.

Valerian

Dunaev et al. *Farmakologyiya I Toksikologiya.* 50:33–37, 1989.

Hobbs C. Valerian—a literature review. *Herbal Gram.* 21, 19–34. Fall, 1989.

Valerian. *Martindale, The Extra Pharmacopoeia,* Twenty-ninth Edition. London: The Pharmaceutical Press, 1628–1989.

Weiss RF. *Valeriana officinalis* (valerian). *Herbal Medicine.* Beaconsfield, England: Beaconsfield Publishers, Ltd., 1988, pp. 281–285.

Wheat Grass/Barley Grass

Hotta Y et al. Studies on the components in barley extracts: Stimulation of the naturally occurring and induced DNA repair in meiotic cells (Report). *Annual Meeting of Japan Pharmaceutical Sciences.* April 1981.

Hotta Y et al. Studies on the components in barley extracts stimulation of DNA repair in human cultured cells (Report). *Annual Meeting of Japan Pharmaceutical Sciences.* April 1982.

Lai C-N. Chlorophyll: The active factor in wheat sprout extract inhibiting the metabolic activation of carcinogens *in vitro. Nutr. Cancer.* 1(3):19–21, 1979.

Lai C-N, Dabney BJ and Shaw CR. Inhibition of *in vitro* metabolic activation of carcinogens by wheat sprout extracts. *Nutr. Cancer.* 1(1):27–30, 1978.

Yohimbine

Reid K et al. Double-blind trial of yohimbine in treatment of psychogenic impotence. *Lancet.* 2:421–423, 1987.

OTHER SUPPLEMENTS

Acidophilus, Yogurt, Kefir, etc.

Friend BA et al. Nutritional and therapeutic aspects of lactobacilli. *Journal of Applied Nutrition.* 36:125–153, 1984.

Gotz V et al. Prophylaxis against ampicillin-associated diarrhea with a lactobacillus preparation. *American Hospital Pharmacy.* 36:754–757, 1979.

Gunston KD and Fairbrothers PF. Treatment of vaginal discharge with yoghurt. *South African Medical Journal.* 49:675–676, 1975.

Hamdan IY et al. Acidolin: An antibiotic produced by *Lactobacillus acidophilus. Journal of Antibiotics.* 27:63–66, 1974.

Hepner B et al. Hypocholesterolemic effect of yogurt and milk. *Am. J. Clin. Nutr.* 32:19–24, 1979.

Kolars JC et al. Yogurt: An autodigesting source of lactose. *N. Eng. J. Med.* 310:1–3, 1984.

Mann GV. Factor in yogurt which lowers cholesteremia in man. *Atherosclerosis.* 26:335–340, 1977.

Retty GV et al. Antitumor activity of yogurt components. *Journal of Food Protection.* 46:8–11, 1983.

Vincent JG, Veomott RC and Riley RF. Antibacterial activity associated with *Lactobacillus acidophilus. Journal of Bacteriology.* 78:477–484, 1959.

Will TW. Lactobacillus overgrowth for treatment of monilary vulvovaginitis (Letter). *Lancet.* 2:482, 1979.

Bioflavonoids

Afanas'ev IB et al. Chelating and free radical scavenging mechanisms of inhibitory action of rutin and quercetin in lipid peroxidation. *Biochemical Pharmacology.* 38:1763–1769, 1989.

Collin-Williams C. Oral use of cromolyn in food allergy. In: Chiaramonte LT, Schneider AT and Lifshitz F (eds.), *Food Allergy: A Practical Approach to Diagnosis and Management.* New York: Marcel Dekker, Inc., 1988, pp. 377–391.

Havsteen B. Flavonoids, a class of natural products of high pharmacological potency. *Biochemical Pharmacology.* 32:1141–1148, 1983.

Kaul TN, Middleton E and Ogra PL. Antiviral effect of flavonoids on human viruses. *Journal of Medical Virology.* 15:71–79, 1985.

Middleton EJ. The flavonoids. *Trends in Pharmacological Sciences.* 335–338, August 1984.

Middleton EJ, Drzewiecki G and Tatum J. The effects of citrus flavonoids on human basophil and neutrophil function. *Planta Medica.* 53:325–328, 1987.

Spedding G, Ratty A and Middleton EJ. Inhibition of

reverse transcriptases by flavonoids. *Antiviral Research.* 12:99–110, 1989.

Brewer's Yeast/Skin Respiratory Factor

Goodson W et al. Augmentation of some aspects of wound healing by a "skin respiratory factor." *Journal of Surgical Research.* 21:125–129, 1976.

Kaplan JZ. Acceleration of wound healing by a live yeast cell derivative. *Archives of Surgery.* 119:1005–1008, 1984.

Leibovich SJ and Danon D. Promotion of wound repair in mice by application of glucan. *Journal of the Reticuloendothelial Society.* 27:1–11, 1980.

Sinai Y et al. Enhancement of resistance to infectious diseases by oral administration of brewer's yeast. *Infec. Immun.* 9:781–787, 1974.

Coenzyme Q_{10}

Beyer RB. Inhibition by coenzyme Q of ethanol- and carbon tetrachloride-stimulated lipid peroxidation in vivo and catalyzed by microsomal and mitochondrial systems. *Free Radical Biology and Medicine.* 5:297–303, 1989.

Folkers K. Vadhanavikit S and Mortensen SA. Biochemical rationale and myocardial tissue data on the effective therapy of cardiomyopathy with coenzyme Q_{10}. *Proc. Nat. Acad. Sci.* 62:901–904, 1985.

Folkers K, Watanabe T and Kaji M. Critique of coenzyme Q in biochemical and biomedical research and in ten years of clinical research on cardiovascular disease. *Journal of Molecular Medicine.* 2:431–460, 1977.

Folkers K and Wolaniuk A. Research on coenzyme Q_{10} in clinical medicine and in immunomodulation. *Drugs Under Experimental and Clinical Research.* 11:539–546, 1985.

Ishiuama T, Morita Y and Toyama S. A clinical study of the effect of coenzyme Q on congestive heart failure. *Japanese Heart Journal.* 17:32, 1976.

Kamikawa T et al. Effects of coenzyme Q_{10} on exercise tolerance in chronic stable angina pectoris. *Am. J. Cardiol.* 56:247–251, 1985.

Langsjoen PH, Vadhanavikit S and Folkers K. Effective treatment with coenzyme Q_{10} of patients with chronic myocardial disease. *Drugs Under Experimental and Clinical Research.* 11:577–580, 1985.

Nagai S et al. The effects of coenzyme Q_{10} on reperfusion injury in canine myocardium. *Journal of Molecular and Cellular Cardiology.* 17:873, 1985.

Nakamura Y et al. Protection of ischemic myocardium with coenzyme Q_{10}. *Cardiovascular Research.* 16:132–137, 1982.

Dietary Fiber

Abraham ZD and Mehts T. Three-week psyllium-husk supplementation: Effect on plasma cholesterol concentrations, fecal steroid excretion, and carbohydrate absorption in men. *Am. J. Clin. Nutr.* 47:67–74, 1988.

Anderson JW et al. Cholesterol-lowering effects of psyllium hydrophilic mucilloid for hypercholesterolemic men. *Archives of Internal Medicine.* 148:292–296, 1988.

Anderson JW et al. Hypocholesterolemic effects of oat-bran or bean intake for hypercholesterolemic men. *Am. J. Clin. Nutr.* 40:1146–1155, 1984.

Cranston D, McWhinnie D and Collin J. Dietary fibre and gastrointestinal disease. *British Journal of Surgery.* 75:508–512, 1988.

Danielsson A et al. Effect of long term treatment with hydrophilic colloid on serum lipids. *Acta Hepato-Gastroenterologica.* 26:148–153, 1979.

DeCosse JJ, Miller HH and Lesser ML. Effect of wheat fiber and vitamins C and E on rectal polyps in patients with familial adenomatous polyposis. *J.N.C.I.* 81:1290–1297, 1989.

DeGroot AP, Luyken R and Pikaar NA. Cholesterol-lowering effect of rolled oats. *Lancet.* 2:303–304, 1963.

Durrington PN et al. Effect of pectin on serum lipids and lipoproteins, whole-gut transit-time, and stool weight. *Lancet.* 2:394, 1976.

Eastwood MA and Passmore R. Dietary fiber. *Lancet.* 2:202–205, 1983.

Florholmen J et al. The effect of Metamucil on postprandial blood glucose and plasma inhibitory peptide in insulin-dependent diabetics. *Acta Medica Scandinavica.* 212:237–239, 1982.

Garvin JE et al. Lowering of human serum cholesterol by an oral hydrophilic colloid. *Proceedings of the Society for Experimental Biology and Medicine.* 120:744–746, 1965.

Gold KV and Davidson DM. Oat bran as a cholesterol-reducing dietary adjunct in a young, healthy population. *Western Journal of Medicine.* 148:299–302, 1988.

Heaton KW. Dietary fibre in perspective. *Clinical Nutrition.* 37C:151–170, 1983.

Jenkins DJA et al. Decrease in postprandial insulin and glucose concentrations by guar and pectin. *Ann. Intern. Med.* 86:20, 1977.

Jenkins DJA et al. Treatment of diabetes with guar-gum: Reduction of urinary glucose loss in diabetics. *Lancet*. 2:779, 1979.

Judd PA and Truswell AS. Comparison of the effects of high- and low-methoxyl pectins on blood and faecal lipids in man. *British Journal of Nutrition*. 48:451, 1982.

Judd PA and Truswell AS. The effect of rolled oats on blood lipids and fecal steroid excretion in man. *Am. J. Clin. Nutr*. 34:2061–2067, 1981.

Kay RM, Judd PA and Truswell AS. The effect of pectin on serum cholesterol. *Am. J. Clin. Nutr*. 31:562, 1978.

Kirby RW et al. Oat-bran intake selectively lowers serum low-density lipoprotein cholesterol concentrations of hypercholesterolemic men. *Am. J. Clin. Nutr*. 34:824–829, 1981.

Krotkiewski M. Effect of guar gum on body-weight, hunger ratings and metabolism in obese subjects. *British Journal of Nutrition*. 52:97–105, 1984.

Nuovo J. Use of dietary fiber to lower cholesterol. *American Family Physician*. 39(4):137–140, 1989.

Osilesi O et al. Use of xanthan gum in dietary management of diabetes mellitus. *Am. J. Clin. Nutr*. 42:597–603, 1985.

Palmer GH and Dixon DG. Effect of pectin dose on serum cholesterol levels. *Am. J. Clin. Nutr*. 18:437, 1966.

Sartor G, Carlstom S and Schersten B. Dietary supplementation of fibre (lunelax) as a means to reduce postprandial glucose in diabetics. *Acta Medica Scandinavica* (Supplement). 656:51–53, 1981.

Schneeman BO. Dietary fiber and gastrointestinal function. *Nutr. Rev*. 45(5):129–132, 1987.

Slavin JL and Levine AS. Dietary fiber and gastrointestinal disease, I: What is fiber and how much should you take? *Practical Gastroenterology*. 10(3):56–59, 1986.

Slavin JL and Levine AS. Dietary fiber and gastrointestinal disease, II: How to use fiber to treat disease. *Practical Gastroenterology*. 10(4):19–24, 1986.

VanHorn LV et al. Serum lipid response to oat product intake with a fat-modified diet. *Journal of the American Dietetic Association*. 86:759–764, 1986.

Watanabe K et al. Effect of dietary alfalfa, pectin and wheat bran on azoxymethane- or methylnitrosourea-induced colon carcinogenesis in F344 rats. *J.N.C.I*. 63:141, 1979.

Yang P and Banwell JG. Dietary fiber: Its role in the pathogenesis and treatment of constipation. *Practical Gastroenterology*. (6):28–32, 1986.

Enzymes (Including Wobe Mugos)

Ransberger K. Enzyme treatment of immune complex diseases. *Arthritis and Rheumatism*. 8:16–19, 1986.

Steffen C and Menzel J. Basic investigation of enzymatic treatment of immune complex disease. *Wiener Klinische Wochenschrift*. 97:3–11, 1985.

Steffen C and Menzel J. In vivo breakdown of immune complexes in the kidney by oral administration of enzymes. *Wiener Klinische Wochenschrift*. 99:525–531, 1987.

Steffen C et al. Enzyme treatment in comparison with immune complex determinations in rheumatoid arthritis. *Zeitschrift fur Rheumatologie*. 44:51–56, 1985.

L-Carnitine

Bazzato G et al. Myasthenia-like syndrome after DL-but not L-carnitine. *Lancet*. 1:1209, 1981.

Borum PR. Carnitine. *Ann. Rev. Nutr*. 3:233–259, 1983.

Brevetti G et al. Increases in walking distance in patients with peripheral vascular disease treated with L-carnitine: A double-blind, cross over study. *Circulation*. 77:767–773, 1988.

Dipalma JR. Carnitine deficiency. *American Family Physician*. 38(1):243–251, 1988.

Dipalma JR. L-carnitine: Its therapeutic potential. *American Family Physician*. 34(6):127–130, 1986.

Fanelli O. Carnitine and acetyl carnitine: Natural substances endowed with interesting pharmacological properties. *Life Sciences*. 23:2563, 1978.

Ferrari R, Cucchini F and Visioli O. The metabolic effects of L-carnitine in angina pectoris. *International Journal of Cardiology*. 5:213, 1984.

Folts JD et al. Protection of the ischemic myocardium with L-carnitine. *Am. J. Cardiol*. 41:1209, 1978.

Gorostiaga EM, Maurer CA and Eclache JP. Decrease in respiratory quotient during exercise following L-carnitine supplementation. *International Journal of Sports Medicine*. 10:169–174, 1989.

Kamikawa T et al. Effects of L-carnitine on exercise tolerance in patients with stable angina pectoris. *Japanese Heart Journal*. 25:587, 1984.

Kosolcharoen P et al. Improved exercise tolerance of administration of carnitine. *Curr. Ther. Res*. 30:753, 1981.

Maebashi M et al. Lipid-lowering effect of carnitine in patients with type IV hyperlipoproteinemia. *Lancet*. 2:805–807, 1978.

Marconi C, Sassi G and Cerrettilli P. Effects of L-carnitine on the aerobic and anaerobic performance of endurance athletes. *European Journal of Applied Physiology*. 54:131, 1985.

Opie LH. Role of carnitine in fatty acid metabolism of normal and ischemic myocardium. *Am. Heart J*. 97:375–388, 1979.

Pola P et al. Carnitine in the therapy of dyslipidemic patients. *Cur. Ther. Res*. 27:208–216, 1980.

Rebouche CJ and Engel AG. Carnitine metabolism and deficiency syndromes. *Mayo Clinic Proceedings.* 58:533–540, 1983.

Rossi CS and Siliprandi N. Effect of carnitine on serum HDL-cholesterol: Report of two cases. *Johns Hopkins Medical Journal.* 150:51–54, 1982.

Sachan DS, Rhew TH and Ruark RA. Ameliorating effects of carnitine and its precursors on alcohol-induced fatty liver. *Am. J. Clin. Nutr.* 39:738–744, 1984.

Thomsen JH et al. Improved stress tolerance of the ischemic human myocardium after carnitine administration. *Am. J. Cardiol.* 39:289, 1977.

Lipoic Acid

Natraj CV, Gandhi VM and Menon KKG. Lipoic acid and diabetes: Effect of dihydrolipoic acid administration in diabetic rats and rabbits. *Journal of Bioscience.* 6:37–46, 1984.

Ohmari H, Yamauchi T and Yamamoto I. Augmentation of the antibody response by lipoic acid in mice, II: Restoration of the antibody response in immunosuppressed mice. *Japanese Journal of Pharmacology.* 42:275–280, 1986.

Sachse G and Willms B. Efficiency of thioctic acid in the therapy of peripheral diabetic neuropathy. *Hormone and Metabolic Research* (Supplement). 9:105, 1980.

Shih JCH. Atherosclerosis in Japanese quail and the effect of lipoic acid. *Fed. Proc.* 42:2494–2497, 1983.

Wagh SS, Natraj CV and Menon KKG. Mode of action of lipoic acid in diabetes. *Journal of Bioscience.* 11:59–74, 1987.

Pangamic Acid/DMG ("Vitamin B$_{15}$")

Gerlernt MD and Herbert V. Mutagenicity of diisopropylamine dichloroacetate, the "active constituent" of vitamin B$_{15}$ (pangamic acid). *Nutr. Cancer.* 3(3):129–133, 1982.

Gray ME and Titlow LW. The effect of pangamic acid on maximal treadmill performance. *Medicine and Science in Sports and Exercise.* 14:424–427, 1982.

Harpaz M, Otto RM and Smith TK. The effect of N,-N,dimethylglycine ingestion upon aerobic performance. *Medicine and Science in Sports and Exercise.* 17:287, 1985.

Seaweeds and Derivatives

Barnett SE and Varley SJ. The effects of calcium alginate on wound healing. *Annals of the Royal College of Surgeons of England.* 69:153–155, 1987.

Besterman EMM and Evans J. Antilipaemic agent without anticoagulant action. *Br. Med. J.* 310–312, February 9, 1957.

Blaine G. Experimental observations on absorbable alginate products in surgery. *Ann. Surg.* 125:102–114, 1947.

Ehresmann DW, Deig EF and Hatch MT. Antiviral properties of algal polysacchorides and related compounds. In: Hoppe HA, Levring T and Tanaka Y (eds.), *Marine Algae in Pharmaceutical Science.* Berlin, New York: Walter de Gruyter, 1979, pp. 293–302.

Ford, R and Anderson J. *Sea Green Primer: A Beginner's Book of Sea Weed Cookery.* Berkeley, Calif.: Creative Arts Book Company, 1983.

Fraser R and Gilchrist T. Sorbsan calcium alginate fibre dressings in footcare. *Biomaterials.* 4:222–224, 1983.

Gilchrist T and Martin AM. Wound treatment with sorbsan: An alginate fiber dressing. *Biomaterials.* 4:317–320, 1983.

Gonzalez ME, Alarcon B and Carrasco L. Polysaccharides as antiviral agents: Antiviral activity of carrageenan. *Antimicrobial Agents and Chemotherapy.* 31(9):1388–1393, 1987.

Graves AR and Lawrence JC. Alginate dressing as a donor site hemostat. *Annals of the Royal College of Surgeons of England.* 68:27–28, 1986.

Hoppe HA and Levring T (eds.). *Marine Algae in Pharmaceutical Science,* Vol. 2. Berlin, New York: Walter de Gruyter, 1982.

Hoppe HA, Levring T and Tanaka Y (eds.). *Marine Algae in Pharmaceutical Science.* Berlin, New York: Walter de Gruyter, 1979.

Kelly SA, Dickson MG and Sharpe DT. Calcium alginate as a temporary recipient bed dressing prior to the delayed application of split skin grafts. *British Journal of Plastic Surgery.* 41:445, 1988.

Nakashima H et al. Antiretroviral activity in a marine red alga: Reverse transcriptase inhibition by an aqueous extract of *Schizymenia pacifica. Journal of Cancer Research and Clinical Oncology.* 113:413–426, 1987.

Nakashima H et al. Purification and characterization of an avian myeloblastosis and human immunodeficiency virus reverse transcriptase inhibitor, sulfated polysaccharides extracted from sea algae. *Antimicrobial Agents and Chemotherapy.* 31(10):1524–1528, 1987.

Neushul M. Method for the treatment of AIDS virus and other retroviruses. United States Patent: 4,783,446, November 8, 1988.

Odugbesan O and Barnett AH. Use of a seaweed-based dressing in management of leg ulcers in diabetics: A case report. *Practical Diabetes.* 4(1):46–47, 1987.

Stein JR and Borden CA. Causative and beneficial algae in human disease conditions: A review. *Phycologia.* 23(4):485–501, 1984.

Tanaka Y and Stara JF. Algal polysaccharides: Their potential use to prevent chronic metal poisoning. In: Hoppe HA, Levring T and Tanaka Y (eds.), *Marine Algae in Pharmaceutical Science.* Berlin, New York: Walter de Gruyter, 1979, pp. 525–543.

Thomas S. Use of a calcium alginate dressing. *Pharmaceutical Journal.* 235:188–190, 1985.

Yamamoto and Maruyama H. Effect of dietary seaweed preparations on 1,2-dimethylhydrazine-induced intestinal carcinogenesis in rats. *Cancer Letters.* 26:241–251, 1985.

Spirulina and Chlorella

Schwartz J and Shklar G. Growth inhibition and destruction of oral cancer cells by extracts of spirulina. *American Academy of Oral Pathology Abstracts.* 40:23, 1986.

Schwartz J and Shklar G. Regression of experimental hamster cancer by beta carotene and algae extracts. *Journal of Oral and Maxillofacial Surgery.* 45:510–515, 1987.

Schwartz J, Troxler RF and Saffer BG. Algae derived phycocyanin is both cytostatic and cytotoxic to oral squamous cell carcinoma (human or hamster). *Journal of Dental Research.* 66:160, 1987.

Wheat Germ, Wheat Germ Oil, and Octacosanol

Goettsch M and Ritzman J. The preventive effect of wheat germ oils and of alpha-tocopherol in nutritional muscular dystrophy of young rats. *J. Nutr.* 17:371–381, 1939.

Rabinovitch R, Gibson WC and McEachern D. Neuromuscular disorders amenable to wheat germ oil

therapy. *Journal of Neurology, Neurosurgery and Psychiatry.* 14:95–100, 1951.

Mushrooms: Shiitake and Rei-Shi

Aoki T et al. Antibodies to HTLVI and III in sera from two Japanese patients, one with possible pre-AIDS. *Lancet.* 2:936–937, 1984.

Cheng HH et al. The anti-tumor effect of cultivated *Ganoderma lucidum* extract. *Journal of the Chinese Oncology Society.* 1:12–16, 1982.

Chihara G et al. Fractionation and purification of the polysaccharides with marked anti-tumor activity, especially lentinan, from *Lentinus edodes* (an edible mushroom). *Ca. Res.* 30:2776–2781, 1980.

Chihara G et al. Inhibition of mouse sarcoma 180 by polysaccharides from *Lentinus edodes. Nature.* 222:637–638, 1969.

Miyakoshi H, Aoki T and Mizukoshi M. Acting mechanisms of lentinan in humans, II: Enhancement of non-specific cell-mediated cytotoxicity as an interferon inducer. *International Journal of Immunopharmacology.* 6:173–179, 1984.

Shimizu A et al. Isolation of an inhibitor of platelet aggregation from a fungus, *Ganaderma lucidum. Chemical and Pharmaceutical Bulletin.* 33:3012–3015, 1985.

Sone Y et al. Structures and anti-tumor activities of the polysaccharides isolated from fruiting body and the growing *Ganaderma lucidum. Agricultural and Biological Chemistry.* 49:2641–2653, 1985.

Tochikura TS et al. Inhibition (in vitro) of replication and of the cytopathic effect of the human immunodeficiency virus by an extract of culture medium of *Lentinus edodes* mycelia. *Microbiology and Immunology.* 177:235–244, 1988.

Yoshida O et al. Sulfation of the immunomodulating polysaccharide lentinan: A novel strategy for antivirals to human immunodeficiency virus (HIV) *Biochemical Pharmacology.* 37:2887–2891, 1988.

OTHER SUBSTANCES

Aspirin

Antiplatelet Trialists' Collaboration. Secondary prevention of vascular disease by prolonged antiplatelet treatment. *Br. Med. J.* 296:320–331, 1988.

Aspirin for prevention of myocardial infarction and stroke. *Medical Letter.* 31:77–79, 1989.

Baudoin C et al. Effect of aspirin alone and aspirin plus dipyridamole in early diabetic retinopathy: A multicenter randomized controlled clinical trial. *Diabetes.* 38:491–498, 1989.

Cairns JA et al. Aspirin, sulfinpyrazone, or both in unstable angina: Results of a Canadian multicenter trial. *N. Eng. J. Med.* 313:1369–1375, 1985.

Fuster V, Cohen M and Halperin J. Aspirin in the prevention of coronary disease (Editorial). *N. Eng. J. Med.* 321:183–185, 1989.

Huang RTC and Dietsch E. Anti-influenza viral activity of aspirin in cell culture (Letter). *N. Eng. J. Med.* 319:797, 1988.

ISIS-2 (Second International Study of Infarct Survival) Collaborative Group. Randomized trial of intravenous streptokinase, oral aspirin, both, or neither among 17,187 cases of suspected acute myocardial infarction: ISIS-2. *Lancet.* 2:349–360, 1988.

Lewis HD Jr. et al. Protective effects of aspirin against acute myocardial infarction and death in men with unstable angina: Results of a Veterans Administration cooperative study. *N. Eng. J. Med.* 309:396–403, 1983.

Meyer JS et al. Randomized clinical trial of daily aspirin therapy in multi-infarct dementia: A pilot study. *Journal of the American Geriatrics Society.* 37:549–555, 1989.

Steering Committee of the Physicians' Health Study Research Group. Final report on the aspirin component of the ongoing physicians' health study. *N. Eng. J. Med.* 321:129–135, 1989.

Steering Committee of the Physicians' Health Study Research Group. Preliminary report: Findings from the aspirin component of the ongoing physicians' health study. *N. Eng. J. Med.* 318:262–264, 1988.

Theroux P et al. Aspirin, heparin, or both to treat acute unstable angina. *N. Eng. J. Med.* 319:1105–1111, 1988.

UK-TIA Study Group. United Kingdom transient ischaemia attack (UK-TIA) aspirin trial: Interim results. *Br. Med. J.* 296:316–320, 1988.

United States Prevention Services Task Force. Aspirin prophylaxis for cardiovascular disease. *American Family Physician.* 40:117–120, 1989.

Bee and Flower Pollen

Chandler JV and Hawkins JD. The effect of bee pollen on physiological performance. *Medicine and Science in Sports and Exercise.* 17:287, 1985.

Cohen SH et al. Acute allergic reactions after composite pollen ingestion. *Journal of Allergy and Clinical Immunology.* 64:270–274, 1979.

Mansfield LE and Goldstein GB. Anaphylactic reaction after ingestion of local bee pollen. *Annals of Allergy.* 47:154–156, 1981.

Mirkin GB. Bee pollen. *Physician and SportsMedicine.* 13:159–160, 1985.

Steben RE and Boudreaux P. The effects of pollen and protein extracts on selected blood factors and performance of athletes. *Journal of Sports Medicine and Physical Fitness.* 18:221–226, 1978.

BHA and BHT

Babich H. Butylated hydroxytoluene (BHT): A review. *Environmental Research.* 29:1–29, 1982.

Charcoal

Friedman EA et al. Charcoal-Induced lipid reduction in uremia. *Kidney International.* 13 (Supplement 8):S-170, 1978.

Jain NK, Patel VP and Pitchumoni CS. Activated charcoal, simethicone, and intestinal gas: A double-blind study. *Ann. Intern. Med.* 105:61–62, 1986.

Jain NK, Patel VP and Pitchumoni CS. Efficiency of activated charcoal in reducing intestinal gas: A double-blind clinical trial. *American Journal of Gastroenterology.* 81:532–535, 1986.

Kuusista P et al. Effect of activated charcoal on hypercholesterolemia. *Lancet.* 2:366–367, 1986.

Chondroitin Sulfate

Morrison LM and Enrick L. Coronary heart disease: Reduction of death rate by chondroitin sulfate A. *Angiology.* 24:269–287, 1973.

Morrison LM et al. Prevention of vascular lesions by chondroitin sulfate A in the coronary artery and aorta of rats induced by a hypervitaminosis D, cholesterol-containing diet. *Atherosclerosis.* 16:105–118, 1972.

Nakazawa K and Murato K. The therapeutic effect of chondroitin polysulfate in elderly atherosclerotic patients. *Journal of International Medical Research.* 6:217–225, 1978.

Deaner [DMAE]

Cherkin A and Eckhardt MJ. Effects of dimethylaminoethanol upon life span and behavior of aged Japanese quail. *Journal of Gerontology.* 32:38–45, 1977.

Ferris SH et al. Senile dementia: Treatment with Deanol. *Journal of the American Geriatric Society.* 25:241–244, 1977.

Kostopoulos GK and Phyllis JW. The effect of dimethylaminoethanol (Deanol) on cerebral cortical neurons. *Psychopharmacology Communications.* 1:339–347, 1975.

Stafford JR and Farr WE. Deanol acetamidobenzoate (Deaner) in tardive dyskinesia. *Diseases of the Nervous System.* 38:3–6, 1977.

Dextran Sulfate (With a Note on Heparin)

Abrams DI et al. Oral dextran sulfate (UA001) in the treatment of the Acquired Immunodeficiency Syndrome (AIDS) and AIDS-related complex. *Ann. Intern. Med.* 110:183–188, 1989.

Baba M et al. Pentosan polyphosphate, a sulfated oligosaccharide is a potent and selective anti-HIV agent in vitro. *Antiviral Research.* 9:335–343, 1988.

Engleberg H. Can heparin help prevent the complications of AIDS. *Internal Medicine.* 9(10):82–89, 1988.

Engleberg H. Heparin and the atherosclerotic process. *Pharmacological Reviews.* 36:91–110, 1984.

Ito M et al. Inhibitory effect of dextran sulfate and heparin on the replication of human immunodeficiency virus (HIV) in vitro. *Antiviral Research.* 7:361–367, 1987.

Lorentsen KJ et al. Dextran sulfate is poorly absorbed after oral administration. *Ann. Intern. Med.* 111:561–566, 1989.

Mitsuya H et al. Dextran sulfate suppression of viruses in the HIV family: Inhibition of virion budding to $CD4^+$ cells. *Science.* 240:646–649, 1988.

Ueno R and Kuno S. Anti-HIV syngergism between dextran sulfate and zidovudine (Letter). *Lancet.* 2:796–797, 1987.

Ueno R and Kuno S. Dextran sulfate, a potent anti-HIV agent in vitro having syngergism with zidovudine (Letter). *Lancet.* 1:1379, 1987.

DHEA

Barrett-Conner E, Khaw K-T and Yen SSC. A prospective study of dehydroepiandrosterone sulfate, mortality, and cardiovascular disease. *N. Eng. J. Med.* 315:1519–1524, 1986.

Bologna L, Sharma J and Roberts E. Dehydroepiandrosterone and its sulfated derivative reduce neuronal death and enhance astrocytic differentiation in brain cell cultures. *Journal of Neuroscience Research.* 17:225–234, 1987.

Coleman DL, Schwizer RW and Leiter EH. Effect of genetic background on the therapeutic effects of dehydroepiandrosterone (DHEA) in diabetes-obesity mutants and in aged normal mice. *Diabetes.* 33:26–32, 1984.

Flood, JF and Roberts E. Dehydroepiandrosterone sulfate improves memory in aging mice. *Brain Research.* 448:178–181, 1988.

Flood JF, Smith GE and Roberts E. Dehydroepiandrosterone and its sulfate enhance memory retention in mice. *Brain Research.* 447:267–278, 1988.

Gordon GB, Bush DE and Weisman HF. Reduction of atherosclerosis by administration of dehydroepiandrosterone. *Journal of Clinical Investigation.* 82:712–720, 1988.

Gordon GB, Shantz LM and Talalay P. Modulation of growth, differentiation and carcinogenesis by dehydroepiandrosterone. *Advances in Enzyme Regulation.* 26:355–383, 1987.

Loria RM et al. Protection against acute lethal viral infections with the native steroid dehydroepiandrosterone (DHEA). *Journal of Medical Virology.* 26:301–314, 1988.

Nestler JE et al. Dehydroepiandrosterone reduces serum low density lipoprotein levels and body fat but does not alter insulin sensitivity in normal men. *Journal of Clinical Endocrinology and Metabolism.* 66:57–61, 1988.

Orentreich N et al. Age changes and sex differences in serum dehydroepiandrosterone sulfate concentrations throughout adulthood. *Journal of Clinical Endocrinology and Metabolism.* 59:551–555, 1984.

Regelson W, Loria R and Kalim M. "Hormonal intervention," "buffer hormones" or "state dependency": The role of dehydroepiandrosterone (DHEA), thyroid hormone, estrogen and hypophysectomy in aging. *Ann. N.Y. Acad. Sci.* 521:260–273, 1988.

Schwartz A et al. Dehydroepiandrosterone: An antiobesity and anti-carcinogenic agent. *Nutr. Cancer.* 3(1):46–53, 1981.

Schwartz AG, Lewbart ML and Pashko LL. Novel dehydroepiandrosterone analogues with enhanced biological activity and reduced side effects in mice and rats. *Ca. Res.* 48:4817–4822, 1988.

Schwartz AG, Pashko L and Whitcomb JM. Inhibition of tumor development by dehydroepiandrosterone and related steroids. *Toxicol. Path.* 14:357–362, 1986.

Sunderland T et al. Reduced plasma dehydroepiandrosterone concentrations in Alzheimer's disease (Letter). *Lancet.* 2:570, 1989.

DMSO

Carson JD and Percy EC. The use of DMSO in tennis elbow and rotator cuff tendonitis: a double-blind study. *Medicine and Science in Sports and Exercise.* 13:215–219, 1981.

De la Torre JC et al. Dimethyl sulfoxide in central nervous system trauma. *Ann. N.Y. Acad. Sci.* 243:362–389, 1975.

Ek A et al. The use of dimethyl sulfoxide in the treatment of interstitial cystitis. *Scandinavian Journal of Urology and Nephrology* (supplement) 12:129–131, 1978.

Jacob SW and Herschler R. Biological actions of dimethyl sulfoxide. *Ann. N.Y. Acad. Sci.* 243:1975.

Martin ML. Pharmacologic therapeutic modalities: phenytoin, dimethyl sulfoxide, and calcium channel blockers. *Critical Care Quarterly* pp. 72–81, March 1983.

Milner LS et al. Amelioration of murine lupus nephritis by dimethylsulfoxide. *Clinical Immunology and Immunopathology* 45:259–267, 1987.

Experimental Immunomodulators

Bihari B et al. Low dose naltrexone in the treatment of AIDS: Long term follow-up results. *Abstracts of the 5th International Conference on AIDS*. P. 552, 1989.

Delepine N et al. Sodium diethyldithiocarbamate inducing long-lasting remission in a class of juvenile systemic lupus enythematosus. *Lancet*. 2:1246, 1985.

Lang J-M et al. Immunomodulation with diethyldithiocarbomate in patients with AIDS-related complex. *Lancet*. 2:1066, 1985.

Pompidou A et al. Two potentially active compounds in patients with AIDS related complex syndrome. *Ca. Res.* (Supplement). 45:4671, 1985.

Pompidou A et al. The generation and regulation of human T lymphocytes by Imuthiol: Evidence from an in vitro differentiation induction system. *International Journal of Immunopharmacology*. 7:561, 1985.

Pompidou A et al. In vitro inhibition of LAV/HTLV-III infected lymphocytes by dithiocarbomate and inosine pranobex. *Lancet*. 2:1423, 1985.

Prieto J et al. Naloxone-reversible monocyte dysfunction in patients with chronic fatigue syndrome. *Scandinavian Journal of Immunology*. 30:13–20, 1989.

Fruit Acids

Van Scott EJ. Control of keratinization with alpha-hydroxy acids and related compounds. *Archives of Dermatology*. 110:586–590, 1974.

Gerovital H3

Fuller RW and Roush BW. Procaine hydrochloride as a monoamine oxidase inhibitor: Implications for geriatric therapy. *Journal of the American Geriatric Society*. 25:90–93, 1977.

Jarvik LF and Milne JF. Gerovital-H3: A review of the literature. In: Gershon S and Raskin A (eds.), *Aging*. New York: Raven Press, 1975, 2:203–227.

Kent S. A look at gerovital—The "youth" drug. *Geriatrics*. 31:95–102, 1976.

MacFarlane MD. Procaine HCl (Gerovital H3), a weak, reversible, fully competitive inhibitor of monoamine oxidase. *Fed. Proc.* 34:108–110, 1975.

Olsen EJ, Bank L and Jarvik LF. Gerovital-H3: A clinical trial as an antidepressant. *Journal of Gerontology*. 33:514–520, 1978.

Ostfeld A, Smith CM and Stotsky BA. The systemic use of procaine in the treatment of the elderly: A review. *Journal of the American Geriatrics Society*. 25:1–19, 1977.

Hyaluronic Acid

Bourne WM et al. The effect of sodium hyaluronate on endothelial cell damage during extracapsular cataract extraction and posterior chamber lens implantation. *American Journal of Ophthalmology*. 98:759–762, 1984.

DeLuise VP and Peterson WS. The use of topical Healon tears in the management of refractory dry eye syndrome. *Annals of Ophthalmology*. 16:823–824, 1984.

Limberg MB et al. Topical application of hyaluronate acid chondroitin acid sulfate in the treatment of dry eyes. *American Journal of Ophthalmology*. 103:194–197, 1987.

Nelson JD and Farris RL. Sodium hyaluronate and polyvinyl alcohol tear preparations. *Archives of Ophthalmology*. 106:484–487, 1988.

Pape LG and Balazs EA. The use of sodium hyaluronate (Healon) in human anterior segment surgery. Ophthalmology. 87:699–705, 1980.

Polack FM and McNiece MT. The treatment of dry eyes with NA hyaluronate (Healon). *Cornea*. 1:133–136, 1982.

Hyperbaric Oxygen

Gabb G and Robin ED. Hyperbaric oxygen: A therapy in search of diseases. *Chest*. 92:1074–1082, 1987.

Memory Enhancers

Exton-Smith AN et al. Clinical experience with ergot alkaloids. In: *Aging*. 23:323–328, 1983.

Giurgia C. Piracetam: Nootropic pharmacology of neurointegrative activity. In: Esman WB and Valzelli I (eds.), *Current Developments in Psychopharmacology*. 3:221–276, 1976.

Hollister LE and Yesavage J. Ergoloid mesylates for senile dementias: Unanswered questions. *Ann. Int. Med.* 100:894–898, 1984.

Moos WH and Hershenson FM. Potential therapeutic strategies for senile cognitive disorders. *Drug News and Perspectives*. 2(7):397–409, 1989.

Neshkes RE and Jarvik LF. Pharmacologic approach to the treatment of senile dementia. *Psychiatric Annals*. 13(1):14–30, 1983.

Oliveras JC et al. Vasopressin in amnesia (Letter). *Lancet*. 1:42, 1978.

Porslot RD. The silent epidemic: The search for treatment of age-related memory impairment. *Trends in Pharmacological Science*. 10:3–6, January 1989.

Reisberg B et al. Effects of naloxone in senile dementia: A double-blind trial (Letter). *N. Eng. J. Med.* 308:721–722, 1983.

Scott FL. A review of some current drugs used in the pharmacology of organic brain syndrome. In: Cherkin A et al. (eds.), *Aging*. New York: Raven Press, 1979, 8:151–184.

Tennant FS Jr. Preliminary observations on naltrexone for treatment of Alzheimer's type dementia. *Journal of the American Geriatrics Society*. 35:369–370, 1987.

Minoxidil and Other Baldness Remedies

Groveman HD, Ganiats R and Klauber MR. Lack of efficacy of polysorbate 60 in the treatment of male pattern baldness. *Archives of Internal Medicine*. 145:1454–1458, 1985.

Millikan LE. Treatment of male pattern baldness. *Drug Therapy*. Pp. 62–73, March 1989.

Olsen EA et al. Topical minoxidil in early male pattern baldness. *J. Am. Acad. Derm*. 13:185–192, 1985.

Price VH (ed.). Rogaine (topical minoxidil 2%) in the management of male pattern baldness and alopecia areata. *J. Am. Acad. Derm*. (Supplement). 16(3) Part 2:647–750, 1987.

Other Oxygen "Therapies"

Knighton DR, Halliday B and Hunt TK. Oxygen as an antibiotic. *Archives of Surgery*. 119:119–204, 1984.

Love IN. Peroxide of hydrogen as a remedial agent. *J. Am. Med. Assoc*. 10:262–265, 1988.

Wilson BA, Welch HG and Lile JN. Effects of hyperoxic gas mixtures on energy during prolonged work. *Journal of Applied Physiology*. 39:267–271, 1975.

Winter FD, Snell PG and Stray-Gunfrtdren. Effects of 100% oxygen on performance of professional soccer players. *J. Am. Med. Assoc*. 263:227–229, 1989.

Sanguinaria, Chlorhexidine and Other Mouthwashes

Loe HC (ed.). Chlorhexidine in the prevention and treatment of gingivitis. *Journal of Periodontal Research* (Supplement, No. 16). Volume 21, 1986.

Southard G et al. Sanguinarine, a new antiplaque agent: Retention and plaque specificity. *Journal of the American Dental Association*. 108:338–341, 1984.

Superoxide Dismutase

Baillet F et al. Treatment of radiofibrosis with liposomal superoxide dismutase: Preliminary results of 50 cases. *Free Radical Research Communications*. 1:387–394, 1986.

McCord JM. Superoxide dismutase: Rationale for use in reperfusion injury and inflammation. *Journal of Free Radicals in Biology and Medicine*. 2:307–310, 1986.

Michelson AM. Medical aspects of superoxide dismutase. *Life Chemistry Reports*. 6:1–140, 1987.

Rotilio G (ed.). *Superoxide and Superoxide Dismutase in Chemistry, Biology and Medicine*. Amsterdam: Elsevier, 1986.

Testosterone and Steroids

Alen M. Androgenic steroid effects on liver and red cells. *British Journal of Sports Medicine*. 19(1):15–20, 1985.

Ammus SS. The role of androgens in the treatment of hematologic disorders. *Advances in Internal Medicine*. 34:191–208, 1989.

Hallagan JB, Hallagan LF and Snyder MB. Anabolic-androgenic steroid use by athletes. *N. Eng. J. Med*. 321:1042–1045, 1989.

Haupt HA and Rovere GD. Anabolic steroids: A review of the literature. *American Journal of Sports Medicine*. 12:469–484, 1984.

Jackson JA, Waxman J and Spiekerman M. Prostatic complications of testosterone replacement therapy. *Archives of Internal Medicine*. 149:2365–2366, 1989.

Ottenweller JE et al. Aging, stress, and chronic disease interact to suppress plasma testosterone in Syrian hamsters. *Journal of Gerontology*. 43:M175–M180, 1988.

Swartz CM. Low serum testosterone: A cardiovascular risk in elderly men. *Geriatric Medicine Today*. 7(12):39–49, 1988.

Swartz CM and Young MA. Low serum testosterone and myocardial infarction in geriatric male patients. *Journal of the American Geriatric Society*. 35:39–44, 1987.

Wilson JD. Androgen abuse by athletes. *Endocrine Reviews*. 9:181–199, 1988.

Thymic Therapies

Beatty DW et al. A controller trial of treatment of acquired immunodeficiency in severe measles with thymic humoral factor. *Clinical and Experimental Immunology*. 56:479, 1984.

Chretien PB et al. Effects of thymosin in vitro in cancer patients and correlation with clinical course after thymosin immunotherapy. *Ann. N.Y. Acad. Sci*. 332:135–147, 1979.

Clumeck N et al. Thymopentin treatment in AIDS and pre-AIDS patients. *Survey of Immunologic Research.* 4:58, 1985.

Goldstein AL. Current status of thymosin and other hormones of the thymus gland. *Recent Progress in Hormone Research.* 37:369–415, 1981.

Lin C-Y et al. Treatment of combined immunodeficiency with thymic extract (Thymostimulin). *Annals of Allergy.* 58:379–384, 1987.

Oates KK and Goldstein AL. Thymosins: Hormones of the thymus gland. *Trends in Pharmacological Sciences.* 5:347–351, 1984.

Shoham J et al. Enhancement of the immune system of chemotherapy treated cancer patients by simultaneous treatment with thymic extract. *Cancer Immunology and Immunotherapy.* 9:173, 1980.

Wada S et al. Thymus lymphocytes in rats during induction of bladder tumors and effects of thymosin fraction 5 in vitro. *J.N.C.I.* 74:659–664, 1985.

Transfer Factor

Carey JT et al. Augmentation of skin test reactivity and lymphocyte blastogenesis in patients with AIDS treated with transfer factor. *J. Am. Med. Assoc.* 257:651–655, 1987.

Dundas SAC and Clark A. The effect of transfer factor on lymph node morphology in murine toxoplasmosis. *British Journal of Experimental Pathology.* 67:181–190, 1986.

Jose DG, Ford GW and Welch JS. Therapy with parent's lymphocyte transfer factor in children with infection and malnutrition. *Lancet.* 1:263–265, 1976.

Kirkpatrick CH. Transfer factor. *Journal of Allergy and Clinical Immunology.* 81:803–813, 1988.

Louie E et al. Treatment of cryptosporidiosis with oral bovine transfer factor. *Clinical Immunology and Immunopathology.* 44:329–324, 1987.

Massicot JG and Goldstein RA. Transfer factor. *Annals of Allergy.* 49:326–329, 1982.

Motszko CS et al. A randomized trial of transfer factory therapy in the treatment of herpes zoster infections. *Immunology and Allergy Practice.* 7(1):37–42, 1985.

Shulman ST et al. A double-blind evaluation of transfer factor therapy of HBsAg-positive chronic aggressive hepatitis: Preliminary report of efficacy. *Cellular Immunology.* 43:353–361, 1979.

Steele RW, Myers MG and Vincent MM. Transfer factor for the prevention of varicella-zoster infection in childhood leukemia. *N. Eng. J. Med.* 303:355–359,1980.

Tsang KY and Fudenberg HH. Transfer factor and other T cell products. *Springer Seminars in Immunopathology.* 9:19–32, 1986.

Viza D et al. Specific transfer factor protects mice against lethal challenge with herpes simplex virus. *Cellular Immunology.* 100:555–561, 1986.

Index